T0226870

Echocardiography in Diagnosis and Management of Mitral Valve Disease

Editors

JUDY W. HUNG
TIMOTHY C. TAN

CARDIOLOGY CLINICS

www.cardiology.theclinics.com

Consulting Editors
ROSARIO FREEMAN
JORDAN M. PRUTKIN
DAVID SHAVELLE
AUDREY H. WU

May 2013 • Volume 31 • Number 2

ELSEVIER

1600 John F. Kennedy Boulevard • Suite 1800 • Philadelphia, Pennsylvania, 19103-2899

http://www.theclinics.com

CARDIOLOGY CLINICS Volume 31, Number 2

May 2013 ISSN 0733-8651, ISBN-13: 978-1-4557-7070-0

Editor: Barbara Cohen-Kligerman
Developmental Editor: Teia Stone

© **2013 Elsevier Inc. All rights reserved.**

This periodical and the individual contributions contained in it are protected under copyright by Elsevier, and the following terms and conditions apply to their use:

Photocopying
Single photocopies of single articles may be made for personal use as allowed by national copyright laws. Permission of the Publisher and payment of a fee is required for all other photocopying, including multiple or systematic copying, copying for advertising or promotional purposes, resale, and all forms of document delivery. Special rates are available for educational institutions that wish to make photocopies for non-profit educational classroom use. For information on how to seek permission visit www.elsevier.com/permissions or call: (+44) 1865 843830 (UK)/(+1) 215 239 3804 (USA).

Derivative Works
Subscribers may reproduce tables of contents or prepare lists of articles including abstracts for internal circulation within their institutions. Permission of the Publisher is required for resale or distribution outside the institution. Permission of the Publisher is required for all other derivative works, including compilations and translations (please consult www.elsevier.com/permissions).

Electronic Storage or Usage
Permission of the Publisher is required to store or use electronically any material contained in this periodical, including any article or part of an article (please consult www.elsevier.com/permissions). Except as outlined above, no part of this publication may be reproduced, stored in a retrieval system or transmitted in any form or by any means, electronic, mechanical, photocopying, recording or otherwise, without prior written permission of the Publisher.

Notice
No responsibility is assumed by the Publisher for any injury and/or damage to persons or property as a matter of products liability, negligence or otherwise, or from any use or operation of any methods, products, instructions or ideas contained in the material herein. Because of rapid advances in the medical sciences, in particular, independent verification of diagnoses and drug dosages should be made.

Although all advertising material is expected to conform to ethical (medical) standards, inclusion in this publication does not constitute a guarantee or endorsement of the quality or value of such product or of the claims made of it by its manufacturer.

Cardiology Clinics (ISSN 0733-8651) is published quarterly by Elsevier Inc., 360 Park Avenue South, New York, NY 10010-1710. Months of issue are February, May, August, and November. Business and Editorial Offices: 1600 John F. Kennedy Blvd., Ste. 1800, Philadelphia, PA 19103-2899. Customer Service Office: 3251 Riverport Lane, Maryland Heights, MO 63043. Periodicals postage paid at New York, NY and additional mailing offices. Subscription prices are $305.00 per year for US individuals, $508.00 per year for US institutions, $149.00 per year for US students and residents, $373.00 per year for Canadian individuals, $630.00 per year for Canadian institutions, $432.00 per year for international individuals, $630.00 per year for international institutions and $211.00 per year for Canadian and international students/residents. To receive student/resident rate, orders must be accompanied by name of affiliated institution, data of term, and the *signature* of program/residency coordinator on institution letterhead. Orders will be billed at individual rate until proof of status is received. Foreign air speed delivery is included in all *Clinics* subscription prices. All prices are subject to change without notice. **POSTMASTER:** Send address changes to *Cardiology Clinics*, Elsevier Health Sciences Division, Subscription Customer Service, 3251 Riverport Lane, Maryland Heights, MO 63043. **Customer Service: 1-800-654-2452 (U.S. and Canada); 314-447-8871 (outside U.S. and Canada). Fax: 314-447-8029. E-mail: journalscustomerservice-usa@ elsevier.com (for print support); journalsonlinesupport-usa@elsevier.com (for online support).**

Reprints. For copies of 100 or more, of articles in this publication, please contact the Commercial Reprints Department, Elsevier Inc., 360 Park Avenue South, New York, NY 10010-1710. Tel.: 212-633-3812; Fax: 212-462-1935; E-mail: reprints@elsevier.com.

Cardiology Clinics is also published in Spanish by McGraw-Hill Interamericana Editores S. A., P.O. Box 5-237, 06500, Mexico D. F., Mexico; in Portuguese by Reichmann and Alfonso Editores Rio de Janeiro, Brazil; and in Greek by Dimitrios P. Lagos, 8 Pondon Street, GR115-28 Ilissia, Greece.

Cardiology Clinics is covered in *MEDLINE/PubMed (Index Medicus)*, *Excerpta Medica*, *The Cumulative Index to Nursing and Allied Health Literature* (CINAHL).

Printed and bound by CPI Group (UK) Ltd, Croydon, CR0 4YY

Transferred to digital print 2012

Contributors

EDITORIAL BOARD

ROSARIO FREEMAN, MD, MS, FACC
Associate Professor of Medicine, Director,
Coronary Care Unit; Director,
Echocardiography Laboratory, University of
Washington Medical Center, Seattle,
Washington

JORDAN M. PRUTKIN, MD, MHS, FHRS
Assistant Professor of Medicine, Division of
Cardiology/Electrophysiology, University of
Washington Medical Center, Seattle,
Washington

DAVID SHAVELLE, MD, FACC, FSCAI
Associate Professor of Clinical Medicine,
Keck School of Medicine at USC; Director,
Los Angeles County/USC Cardiac
Catheterization Laboratory; Director,
Interventional Cardiology Fellowship,
Los Angeles County/USC Medical Center,
Los Angeles, California

AUDREY H. WU, MD
Assistant Professor, Internal Medicine,
University of Michigan, Ann Arbor, Michigan

EDITORS

JUDY W. HUNG, MD
Associate Director, Echocardiography,
Massachusetts General Hospital; Associate
Professor, Harvard Medical School, Boston,
Massachusetts

TIMOTHY C. TAN, MD, PhD
Clinical and Research Fellow,
Echocardiography, Division of Cardiology,
Massachusetts General Hospital, Harvard
Medical School, Boston, Massachusetts

AUTHORS

MICHAEL N. ANDRAWES, MD
Instructor, Department of Anesthesia, Critical
Care, and Pain Medicine, Massachusetts
General Hospital, Boston, Massachusetts

ROY BEIGEL, MD
The Heart Institute, Cedars Sinai Medical
Center, Los Angeles, California; The Leviev
Heart Center, Sheba Medical Center,
Tel-Hashomer, Israel; Sackler School of
Medicine, Tel Aviv University, Tel Aviv, Israel

JACOB P. DAL-BIANCO, MD
Instructor in Medicine, Division of Cardiology,
Department of Medicine, Massachusetts
General Hospital, Harvard Medical School,
Boston, Massachusetts

MAURICE ENRIQUEZ-SARANO, MD
Division of Cardiovascular Diseases and
Internal Medicine, Mayo Clinic, Rochester,
Minnesota

JARED W. FEINMAN, MD
Fellow, Cardiothoracic Anesthesiology,
Department of Anesthesia, Critical Care,
and Pain Medicine, Massachusetts General
Hospital, Boston, Massachusetts

BENJAMIN H. FREED, MD
Northwestern Memorial Hospital, Chicago,
Illinois

REBECCA T. HAHN, MD, FACC, FASE
Columbia University Medical Center,
New York-Presbyterian Hospital, New York,
New York

JUDY W. HUNG, MD
Associate Director, Echocardiography,
Massachusetts General Hospital; Associate
Professor, Harvard Medical School, Boston,
Massachusetts

SONIA JAIN, MBBS
Division of Cardiovascular Diseases,
Department of Medicine, Mayo Clinic College
of Medicine, Rochester, Minnesota

PATRIZIO LANCELLOTTI, MD, PhD, FACC
Department of Cardiology, GIGA
Cardiovascular Sciences, Heart Valve Clinic,
University Hospital Sart Tilman, University of
Liège, Liège, Belgium

ROBERTO M. LANG, MD
University of Chicago Medical Center,
Chicago, Illinois

ROBERT A. LEVINE, MD
Professor of Medicine, Cardiac Ultrasound
Laboratory, Massachusetts General Hospital,
Harvard Medical School, Boston,
Massachusetts

GERARD LOUGHLIN, MD
Department of Cardiology, Hospital General
Universitario Gregorio Marañón, Madrid, Spain

JULIEN MAGNE, PhD
Department of Cardiology, GIGA
Cardiovascular Sciences, Heart Valve Clinic,
University Hospital Sart Tilman, University of
Liège, Liège, Belgium

SUNIL V. MANKAD, MD
Division of Cardiovascular Diseases,
Department of Medicine, Mayo Clinic College
of Medicine, Rochester, Minnesota

DAVID MESSIKA-ZEITOUN, MD, PhD
Department of Cardiology, AP-HP, Bichat
Hospital; University Paris 7, Diderot, Paris,
France

LAILA A. PAYVANDI, MD
Instructor of Medicine, Division of Cardiology,
Department of Medicine, Bluhm

Cardiovascular Institute, Northwestern
University Feinberg School of Medicine,
Chicago, Illinois

LUC A. PIÉRARD, MD, PhD, FACC
Department of Cardiology, GIGA
Cardiovascular Sciences, Heart Valve Clinic,
University Hospital Sart Tilman, University of
Liège, Liège, Belgium

VICTORIA PIRO, MD
Division of Cardiology, Massachusetts General
Hospital, Boston, Massachusetts

VERA H. RIGOLIN, MD
Associate Professor of Medicine, Division of
Cardiology, Department of Medicine, Bluhm
Cardiovascular Institute, Northwestern
University Feinberg School of Medicine,
Chicago, Illinois

ROBERT J. SIEGEL, MD, FACC
The Heart Institute, Cedars Sinai Medical
Center, Los Angeles, California

JORGE SOLIS, MD
Department of Cardiology, Hospital General
Universitario Gregorio Marañón; Assistant
Professor, Complutense Medical School,
Madrid, Spain

YAN TOPILSKY, MD
Division of Cardiology, Tel-Aviv Medical
Center, Tel-Aviv, Israel

WENDY TSANG, MD
Division of Cardiology, Toronto General
Hospital, University Health Network, University
of Toronto, Toronto, Ontario, Canada

**JOSE ANTONIO VAZQUEZ DE PRADA,
MD, PhD**
Department of Cardiology, Hospital
Universitario Marques de Valdecilla; Marques
de Valdecilla Research Institute (IFIMAV),
Santander, Spain

NINA C. WUNDERLICH, MD
Cardiovascular Center, Darmstadt, Germany;
University Hospital, Mainz, Germany

Contents

assessment of patient candidacy for percutaneous balloon valvuloplasty versus surgery. Baseline echocardiographic features are strong independent predictors of procedural success and long-term outcome. Evolving technology such as 3-dimensional echo has the potential to improve the understanding and management of this globally relevant disease.

CARDIOLOGY CLINICS

DOWNLOAD Free App!

Review Articles
THE CLINICS

NOW AVAILABLE FOR YOUR iPhone and iPad

Preface

Echocardiography in Mitral Valve Disease

Mitral valve disease has widespread global impact, contributing significantly to cardiovascular morbidity and mortality. According to the American Heart Association, in the United States alone over 4 million people are affected with some form of mitral valve disease. The spectrum of disease affecting the mitral valve is diverse and stems from a wide range of causes that include infectious causes, such as rheumatic mitral valve disease, degenerative disease, and secondary causes, such as mitral valve regurgitation due to cardiac ischemia.

Echocardiography plays a major role in the diagnosis and management of mitral valve disease. While its many advantages—including accessibility, reasonable low cost, and noninvasive nature—make it an ideal imaging tool for the diagnosis and long-term monitoring of patients with mitral valve disease, its ability to provide hemodynamic information in real-time is what makes it most suitable for use in this disease entity. In addition, the development of novel ultrasound technology, such as three-dimensional echocardiography, has broadened the application of this imaging modality to now include guidance for interventional approaches to management of this disease.

The diverse manifestations of mitral disease and the significant advances made in the understanding of the disease process, in combination with all the developments in the area of diagnosis and management of this condition, are the basis for this issue of *Cardiology Clinics*. Our aim is to provide clinicians with a comprehensive yet concise overview of mitral valve disease, featuring the role of echocardiography in current diagnostic criteria and management strategies. We have put together a panel of renowned experts who have made significant and original contributions to mitral valve disease and echocardiography.

This issue of *Cardiology Clinics* provides clinicians with important insight into the broad spectrum of mitral valve disease and critical role of echocardiography in this context. The content is headed by an article on the anatomy of the mitral valve apparatus and the contributions of two-dimensional and three-dimensional echocardiography toward the current understanding of the way the mitral valve functions. This is followed by two articles discussing mitral stenosis, including the various causes, demographics, mechanism of underlying disease, and the echocardiographic methods for assessing severity. Subsequently, there are articles discussing mitral regurgitation and the various qualitative and quantitative echocardiographic methods for assessing mitral regurgitation followed by articles covering common causes for mitral regurgitation. To round off this issue of *Cardiology Clinics*, we have chosen to focus on some of the important applications for echocardiography in the management of mitral valve disease, including stress echocardiography for assessment of the functional impact of mitral valve disease and the role of echocardiography in percutaneous interventions, presurgical, and postsurgical intervention.

This issue of *Cardiology Clinics* addresses an important valve problem that is dynamic and evolving, addressing many key concepts that will be of benefit to all physicians, whether cardiologists or non-cardiologists. We sincerely hope that the reader would not only take away from this issue a comprehensive overview of this disease but also an appreciation for the value of echocardiography in the diagnosis and management of this condition that cannot be afforded by any other cardiac imaging modalities.

We would like to sincerely thank all the distinguished authors who contributed to this issue of *Cardiology Clinics* for their invaluable contributions

Cardiol Clin 31 (2013) ix–x
http://dx.doi.org/10.1016/j.ccl.2013.05.001
0733-8651/13/$ – see front matter © 2013 Published by Elsevier Inc.

by way of their time and in providing outstanding articles. Last, we would also like to thank Barbara Cohen Kligerman and Elsevier for supporting this work.

Judy W. Hung, MD
Echocardiography
Massachusetts General Hospital
Harvard Medical School
Cardiac Ultrasound Laboratory, YAW 5E
55 Fruit Street
Boston, MA 02114-2696, USA

Timothy C. Tan, MD, PhD
Echocardiography
Division of Cardiology
Massachusetts General Hospital
Harvard Medical School
Cardiac Ultrasound Laboratory, YAW 5E
55 Fruit Street
Boston, MA 02114-2696, USA

E-mail addresses:
jhung@partners.org (J.W. Hung)
TCTan@partners.org (T.C. Tan)

Anatomy of the Mitral Valve Apparatus
Role of 2D and 3D Echocardiography

Jacob P. Dal-Bianco, MD[a], Robert A. Levine, MD[b],*

KEYWORDS

- Mitral valve apparatus • Mitral valve • Mitral annulus • Papillary muscles • Chordae tendineae
- Mitral regurgitation • Echocardiography

KEY POINTS

- The mitral valve apparatus is a complex 3-dimensional functional unit that is critical to unidirectional heart pump function.
- The main mitral valve apparatus components are (1) mitral annulus, (2) mitral valve leaflets, (3) chordae tendineae, and (4) papillary muscles.
- Tight-sealed mitral leaflet coaptation depends on the balance of systolic tethering and closing forces on the valve and on the amount of leaflet tissue available.
- Echocardiography is ideally suited to examine the mitral valve apparatus and has provided insights into the mechanism of mitral valve disease.
- Understanding normal mitral valve apparatus function is essential to comprehend alterations in mitral valve disease and the rationale for repair strategies.

INTRODUCTION

The normal mitral valve apparatus is a dynamic 3-dimensional (3D) system that allows brisk left ventricular (LV) blood-inflow during diastole and ensures unidirectional heart pump function by sealing the left atrium from the LV during systole. Key components are the mitral annulus (MA), the mitral valve leaflets, the chordae tendineae, and the LV wall with its attached papillary muscles (PMs) (**Fig. 1**). Proper valve function is dependent on the integrity and harmonious interplay of these components; an imbalance can result in a leaking (regurgitant, insufficient, incompetent), stenotic, or combined regurgitant and stenotic valve dysfunction. A detailed understanding of mitral valve apparatus development, anatomy, and function is important for cardiac imaging interpretation, for disease diagnosis, and for comprehending the rationale for repair strategies. Repair of the diseased mitral valve requires understanding the *dysfunction* caused by the disease *lesion* to restore a normally functioning valve, a lesson learned from one of the foremost pioneers in mitral valve repair, Professor Alain Carpentier.

MITRAL VALVE APPARATUS DEVELOPMENT

Mitral valve development is complex and still under investigation.[1] The developing heart tube consists of extracellular matrix sandwiched by myocardial and endothelial layers, and has folded into a basic

Financial Support: This work is supported in part by grant 07CVD04 of the Leducq Foundation, Paris, France, for the Leducq Transatlantic MITRAL Network, and by National Institutes of Health grants K24 HL67434, R01 HL72265, and HL109506.
Financial Disclosure: The authors have nothing to disclose.

[a] Division of Cardiology, Department of Medicine, Massachusetts General Hospital, Harvard Medical School, 55 Fruit Street, Yawkey 5B, Boston, MA 02114, USA; [b] Cardiac Ultrasound Laboratory, Massachusetts General Hospital, Harvard Medical School, 55 Fruit Street, Yawkey 5E, Boston, MA 02114, USA
* Corresponding author.
E-mail address: rlevine@partners.org

cardiology.theclinics.com

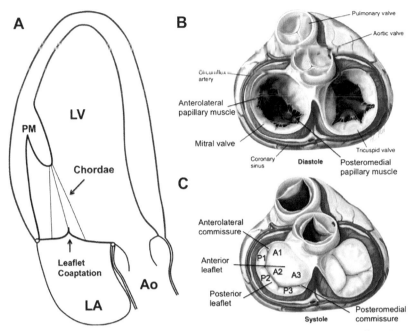

Fig. 1. (*A*) Schematic apical long-axis view of the heart in systole with the apex on top. There is normal function and spatial relationship of the LV myocardium, the PM, chordae, leaflets, and MA. The tethering force–closing force balance relationship is normal; both leaflets are normally configured, concave toward the LV, and coapt without mitral regurgitation. (*B*) Surgical view of the open mitral valve in diastole with the atrial walls removed. (*C*) Surgical view of the closed mitral valve in systole. A#, anterior leaflet scallop; Ao, aorta; LA, left atrium; LV, left ventricle; P#, posterior leaflet scallop; PM, papillary muscle. ([*B, C*] *From* Carpentier A. Carpentier's reconstructive valve surgery. St. Louis: Saunders/Elsevier;2010; with permission.)

4-chamber configuration by the end of fetal week 4. By week 5, the outer myocardial layer has compacted and trabecular structures start to form within the future LV cavity. At this point, superior, inferior, and lateral cardiac cushions can be detected in the common atrioventricular (AV) canal.[2] These 5 cushions are formed by endothelial cells that migrate into the mesenchyme and change into an interstitial fibroblast cell type, a process termed endothelial–mesenchymal transdifferentiation or transformation (EMT).[1] The superior and inferior cardiac cushions fuse at week 7 to 7 1/2 and divide the common AV canal into right and left portions. The anterior (aortic) leaflet of the mitral valve originates from the fused superior and inferior cushion tissue in the left AV canal and starts to delaminate or separate from the myocardial wall shortly thereafter. The posterior (mural) leaflet forms from the left lateral cushion.[2] Over weeks 8 to 10, the LV intracavitary trabecular bridges compact, and by week 10 small (antero)lateral and (postero)medial PMs can be observed delaminated in the LV cavity. Actually, both are located posteriorly relative to the anterior chest wall: one medial, the other lateral. Both PMs attach directly to both leaflet-forming cushions. From week 11 to

13, the leaflets continue to form, the PMs become more distinct, and rudimentary chordae develop. By week 15, the mitral valve leaflets, chordae, and PMs become developed.[2] The mitral valve apparatus then continues to grow to meet the needs and demands of the developing organism.[3]

MITRAL VALVE APPARATUS ANATOMY AND HISTOLOGY
Mitral Annulus

The MA is defined by the tissue juncture of the left atrium, the left ventricle, and the mitral leaflets. It is a dynamic, anatomically ill-defined structure. En face, the MA resembles a kidney bean; in 3 dimensions it is a nonplanar saddle shape.[4–6]

The anterior flatter portion of the MA is continuous with the aortic annulus, is the elevated (most atrial) "horn" of the saddle shape, and consists of parallel collagen fibers.[4,7] The MA-to-aortic annular angle changes dynamically over the cardiac cycle, with displacement coupled through the fibrous continuum.[8] Reciprocal systolic and diastolic aortic and MA area changes have been observed.[9–11] The posterior part of the MA runs distal to the left (lateral) and right (medial) fibrous trigones and includes the low points of the saddle close to the lateral and medial commissures and the posterior saddle horn. Compared with the anterior portion, the posterior MA is more loosely anchored to the surrounding tissue, allowing it to move freely with myocardial contraction and relaxation.[7] It is basically a junction of leaflet and myocardium. Less static in all dimensions than the anterior MA portion, the posterior MA allows for systolic apical bending along a mediolateral commissure axis, with increased saddle height and circumferential area decrease.[12] The saddle-shaped MA and its dynamic change reduces leaflet tissue stress and is important for coaptation geometry.[13–20] The MA is innervated and supplies blood vessels to the leaflets.[21–23] From week 18 to 24 on to adulthood the MA area increases 25-fold[24] and, contrary to the widely published "normal" mitral annular orifice area of 4 to 6 cm^2, multiple investigations with differing imaging modalities report an average mitral annular area of approximately 10 cm^2 in healthy subjects.[25–30] The MA area can significantly increase in patients with dilated LVs.[27,29,30] This is accompanied by MA flattening[29,31] and decrease and delay of systolic sphincterlike mitral annular area reduction.[29,32] The final result of these changes is altered leaflet stress and unfavorable mitral leaflet remodeling (Table 1). MA flattening has also been recently described in myxomatous valve disease, associated with more severe MR and chordal rupture, potentially related to increased out-of-plane stresses.[20,33]

Mitral Valve Leaflets

The mitral valve has anterior and posterior leaflets and variable commissural scallops to occlude medial and lateral gaps (see Fig. 1C; Fig. 2). Leaflet tissue circumferentially attaches to the MA with a minimum tissue length of 0.5 to 1.0 cm.[34] Redundant leaflet tissue is critically important for leaflet apposition and tight leaflet coaptation. In normal and dilated LVs, a leaflet-to-MA area ratio of 1.5 to 2.0 has been found sufficient to prevent

significant mitral regurgitation.[30,34] The atrial surface of the leaflets is smooth and the leaflet body translucent (see Fig. 2). A hydrophilic protein-rich zone, termed rough zone, starts approximately 1 cm from the distal leaflet edge. When the leaflets coapt, the irregular, soft surface of this zone helps to maintain and ensure a seal (see Fig. 2, coaptation zone). The ventricular surface of especially the anterior leaflet is a basket-weave of crisscrossed collagen strands that originate at the chordal insertion and continue into the annulus.[35,36] Secondary chordae insert close to the rough zone, whereas primary chordae insert at the free leaflet tips.[35,37]

The anterior (also labeled aortic or septal) mitral leaflet is trapezoid-shaped or dome-shaped, anchored to the fibrous portion of the MA, and shares a fibrous tissue continuity mainly with the noncoronary cusp of the aortic valve (see Fig. 2). Its collagen fiber orientation suggests tight anchoring into the left (anterolateral) and right (posteromedial) fibrous trigones.[38] The anterior leaflet is larger, longer, and thicker than the posterior leaflet (see Fig. 2, Table 2). To facilitate diagnostic and therapeutic medical communication, the anterior leaflet can be divided into lateral (A1), central (A2), and medial scallops (A3). For the anterior leaflet, this nomenclature does not represent anatomically distinct structures (see Fig. 1C).

The posterior (mural) leaflet is crescentic with a long circumferential base (~5 cm vs ~3 cm anterior leaflet[39]) and relatively short radial length (see Figs. 1C and 2, see Table 1). It is attached to the posterior portion of the MA. Similar to the anterior leaflet, the posterior leaflet can be divided into lateral (P1), central (P2), and medial scallops (P3). Slits and indentations within the posterior mitral tissue demarcate these scallops (see Fig. 1C).[37]

Additional leaflet tissue, termed commissural, accessory, or junctional, can be found at the anterolateral (A1-P1) and posteromedial (A3-P3) commissures (see Fig. 1B and C; Fig. 2). Their tissue length measured from annular insertion varies from 0.5 to 1.0 cm.[34,35]

The mitral valve leaflets fully open in less than 100 ms 3 billion times throughout a lifetime and

Table 1
Mitral annulus dimensions in normal human hearts and patients with dilated cardiomyopathy

	Normal	Dilated Cardiomyopathy
Nonplanar mitral annulus shape	Present[4,5]	Reduced, flattened[29,31]
Area, cm^2	~7–12[25–30]	~11–20[27,29,30]
Circumference, cm	7–11[35,129]	8–18[129]
% Area change diastole/systole	~20–42[27–29,32,130]	13–23[29,32]

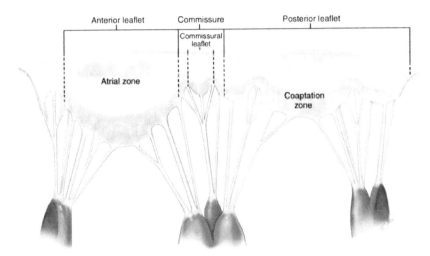

Fig. 2. The mitral valve is unfolded and the atrial leaflet surface exposed. The papillary muscles have been dissected and the heads remain attached via chordae tendineae to the anterior, posterior, and commissural leaflets. (*From* Carpentier A. Carpentier's reconstructive valve surgery. St. Louis: Saunders/Elsevier;2010; with permission.)

are exposed to a wide range of LV pressures.[40] Despite this demanding environment, significant mitral valve disease is uncommonly seen in patients younger than 65 years.[41] Influenced by the immediate environment and mechanical needs, the mitral valve leaflet tissue is trilaminar, consisting of fibrosa/ventricularis, spongiosa, and atrialis layers. Valvular endothelial cells cover the blood-interfacing surfaces. Each layer has unique extracellular matrix (ECM) characteristics: hemodynamically exposed to LV pressures, the fibrosa/ventricularis is composed of dense collagen, which is important for mechanical stability. The spongiosa has less organized collagen, but especially at the leaflet tip rough zone, is rich in water absorbent proteins. This protects the leaflet edges and ensures a tight seal. The atrialis contains a network of collagen and elastin and appears to play a critical role in leaflet remodeling and adaptation.[42] Although trilaminar, the layer distribution of the anterior and posterior leaflets differs significantly: much of the anterior leaflet thickness is due to a dominant fibrosa

layer, which allows this leaflet to withstand a significantly higher tensile load without tissue disruption.[43,44] The posterior leaflet is thinner and more flexible.[43,44] The anterior mitral leaflet has an especially dense innervation, and nerve terminals close to smooth muscle cells and fibroblasts suggest a potential neural feedback or regulatory mechanism.[45] Interestingly, but of unknown significance, this neural innervation greatly diminishes with age.[45,46] Cardiac muscle cells can be detected in both leaflets close to the annulus. This tissue is excitable via the atria, isolated from LV excitation, and resembles atrial myocardium.[36] The healthy, mature mitral valve has a very rudimentary vascular and lymphatic system,[23,47] interstitial cells are mostly dormant, and the ECM turnover is slow. Physiologic-induced or pathologic-induced leaflet stress can induce prominent EMT, interstitial cell activation and proliferation, ECM remodeling, and neovascularization.[3,42,48,49] Regulation of mitral leaflet adaptation is not well understood, but the wide range of total leaflet area (see **Table 2**) suggests a potent

Table 2
Mitral valve leaflet dimensions in healthy subjects, patients with dilated CMP and HCM

	Normal	Dilated CMP	HCM
Anterior leaflet area, cm^2	4–7[34,124,131,132]	7[131]	6–14[124,131,132]
Posterior leaflet area, cm^2	2–3[34,131,132]	2[131]	3–7[124,131,132]
Total leaflet area, cm^2	9–15[34,131,132]	12–20[30,131]	13–21[124,131,132]
Anterior leaflet length, mm	18–24[30,35,39,131,132]	24[30,131]	22[131,132]
Posterior leaflet length, mm	11–14[30,39,131,132]	13–14[30,131]	14[131,132]

Abbreviations: CMP, cardiomyopathy; HCM, hypertrophic cardiomyopathy.

adaptation mechanism that has to be further explored and therapeutically targeted.

Chordae Tendineae

The chordae tendineae are fibrous strings that originate with highly variable branching from the PM tips (heads) and insert fanlike into the ventricular aspects of the anterior, posterior, and commissural leaflets (see **Fig. 1**B and C; **Fig. 2**).[37,50] Occasionally, chordae originate from the basal posterior myocardium and insert directly into the posterior leaflet.[34] Two main types of chordae can be distinguished based on leaflet insertion: primary (marginal) chordae, which attach to the leaflet-free edges, and secondary (basal) chordae, which insert into the anterior leaflet edge rough zone and throughout the posterior leaflet body.[51] Chordae are composed of an interfacing, tightly linked collagen and elastin network that dampens PM-leaflet force transmission.[50]

Secondary chordae are thicker than primary chordae and have more tightly crimped collagen, making them more extensible.[52] Commonly, a pair of thick secondary chordae, termed strut chordae, insert at 4 and 8 PM into the ventricular aspect of the anterior leaflet; additional strut chords, including to the posterior leaflet have been described. Basket-woven collagen fibers distribute chordal force over the leaflet surface from insertion to the annulus.[34,36,51] To relieve pathologic apical leaflet tethering and restore mitral leaflet coaptation in patients with functional/ischemic mitral regurgitation, selected secondary chordae can be cut without deleterious effects on LV function.[53–55]

Primary chordae are thinner, insert at the leaflet tips, and have limited extensibility because of higher collagen fibril density and reduced crimping.[52] These characteristics prevent leaflet edge eversion (=flail leaflet).[56] There is a wide variability in chordal anatomy and branching patterns,[37] which makes correct anatomic labeling and measurement comparisons difficult. Most consistent and reproducible results are available for the anterior strut chordae. Their normal average length and thickness are reported at approximately 20 mm and 1 to 2 mm, respectively.[37,39,42,51] Similar to mitral leaflets, chordae adapt to altered loading conditions.[42]

Papillary Muscles

The PMs are labeled by their projected relationship to the mitral commissures as lateral and medial (see **Fig. 1**B and C).[35] Their bodies originate from the apical one-third of the LV and protrude finger-like into the cavity.[2] Chordal fans extend from the PM heads to the corresponding anterior, posterior, and commissural leaflet portions (see **Fig. 2**).[34] The lateral PM in most cases has a single head and dual blood supply from the left circumflex and left anterior descending artery. The medial PM most commonly has 2 heads and is either supplied by the right or circumflex coronary artery based on dominance.[34,35,57] The PM-chordal system is finely tuned so that PM contraction maintains the systolic spatial relationship between the MA and the PM heads as the intervening myocardium contracts, akin to a shock absorber, thereby preventing leaflet prolapse.[58–60] The PM head positions and relative distance to each other keep both leaflets under outwardly directed tension and therefore posteriorly restrained to prevent anterior motion (see the Hypertrophic Cardiomyopathy section, later in this article). The anterior, posterior, and commissural leaflets are therefore in optimal position and configuration to form an effective systolic coaptation seal.[61]

TWO-DIMENSIONAL AND 3D ECHOCARDIOGRAPHY OF THE MITRAL VALVE APPARATUS

Echocardiography is the clinical tool of choice for diagnosing, assessing, and following patients with valvular heart disease.[62] It is a noninvasive, nonionizing imaging test with excellent spatial and temporal resolution. Two-dimensional and 3D echocardiography (Echo) provides detailed morphologic and functional assessment, whereas Doppler echocardiography evaluates hemodynamics. Indeed, the functional mechanisms of mitral regurgitation in many conditions were first clearly defined by Echo. Constant advances in information technology make Echo very portable[63] and an increasingly important tool to guide minimally invasive percutaneous valve repairs.[64]

Three-dimensional Echo has been pivotal to today's understanding of the normal and diseased mitral valve apparatus: 3D Echo established the saddle-shaped, nonplanar shape of the MA,[4,6] helped explore the complex geometric relationship of PM and leaflet position relative to the MA and LV outflow tract,[61,65–67] and recently made it possible to measure mitral leaflet size in the beating heart.[20,30,42,68] Consequences have been the development of nonplanar mitral annuloplasty rings,[69] and a detailed understanding of the mechanisms of ischemic/function mitral regurgitation (MR) and systolic anterior motion (SAM) of the anterior leaflet in hypertrophic cardiomyopathy (HCM),[61,65–67] a redefinition of the diagnostic criteria of mitral valve prolapse (MVP),[70,71] and recent evidence of mitral valve adaptation and leaflet growth.[30,42,68]

Correct diagnosis of mitral valve disease is dependent on optimally acquired 2D Echo views. A 3D cardiac anatomic understanding is paramount for 2D image acquisition and interpretation. **Fig. 3** shows the LV and mitral valve in a schematic short-axis view and the Echo beam planes for the most common 2D Echo views. Following the projected 4-chamber view (4C) Echo beam helps to understand that the mitral valve scallops A3, A2, and P1 are typically shown in this very common

Echo view. One can, however, also appreciate that a slight Echo probe and beam angulation will image a different plane and set of scallops while presenting an apparently similar image.[72] The 3D Echo controls for such uncertainty, as the acquired 3D data can be precisely sliced in every dimension until the optimal and desired 2D view is obtained.[73] The middle panel in **Fig. 4** shows a 3D-rendered mitral valve from the surgical perspective (compare with **Fig. 1**C). Slicing the 3D image set perpendicular (red line) to a mediolateral commissural axis (green line) will create

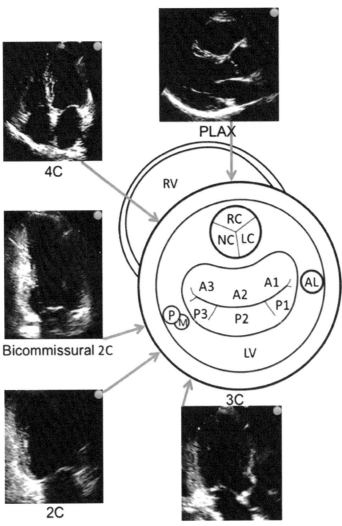

Fig. 3. The central schematic shows the left ventricle in short axis view seen from the apex. The approximate locations of the aortic valve, mitral valve, and PMs are projected. The most common and standardized 2D Echo views are arranged around the schematic. The *blue arrows* indicate the direction of the Echo beam and are connected to the corresponding Echo views. The *blue dots* on the Echo images relate to the orientation of the *blue arrows*. Extrapolating the Echo beam lines allows to estimate the 2D Echo mitral scallops represented in the corresponding Echo views. 2C, 2-Chamber view; 4C, 4-Chamber view; AL, anterolateral papillary muscle; LC, left aortic cusp; LV, left ventricle; NC, noncoronary aortic cusp; PLAX, parasternal long axis view; PM, posterolateral papillary muscle; RC, right coronary cusp; RV, right ventricle.

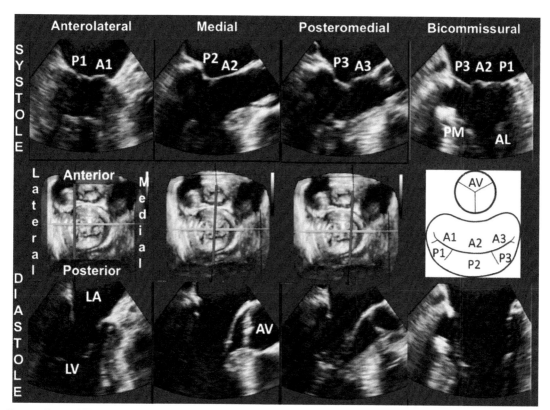

Fig. 4. The *middle panel* shows a 3D-rendered surgical view of the mitral valve. A schematic on the right side of the middle panel helps identify the mitral valve scallops and aortic valve in this view. The *upper panel* shows 2D Echo views of precisely known orientation because they are derived as slices of the 3D mitral valve apparatus in systole. The slice plane is indicated by the *red line* in the middle plane (perpendicular to a bicommissural axis, *green line*). The *lower panel* shows the same slice planes in diastole with the mitral leaflets open. AL, anterolateral papillary muscle; AV, aortic valve; LA, left atrium; LV, left ventricle; PM, posteromedial papillary muscle.

2D Echo views that accurately show the paired leaflet scallops in systole (upper panel) and diastole (lower panel).

NORMAL AND ABNORMAL MITRAL VALVE APPARATUS FUNCTION

Mitral valve anatomy is designed to promote and maintain normal mitral valve apparatus function; perturbations of the normal anatomic relations can result in mitral valve dysfunction (**Table 3**).

Tightly sealed MV leaflet coaptation depends on the balance of systolic tethering and closing forces on the valve and the amount of leaflet tissue available to cover the MA.[74] Tethering forces are transmitted via the LV wall–PM–chordae system and keep the leaflets from prolapsing into the left atrium (see **Fig. 1A**). Closing forces depend on the pressure generated by the LV to close the mitral valve.[67,68,75] Disturbance of this finely tuned spatial and temporal interplay of LV contraction, PMs, mitral valve leaflets, and MA can unsettle the tethering force–closing force balance relationship.

If this leads to a deficit of leaflet area relative to annulus area, coaptation will be impaired and mitral regurgitation will occur.[67,68,75] A vicious cycle may begin: significant MR volume will overload the LV; to restore wall tension, the LV will remodel and dilate. Altered LV geometry will consequently remodel the MA, leaflets, and chordae. MR severity will dynamically change throughout these adaptation processes, which conceivably are aimed to restore the tethering force–closing force balance relationship.[30,42,68] The natural disease course, however, suggests this process is comparable to destructive resonance, with each remodeled component causing disturbance in its relation to all the others. Throughout this, MR severity is a moving target, which, if progressive, will fuel ongoing LV remodeling.

Mitral Valve Prolapse

MVP is defined as mitral leaflet billowing by more than 2 mm above the anterior and posterior horns of the MA during ventricular systole (**Fig. 5A**).[70,71]

Table 3
Mitral valve apparatus components in normal and diseased states

	Normal	Mitral Valve Prolapse	Functional/Ischemic MR	Hypertrophic CMP
Papillary muscles	Parallel to the LV long axis	Superior traction	Apical/posterior/ posterolateral displacement	Hypertrophied, anteriorly displaced, PM heads closer to each other
Chordae tendineae	Normal	Elongated, thick or thin, rupture-prone	Elongated, thick	
Leaflet area/length	Normal	Increased/elongated	Increased/elongated vs thick	Increased/elongated in many
Mitral annulus shape/area	Saddle-shaped/ normal	Flattened/normal - increased	Flattened/Increased	Saddle-shaped/normal - decreased
Leaflet coaptation	At the annular level	At or superior to the annulus	Significantly apical to the annulus	Shifted toward the LVOT in SAM

Abbreviations: CMP, cardiomyopathy; HCM, hypertrophic cardiomyopathy; LV, left ventricle; LVOT, left ventricular outflow tract; MR, mitral regurgitation; PM, papillary muscles; SAM, systolic anterior motion.

MVP is usually diagnosed by echocardiography and is a manifestation of degenerative mitral valve disease. Coaptation geometry is altered because of a combination of leaflet and chordal extensibility, redundancy, and elongation; whether superior papillary muscle displacement or traction is cause or effect has yet to be determined[76,77] (see **Fig. 5**A, dashed line and arrow). The billowing leaflets may appear diffusely thickened (Barlow syndrome) or thin except in flail portions (fibroelastic deficiency).[39] Severe leaflet prolapse or flail leaflets can result in important MR (see **Table 3**). Repair strategies aim to restore effective leaflet coaptation by reducing leaflet redundancy and MA dimensions, and, if needed, implanting artificial chordae. Suitable mitral valve leaflet

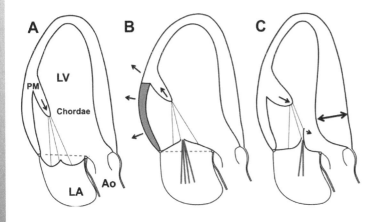

Fig. 5. (*A*) Mitral valve prolapse. The schematic shows bileaflet mitral valve prolapse, with superior displacement of the papillary muscle tip, "tugged" by the leaflets, and excessive leaflet and chordal tissue and mobility. Leaflet coaptation is displaced into the left atrium superior to the annular plane (*dashed line*). (*B*) Functional/ischemic mitral regurgitation. The papillary muscle (medial in inferior myocardial infarction) is displaced posteriorly, laterally and, to the extent allowed by the chords, apically (*arrow*) due to left ventricular local dilatation and remodeling (*arrows*) caused by myocardial infarction (*shaded area*). The LV wall-PM displacement tethers the mitral leaflets apically and limits coaptation. There is often not enough leaflet tissue to compensate for leaflet tenting (area apical to the *dashed line*), resulting in mitral regurgitation (*red lines*). (*C*) Hypertrophic cardiomyopathy. The geometry of the left ventricle and papillary muscles is altered by myocardial hypertrophy (interventricular septum, *double arrow*). The papillary muscles are enlarged and displaced anteriorly (*arrow*) and closer to each other (not shown). This decreases intercommissural leaflet tension and moves the coaptation point and distal leaflets toward the left ventricular outflow tract. Like a sail catching a breeze, the distal anterior leaflet and/or posterior leaflet if elongated, is at risk of being displaced into the LV outflow tract by blood-flow drag. If anterior leaflet displacement is severe enough and posterior leaflet apposition restricted, mitral regurgitation will occur (*red lines*). Ao, aorta; LA, left atrium; LV, left ventricle; PM, papillary muscle.

characteristics may also allow leaflet-free edge approximation at the site of regurgitation (edge-to-edge technique) by a stitch (Alfieri stitch)[78] or a clip (MitraClip, Abbott Vascular, Santa Clara, California).[79] Repair techniques, pioneered by Alain Carpentier, aim to restore leaflet function while preserving the native valve.[80] Mitral valve replacement is not commonly indicated with a skilled surgeon.

Functional/Ischemic Mitral Regurgitation

Functional or ischemic MR is caused by mitral valve leaflet tethering to displaced papillary muscles in the setting of a distorted, remodeled LV (see Fig. 5B). Pathophysiologic changes of LV form or function that increase the distance between PM heads and MA interfere with adequate leaflet co-aptation.[81–84] Key LV changes are LV remodeling with global dilatation and increased LV sphericity,[67,85–88] or localized LV remodeling.[89] If LV remodeling affects the PM-bearing ventricular walls, apical/posterior/posterolateral and outward PM displacement is likely to develop[89–94] (see Fig. 5B, arrows). Subsequent tethering restricts systolic closure motion of the MV leaflets. Affected leaflets stay "tied back" in the LV cavity, and this prevents a tightly sealed MV closure (see Table 3).[66] Repair strategies aim to restore effective leaflet coaptation by reducing leaflet tethering at the PM and mitral annular ends. Therapeutic PM repositioning targets are LV shape[95–97] and function (revascularization,[98–100] gene/cell therapy,[101–103] cardiac resynchronization therapy[104,105]), PM approximation,[106] chordal cutting,[53–55,107] leaflet edge-to-edge approximation technique,[78,79] MA area reduction, or valve replacement. Overall, functional/ischemic MR therapy strategies that deal with the annulus, but not the ventricular tethering, are often limited, with recurrent MR[108–111]; this can be reduced, for example by chordal cutting.[112]

Hypertrophic Cardiomyopathy

HCM is an autosomal dominant disease of myocyte disarray and fibrosis, morphologically characterized by significant LV hypertrophy in the absence of chronically elevated afterload or infiltrative diseases (eg, cardiac amyloidosis) (see Fig. 5C, double arrow).[113] HCM also involves the papillary muscles and mitral leaflets: total mass (twofold) and number of PM heads are increased.[114] The PMs are anteriorly displaced (see Fig. 5C, arrow) and the heads positioned closer to each other.[61,115] This increases leaflet slack, and like a sail catching a breeze, the anterior leaflet is at risk of being displaced into the LV outflow tract by blood-flow drag forces (SAM).[61,116–120] If anterior leaflet

displacement is severe enough to impair posterior leaflet apposition, mitral regurgitation will occur (see Fig. 5C, red lines).[121] Because PM position is a major culprit, septal reduction therapy does not always eliminate SAM.[122] In HCM, the leaflets are also frequently elongated,[123,124] contributing to leaflet slack and positioning the coaptation point anteriorly to increase the flow drag forces on the enlarged "sail." After obstruction begins, LV outflow tract narrowing increases velocity above the valve, propagating SAM through airplanelike lift forces.[125,126] Because of these mechanisms, repair strategies include papillary muscle repositioning and reducing leaflet redundancy (see Table 3).

In summary, therefore, the mitral valve is an elegantly constructed, well-balanced mechanism. Normal anatomic relations maintain the leaflets within the LV, preventing prolapse, and maintain them below LV outflow tract flow and taut, preventing SAM. Altered leaflet length and PM position can lead to MVP and obstructive SAM, which are both related to leaflet excess, as shown by their occurrence in the same patient.[127,128] Conversely, the PM tethering conducive to normal function becomes maladaptive in ischemic MR when the PMs are displaced. Understanding MV anatomic relationships, appreciated by Echo as well as magnetic resonance imaging and computed tomography, is therefore essential to understanding its dysfunction in disease and developing optimal therapies.[80]

REFERENCES

1. Armstrong EJ, Bischoff J. Heart valve development: endothelial cell signaling and differentiation. Circ Res 2004;95:459–70.
2. Oosthoek PW, Wenink AC, Wisse LJ, et al. Development of the papillary muscles of the mitral valve: morphogenetic background of parachute-like asymmetric mitral valves and other mitral valve anomalies. J Thorac Cardiovasc Surg 1998;116:36–46.
3. Schoen FJ. Evolving concepts of cardiac valve dynamics: the continuum of development, functional structure, pathobiology, and tissue engineering. Circulation 2008;118:1864–80.
4. Levine RA, Handschumacher MD, Sanfilippo AJ, et al. Three-dimensional echocardiographic reconstruction of the mitral valve, with implications for the diagnosis of mitral valve prolapse. Circulation 1989;80:589–98.
5. Kopuz C, Erk K, Baris YS, et al. Morphometry of the fibrous ring of the mitral valve. Ann Anat 1995;177:151–4.
6. Levine RA, Triulzi MO, Harrigan P, et al. The relationship of mitral annular shape to the diagnosis of mitral valve prolapse. Circulation 1987;75:756–67.

7. Puff A. Ischemic mitral incompetence. New York: Springer; 1991.

8. Timek TA, Green GR, Tibayan FA, et al. Aorto-mitral annular dynamics. Ann Thorac Surg 2003;76: 1944–50.

9. Lansac E, Lim KH, Shomura Y, et al. Dynamic balance of the aortomitral junction. J Thorac Cardiovasc Surg 2002;123:911–8.

10. Veronesi F, Corsi C, Sugeng L, et al. Quantification of mitral apparatus dynamics in functional and ischemic mitral regurgitation using real-time 3-dimensional echocardiography. J Am Soc Echocardiogr 2008;21:347–54.

11. Hamdan A, Guetta V, Konen E, et al. Deformation dynamics and mechanical properties of the aortic annulus by 4-dimensional computed tomography: insights into the functional anatomy of the aortic valve complex and implications for transcatheter aortic valve therapy. J Am Coll Cardiol 2012;59:119–27.

12. Komoda T, Hetzer R, Oellinger J, et al. Mitral annular flexibility. J Card Surg 1997;12:102–9.

13. Salgo IS, Gorman JH 3rd, Gorman RC, et al. Effect of annular shape on leaflet curvature in reducing mitral leaflet stress. Circulation 2002;106:711–7.

14. Kunzelman KS, Reimink MS, Cochran RP. Annular dilatation increases stress in the mitral valve and delays coaptation: a finite element computer model. Cardiovasc Surg 1997;5:427–34.

15. Jimenez JH, Liou SW, Padala M, et al. A saddle-shaped annulus reduces systolic strain on the central region of the mitral valve anterior leaflet. J Thorac Cardiovasc Surg 2007;134:1562–8.

16. Padala M, Hutchison RA, Croft LR, et al. Saddle shape of the mitral annulus reduces systolic strains on the P2 segment of the posterior mitral leaflet. Ann Thorac Surg 2009;88:1499–504.

17. Reimink MS, Kunzelman KS, Verrier ED, et al. The effect of anterior chordal replacement on mitral valve function and stresses. A finite element study. ASAIO J 1995;41:M754–62.

18. Jensen MO, Jensen H, Smerup M, et al. Saddle-shaped mitral valve annuloplasty rings experience lower forces compared with flat rings. Circulation 2008;118:S250–5.

19. Jensen MO, Jensen H, Levine RA, et al. Saddle-shaped mitral valve annuloplasty rings improve leaflet coaptation geometry. J Thorac Cardiovasc Surg 2011;142:697–703.

20. Jensen MO, Hagege AA, Otsuji Y, et al. The unsaddled annulus: biomechanical culprit in mitral valve prolapse? Circulation 2013;127:766–8.

21. I-Ida T II, Tamura K, Tanaka S, et al. Blood vessels in normal and abnormal mitral valve leaflets. J Nippon Med Sch 2001;68:171–80.

22. Williams TH, Folan JC, Jew JY, et al. Variations in atrioventricular valve innervation in four species of mammals. Am J Anat 1990;187:193–200.

23. Swanson JC, Davis LR, Arata K, et al. Characterization of mitral valve anterior leaflet perfusion patterns. J Heart Valve Dis 2009;18:488–95.

24. Carceller-Blanchard AM, Fouron JC. Determinants of the Doppler flow velocity profile through the mitral valve of the human fetus. Br Heart J 1993; 70:457–60.

25. Maffessanti F, Gripari P, Pontone G, et al. Three-dimensional dynamic assessment of tricuspid and mitral annuli using cardiovascular magnetic resonance. Eur Heart J Cardiovasc Imaging 2013. [Epub ahead of print].

26. Veronesi F, Corsi C, Sugeng L, et al. A study of functional anatomy of aortic mitral valve coupling using 3D matrix transesophageal echocardiography. Circ Cardiovasc Imaging 2009;2:24–31.

27. Alkadhi H, Desbiolles L, Stolzmann P, et al. Mitral annular shape, size, and motion in normals and in patients with cardiomyopathy: evaluation with computed tomography. Invest Radiol 2009;44: 218–25.

28. Ormiston JA, Shah PM, Tei C, et al. Size and motion of the mitral valve annulus in man. I. A two-dimensional echocardiographic method and findings in normal subjects. Circulation 1981;64:113–20.

29. Flachskampf FA, Chandra S, Gaddipatti A, et al. Analysis of shape and motion of the mitral annulus in subjects with and without cardiomyopathy by echocardiographic 3-dimensional reconstruction. J Am Soc Echocardiogr 2000;13:277–87.

30. Chaput M, Handschumacher MD, Tournoux F, et al. Mitral leaflet adaptation to ventricular remodeling: occurrence and adequacy in patients with functional mitral regurgitation. Circulation 2008;118: 845–52.

31. Watanabe N, Ogasawara Y, Yamaura Y, et al. Mitral annulus flattens in ischemic mitral regurgitation: geometric differences between inferior and anterior myocardial infarction: a real-time 3-dimensional echocardiographic study. Circulation 2005;112: 1458–62.

32. Daimon M, Saracino G, Fukuda S, et al. Dynamic change of mitral annular geometry and motion in ischemic mitral regurgitation assessed by a computerized 3D echo method. Echocardiography 2010;27:1069–77.

33. Lee AP, Hsiung MC, Salgo IS, et al. Quantitative analysis of mitral valve morphology in mitral valve prolapse with real-time 3-dimensional echocardiography: importance of annular saddle shape in the pathogenesis of mitral regurgitation. Circulation 2013;127:832–41.

34. Chiechi MA, Lees WM, Thompson R. Functional anatomy of the normal mitral valve. J Thorac Surg 1956;32:378–98.

35. Rusted IE, Scheifley CH, Edwards JE. Studies of the mitral valve. I. Anatomic features of the normal

mitral valve and associated structures. Circulation 1952;6:825–31.

36. Fenoglio JJ Jr, Tuan Duc P, Wit AL, et al. Canine mitral complex. Ultrastructure and electromechanical properties. Circ Res 1972;31:417–30.

37. Lam JH, Ranganathan N, Wigle ED, et al. Morphology of the human mitral valve. I. Chordae tendineae: a new classification. Circulation 1970; 41:449–58.

38. Cochran RP, Kunzelman KS, Chuong CJ, et al. Nondestructive analysis of mitral valve collagen fiber orientation. ASAIO Trans 1991;37:M447–8.

39. Carpentier A, Guerinon J, Deloche A, et al. The mitral valve—a pluridisciplinary approach. Acton (MA): Publishing Sciences Group Inc; 1976.

40. Laniado S, Yellin EL, Miller H, et al. Temporal relation of the first heart sound to closure of the mitral valve. Circulation 1973;47:1006–14.

41. Nkomo VT, Gardin JM, Skelton TN, et al. Burden of valvular heart diseases: a population-based study. Lancet 2006;368:1005–11.

42. Dal-Bianco JP, Aikawa E, Bischoff J, et al. Active adaptation of the tethered mitral valve: insights into a compensatory mechanism for functional mitral regurgitation. Circulation 2009;120:334–42.

43. Kunzelman KS, Cochran RP, Chuong C, et al. Finite element analysis of the mitral valve. J Heart Valve Dis 1993;2:326–40.

44. Kunzelman KS, Cochran RP, Murphree SS, et al. Differential collagen distribution in the mitral valve and its influence on biomechanical behaviour. J Heart Valve Dis 1993;2:236–44.

45. Marron K, Yacoub MH, Polak JM, et al. Innervation of human atrioventricular and arterial valves. Circulation 1996;94:368–75.

46. Jew JY, Williams TH. Innervation of the mitral valve is strikingly depleted with age. Anat Rec 1999;255: 252–60.

47. Noguchi T, Shimada T, Nakamura M, et al. The distribution and structure of the lymphatic system in dog atrioventricular valves. Arch Histol Cytol 1988;51:361–70.

48. Aikawa E, Whittaker P, Farber M, et al. Human semilunar cardiac valve remodeling by activated cells from fetus to adult: implications for postnatal adaptation, pathology, and tissue engineering. Circulation 2006;113:1344–52.

49. Quick DW, Kunzelman KS, Kneebone JM, et al. Collagen synthesis is upregulated in mitral valves subjected to altered stress. ASAIO J 1997;43: 181–6.

50. Millington-Sanders C, Meir A, Lawrence L, et al. Structure of chordae tendineae in the left ventricle of the human heart. J Anat 1998;192(Pt 4):573–81.

51. Degandt AA, Weber PA, Saber HA, et al. Mitral valve basal chordae: comparative anatomy and terminology. Ann Thorac Surg 2007;84:1250–5.

52. Liao J, Vesely I. A structural basis for the size-related mechanical properties of mitral valve chordae tendineae. J Biomech 2003;36:1125–33.

53. Messas E, Guerrero JL, Handschumacher MD, et al. Chordal cutting: a new therapeutic approach for ischemic mitral regurgitation. Circulation 2001; 104:1958–63.

54. Messas E, Pouzet B, Touchot B, et al. Efficacy of chordal cutting to relieve chronic persistent ischemic mitral regurgitation. Circulation 2003; 100(Suppl I):II111–5.

55. Messas E, Yosefy C, Chaput M, et al. Chordal cutting does not adversely affect left ventricle contractile function. Circulation 2006;114:I524–8.

56. Obadia JF, Casali C, Chassignolle JF, et al. Mitral subvalvular apparatus: different functions of primary and secondary chordae. Circulation 1997; 96:3124–8.

57. Victor S, Nayak VM. Variations in the papillary muscles of the normal mitral valve and their surgical relevance. J Card Surg 1995;10:597–607.

58. Komeda M, Glasson JR, Bolger AF, et al. Papillary muscle-left ventricular wall "complex". J Thorac Cardiovasc Surg 1997;113:292–300 [discussion: 300–1].

59. Joudinaud TM, Kegel CL, Flecher EM, et al. The papillary muscles as shock absorbers of the mitral valve complex. An experimental study. Eur J Cardiothorac Surg 2007;32:96–101.

60. Gorman JH 3rd, Gupta KB, Streicher JT, et al. Dynamic three-dimensional imaging of the mitral valve and left ventricle by rapid sonomicrometry array localization. J Thorac Cardiovasc Surg 1996;112:712–26.

61. Jiang L, Levine RA, King ME, et al. An integrated mechanism for systolic anterior motion of the mitral valve in hypertrophic cardiomyopathy based on echocardiographic observations. Am Heart J 1987;113:633–44.

62. Bonow RO, Carabello BA, Kanu C, et al. ACC/AHA 2006 guidelines for the management of patients with valvular heart disease: a report of the American College of Cardiology/American Heart Association Task Force on Practice Guidelines (writing committee to revise the 1998 Guidelines for the Management of Patients With Valvular Heart Disease): developed in collaboration with the Society of Cardiovascular Anesthesiologists: endorsed by the Society for Cardiovascular Angiography and Interventions and the Society of Thoracic Surgeons. Circulation 2006;114:e84–231.

63. Weiner RB, Wang F, Hutter AM Jr, et al. The feasibility, diagnostic yield, and learning curve of portable echocardiography for out-of-hospital cardiovascular disease screening. J Am Soc Echocardiogr 2012;25:568–75.

64. Zamorano JL, Badano LP, Bruce C, et al. EAE/ASE recommendations for the use of echocardiography

in new transcatheter interventions for valvular heart disease. Eur Heart J 2011;32:2189–214.

65. Messas E, Guerrero JL, Handschumacher MD, et al. Paradoxic decrease in ischemic mitral regurgitation with papillary muscle dysfunction: insights from three-dimensional and contrast echocardiography with strain rate measurement. Circulation 2001;104:1952–7.

66. Otsuji Y, Gilon D, Jiang L, et al. Restricted diastolic opening of the mitral leaflets in patients with left ventricular dysfunction: evidence for increased valve tethering. J Am Coll Cardiol 1998;32:398–404.

67. Otsuji Y, Handschumacher MD, Schwammenthal E, et al. Insights from three-dimensional echocardiography into the mechanism of functional mitral regurgitation: direct in vivo demonstration of altered leaflet tethering geometry. Circulation 1997;96:1999–2008.

68. Chaput M, Handschumacher MD, Guerrero JL, et al. Mitral leaflet adaptation to ventricular remodeling: prospective changes in a model of ischemic mitral regurgitation. Circulation 2009;120:S99–103.

69. Carpentier AF, Lessana A, Relland JY, et al. The "physio-ring": an advanced concept in mitral valve annuloplasty. Ann Thorac Surg 1995;60:1177–85 [discussion: 1185–6].

70. Levine RA, Stathogiannis E, Newell JB, et al. Reconsideration of echocardiographic standards for mitral valve prolapse: lack of association between leaflet displacement isolated to the apical four chamber view and independent echocardiographic evidence of abnormality. J Am Coll Cardiol 1988;11:1010–9.

71. Freed LA, Levy D, Levine RA, et al. Prevalence and clinical outcome of mitral valve prolapse. N Engl J Med 1999;341:1–7.

72. King DL, Harrison MR, King DL Jr, et al. Ultrasound beam orientation during standard two-dimensional imaging: assessment by three-dimensional echocardiography. J Am Soc Echocardiogr 1992;5:569–76.

73. Lang RM, Badano LP, Tsang W, et al. EAE/ASE recommendations for image acquisition and display using three-dimensional echocardiography. Eur Heart J Cardiovasc Imaging 2012;13:1–46.

74. Levy MJ, Edwards JE. Anatomy of mitral insufficiency. Prog Cardiovasc Dis 1962;5:119–44.

75. Levine RA, Schwammenthal E. Ischemic mitral regurgitation on the threshold of a solution: from paradoxes to unifying concepts. Circulation 2005;112:745–58.

76. Sanfilippo AJ, Harrigan P, Popovic AD, et al. Papillary muscle traction in mitral valve prolapse: quantitation by two-dimensional echocardiography. J Am Coll Cardiol 1992;19:564–71.

77. Gornick CC, Tobler HG, Pritzker MC, et al. Electrophysiologic effects of papillary muscle traction in the intact heart. Circulation 1986;73:1013–21.

78. Fucci C, Sandrelli L, Pardini A, et al. Improved results with mitral valve repair using new surgical techniques. Eur J Cardiothorac Surg 1995;9:621–6 [discussion: 626–7].

79. Feldman T, Kar S, Rinaldi M, et al. Percutaneous mitral repair with the MitraClip system: safety and midterm durability in the initial EVEREST (Endovascular Valve Edge-to-Edge REpair Study) cohort. J Am Coll Cardiol 2009;54:686–94.

80. Carpentier A. Cardiac valve surgery—the "French correction". J Thorac Cardiovasc Surg 1983;86:323–37.

81. Perloff JK, Roberts WC. The mitral apparatus. Functional anatomy of mitral regurgitation. Circulation 1972;46:227–39.

82. Silverman ME, Hurst JW. The mitral complex. Interaction of the anatomy, physiology, and pathology of the mitral annulus, mitral valve leaflets, chordae tendineae, and papillary muscles. Am Heart J 1968;76:399–418.

83. Godley RW, Wann LS, Rogers EW, et al. Incomplete mitral leaflet closure in patients with papillary muscle dysfunction. Circulation 1981;63:565–71.

84. Ogawa S, Hubbard FE, Mardelli TJ, et al. Cross-sectional echocardiographic spectrum of papillary muscle dysfunction. Am Heart J 1979;97:312–21.

85. Kaul S, Spotnitz WD, Glasheen WP, et al. Mechanism of ischemic mitral regurgitation. An experimental evaluation. Circulation 1991;84:2167–80.

86. Kono T, Sabbah HN, Rosman H, et al. Left ventricular shape is the primary determinant of functional mitral regurgitation in heart failure. J Am Coll Cardiol 1992;20:1594–8.

87. Sabbah HN, Kono T, Stein PD, et al. Left ventricular shape changes during the course of evolving heart failure. Am J Physiol 1992;263:H266–70.

88. Sabbah HN, Rosman H, Kono T, et al. On the mechanism of functional mitral regurgitation. Am J Cardiol 1993;72:1074–6.

89. Yiu SF, Enriquez-Sarano M, Tribouilloy C, et al. Determinants of the degree of functional mitral regurgitation in patients with systolic left ventricular dysfunction: a quantitative clinical study. Circulation 2000;102:1400–6.

90. Otsuji Y, Handschumacher MD, Liel-Cohen N, et al. Mechanism of ischemic mitral regurgitation with segmental left ventricular dysfunction: three-dimensional echocardiographic studies in models of acute and chronic progressive regurgitation. J Am Coll Cardiol 2001;37:641–8.

91. He S, Fontaine AA, Schwammenthal E, et al. Integrated mechanism for functional mitral regurgitation: leaflet restriction versus coapting force: in vitro studies. Circulation 1997;96:1826–34.

92. Gorman RC, McCaughan JS, Ratcliffe MB, et al. Pathogenesis of acute ischemic mitral regurgitation in three dimensions. J Thorac Cardiovasc Surg 1995;109:684–93.

93. Liel-Cohen N, Guerrero JL, Otsuji Y, et al. Design of a new surgical approach for ventricular remodeling to relieve ischemic mitral regurgitation: insights from 3-dimensional echocardiography. Circulation 2000;101:2756–63.

94. Llaneras MR, Nance ML, Streicher JT, et al. Large animal model of ischemic mitral regurgitation. Ann Thorac Surg 1994;57:432–9.

95. Hung J, Chaput M, Guerrero JL, et al. Persistent reduction of ischemic mitral regurgitation by papillary muscle repositioning: structural stabilization of the papillary muscle-ventricular wall complex. Circulation 2007;116:I259–63.

96. Hung J, Guerrero JL, Handschumacher MD, et al. Reverse ventricular remodeling reduces ischemic mitral regurgitation: echoguided device application in the beating heart. Circulation 2002;106:2594–600.

97. Solis J, Levine RA, Johnson B, et al. Polymer injection therapy to reverse remodel the papillary muscles: efficacy in reducing mitral regurgitation in a chronic ischemic model. Circ Cardiovasc Interv 2010;3:499–505.

98. Di Donato M, Frigiola A, Menicanti L, et al. Moderate ischemic mitral regurgitation and coronary artery bypass surgery: effect of mitral repair on clinical outcome. J Heart Valve Dis 2003;12:272–9.

99. Trichon BH, Glower DD, Shaw LK, et al. Survival after coronary revascularization, with and without mitral valve surgery, in patients with ischemic mitral regurgitation. Circulation 2003;108(Suppl 1):II103–10.

100. Tenenbaum A, Leor J, Motro M, et al. Improved posterobasal segment function after thrombolysis is associated with decreased incidence of significant mitral regurgitation in a first inferior myocardial infarction. J Am Coll Cardiol 1995;25:1558–63.

101. Beeri R, Guerrero JL, Supple G, et al. New efficient catheter-based system for myocardial gene delivery. Circulation 2002;106:1756–9.

102. Cittadini A, Monti MG, Iaccarino G, et al. Adenoviral gene transfer of Akt enhances myocardial contractility and intracellular calcium handling. Gene Ther 2006;13:8–19.

103. Hagege AA, Marolleau JP, Vilquin JT, et al. Skeletal myoblast transplantation in ischemic heart failure: long-term follow-up of the first phase I cohort of patients. Circulation 2006;114:I108–13.

104. Kanzaki H, Bazaz R, Schwartzman D, et al. A mechanism for immediate reduction in mitral regurgitation after cardiac resynchronization therapy: insights from mechanical activation strain mapping. J Am Coll Cardiol 2004;44:1619–25.

105. Solis J, McCarty D, Levine RA, et al. Mechanism of decrease in mitral regurgitation after cardiac resynchronization therapy: optimization of the force balance relationship. Circ Cardiovasc Imaging 2009;2:444–50.

106. Matsui Y, Suto Y, Shimura S, et al. Impact of papillary muscles approximation on the adequacy of mitral coaptation in functional mitral regurgitation due to dilated cardiomyopathy. Ann Thorac Cardiovasc Surg 2005;11:164–71.

107. Messas E, Bel A, Szymanski C, et al. Relief of mitral leaflet tethering following chronic myocardial infarction by chordal cutting diminishes left ventricular remodeling. Circ Cardiovasc Imaging 2010;3(6):679–86.

108. Hung J, Papakostas L, Tahta SA, et al. Mechanism of recurrent ischemic mitral regurgitation after annuloplasty: continued LV remodeling as a moving target. Circulation 2004;110:II85–90.

109. Kuwahara E, Otsuji Y, Iguro Y, et al. Mechanism of recurrent/persistent ischemic/functional mitral regurgitation in the chronic phase after surgical annuloplasty: importance of augmented posterior leaflet tethering. Circulation 2006;114:I529–34.

110. Liel-Cohen N, Otsuji Y, Vlahakes G, et al. Functional ischemic mitral regurgitation can persist despite ring annuloplasty: mechanistic insights. Circulation 1997;96:I540.

111. McGee EC, Gillinov AM, Blackstone EH, et al. Recurrent mitral regurgitation after annuloplasty for functional ischemic mitral regurgitation. J Thorac Cardiovasc Surg 2004;128:916–24.

112. Borger MA, Murphy PM, Alam A, et al. Initial results of the chordal-cutting operation for ischemic mitral regurgitation. J Thorac Cardiovasc Surg 2007;133:1483–92.

113. Watkins H, Ashrafian H, Redwood C. Inherited cardiomyopathies. N Engl J Med 2011;364:1643–56.

114. Harrigan CJ, Appelbaum E, Maron BJ, et al. Significance of papillary muscle abnormalities identified by cardiovascular magnetic resonance in hypertrophic cardiomyopathy. Am J Cardiol 2008;101:668–73.

115. Hwang HJ, Choi EY, Kwan J, et al. Dynamic change of mitral apparatus as potential cause of left ventricular outflow tract obstruction in hypertrophic cardiomyopathy. Eur J Echocardiogr 2011;12:19–25.

116. Levine RA, Vlahakes GJ, Lefebvre X, et al. Papillary muscle displacement causes systolic anterior motion of the mitral valve. Experimental validation and insights into the mechanism of subaortic obstruction. Circulation 1995;91:1189–95.

117. Sherrid MV, Chu CK, Delia E, et al. An echocardiographic study of the fluid mechanics of obstruction in hypertrophic cardiomyopathy. J Am Coll Cardiol 1993;22:816–25.

118. Sherrid MV, Gunsburg DZ, Moldenhauer S, et al. Systolic anterior motion begins at low left ventricular outflow tract velocity in obstructive hypertrophic cardiomyopathy. J Am Coll Cardiol 2000;36: 1344–54.

119. Maron BJ, Gottdiener JS, Roberts WC, et al. Left ventricular outflow tract obstruction due to systolic anterior motion of the anterior mitral leaflet in patients with concentric left ventricular hypertrophy. Circulation 1978;57:527–33.

120. Maron BJ, Epstein SE. Hypertrophic cardiomyopathy. Recent observations regarding the specificity of three hallmarks of the disease: asymmetric septal hypertrophy, septal disorganization and systolic anterior motion of the anterior mitral leaflet. Am J Cardiol 1980;45:141–54.

121. Schwammenthal E, Nakatani S, He S, et al. Mechanism of mitral regurgitation in hypertrophic cardiomyopathy: mismatch of posterior to anterior leaflet length and mobility. Circulation 1998;98:856–65.

122. Delling FN, Sanborn DY, Levine RA, et al. Frequency and mechanism of persistent systolic anterior motion and mitral regurgitation after septal ablation in obstructive hypertrophic cardiomyopathy. Am J Cardiol 2007;100:1691–5.

123. Klues HG, Roberts WC, Maron BJ. Morphological determinants of echocardiographic patterns of mitral valve systolic anterior motion in obstructive hypertrophic cardiomyopathy. Circulation 1993; 87:1570–9.

124. Kim DH, Handschumacher MD, Levine RA, et al. In vivo measurement of mitral leaflet surface area and subvalvular geometry in patients with asymmetrical septal hypertrophy: insights into the mechanism of outflow tract obstruction. Circulation 2010;122:1298–307.

125. Hagege AA, Bruneval P, Levine RA, et al. The mitral valve in hypertrophic cardiomyopathy: old versus new concepts. J Cardiovasc Transl Res 2011;4: 757–66.

126. He S, Hopmeyer J, Lefebvre XP, et al. Importance of leaflet elongation in causing systolic anterior motion of the mitral valve. J Heart Valve Dis 1997;6: 149–59.

127. Maslow AD, Regan MM, Haering JM, et al. Echocardiographic predictors of left ventricular outflow tract obstruction and systolic anterior motion of the mitral valve after mitral valve reconstruction for myxomatous valve disease. J Am Coll Cardiol 1999;34:2096–104.

128. Jebara VA, Mihaileanu S, Acar C, et al. Left ventricular outflow tract obstruction after mitral valve repair. Results of the sliding leaflet technique. Circulation 1993;88:II30–4.

129. Bulkley BH, Roberts WC. Dilatation of the mitral annulus. A rare cause of mitral regurgitation. Am J Med 1975;59:457–63.

130. Komoda T, Hetzer R, Uyama C, et al. Mitral annular function assessed by 3D imaging for mitral valve surgery. J Heart Valve Dis 1994;3:483–90.

131. Mautner SL, Klues HG, Mautner GC, et al. Comparison of mitral valve dimensions in adults with valvular aortic stenosis, pure aortic regurgitation and hypertrophic cardiomyopathy. Am J Cardiol 1993;71:949–53.

132. Klues HG, Maron BJ, Dollar AL, et al. Diversity of structural mitral valve alterations in hypertrophic cardiomyopathy. Circulation 1992;85:1651–60.

Echocardiographic Assessment of Mitral Regurgitation
General Considerations

Jorge Solis, MD[a,b,*], Victoria Piro, MD[c],
Jose Antonio Vazquez de Prada, MD, PhD[d,e],
Gerard Loughlin, MD[a]

KEYWORDS

• Mitral valve • Mitral regurgitation mitral • Echo Doppler • 3D echocardiography

KEY POINTS

• Mitral regurgitation (MR) is diagnosed based on findings provided by Doppler echocardiography.
• Careful quantification of MR is critical for clinical decision making and to determine whether surgery is needed.
• M-Mode, 2-dimensional (2D), and 3D echocardiography provide additional information of the impact of MR on the remaining cardiac structures.
• A combination of qualitative and quantitative methods is needed for assessment of the severity of mitral valve regurgitation.

INTRODUCTION

Echocardiography is undoubtedly one of the main tools used in assessment of mitral regurgitaiton (MR) because it allows characterization of valvular morphology, assessment of the severity of the regurgitation, and its secondary effects. In this article we present an overview of the echocardiographic assessment of MR.

MITRAL VALVE ANATOMY AND CHAMBER QUANTIFICATION

Mitral valve anatomy analysis should always be part of the assessment of MR severity. The mitral valve, as a whole, includes left atrial (LA) walls, the annulus, the anterior and posterior leaflets, chordae, papillary muscles, and the left ventricular (LV) myocardium underlying the papillary muscles (PMs). Two-dimensional transthoracic echocardiography (2D TTE) is the imaging modality of choice for this assessment, whereas 2D transesophageal echocardiography (2D TEE) should be performed in nondiagnostic cases or where further anatomic and functional information is required. Three-dimensional echocardiography (3DE) enables the direct anatomic visualization of the mitral valve apparatus and the size, shape, and space orientation of the MR jet. For this reason, 3D-TTE or 3D-TEE imaging is recommended in complex mitral valve lesions when available.

[a] Department of Cardiology, Hospital General Universitario Gregorio Marañón, Doctor Esquerdo 46, Madrid 28007, Spain; [b] Complutense Medical School, Doctor Esquerdo 46, Madrid 28007, Spain; [c] Division of Cardiology, Massachusetts General Hospital, Blake 2, 55 Fruit Street, Boston, MA 02114, USA; [d] Department of Cardiology, Hospital Universitario Marques de Valdecilla, Avda. de Valdecilla s/n, Santander 39008, Spain; [e] Marques de Valdecilla Research Institute (IFIMAV), Avda. de Valdecilla s/n, Santander 39008, Spain
* Corresponding author. Department of Cardiology, Hospital General Universitario Gregorio Marañón, Doctor Esquerdo 46, Madrid 28007, Spain.
E-mail address: jsolismartin@yahoo.es

Cardiol Clin 31 (2013) 165–168
http://dx.doi.org/10.1016/j.ccl.2013.04.001
0733-8651/13/$ – see front matter © 2013 Elsevier Inc. All rights reserved.

Table 1
Mitral valve information that should be in the echo report and TTE-TEE recommendations

Valve analysis:
- Distinction between primary and secondary MR
- Etiology and mechanism information
- Diameter of MV annulus

Recommendation:
- TTE: First-line imaging modality
- TEE: TTE non diagnostic or further information is required (Planning MV surgery)

The evaluation of LA dimensions (diameters, area, or volume) is important, as LA dimensions provide additional information about MR severity and its natural history. An enlarged LA is usually associated with more severe MR (unless the onset of MR is acute) and is reflective of a chronic lesion, as opposed to acute-onset MR, in which LA dimensions are usually found to be within normal limits, because the hemodynamic overload on the left chambers and remodeling have not yet occurred. The assessment of the LV size and function is also very important, as measures of LV size and function are used to determine the timing of surgery, particularly in asymptomatic patients. Most recent European Association of Echocardiography/American Society of Echocardiography guidelines recommend the use of 3DE over the use of 2DE in this setting because of its greater reproducibility and accuracy.[1–29]

Table 1 summarizes the anatomic and functional information that should be included in the echo report.

ETIOLOGY OF MR

The starting point for the assessment of MR should be an evaluation of the mitral valve as a whole within its environment. It is important to distinguish between organic (primary) MR, in which the valve tissue is originally affected, and functional (secondary) MR, in which LV remodeling as the clinical course and clinical decision making depends on the etiology of MR. In industrialized countries, myxomatous degeneration (60%) is the leading cause of MR, followed by functional MR (20%), infective endocarditis (2%–5%), and rheumatic valve disease (2%–5%).[1] These and other less frequent causes of MR are outlined in **Table 2**. The various mechanisms of valve dysfunction brought on by the different causes of MR are described in Carpentier's functional classification of MR: type I (normal leaflet motion), type II (excessive leaflet motion), type IIIa (restricted diastolic leaflet motion), and type IIIb (restricted systolic leaflet motion).[2]

ACUTE AND CHRONIC ISCHEMIC MITRAL REGURGITATION

Color Doppler and Doppler profiles are helpful in distinguishing acute and chronic ischemic MR. Color Doppler imaging in acute ischemic MR frequently reveals smaller jets and a triangular-shaped continuous wave (CW) Doppler profile. It is now established that in functional MR, the mitral valve and LV remodeling result in a non–vena contracta and effective regurgitant orifice area that are noncircular in shape (**Fig. 1**), which may lead to substantial errors, particularly when calculating these parameters by the 2D method, leading to an underestimation or overestimation of the flow rate.

The assessment of the alteration of mitral valve geometry over time, as expressed by an increase in tenting and annular area, might also provide

Table 2
Etiology and mechanism of mitral regurgitation (MR)

	Primary MR (Organic)		Secondary MR
Type I	Type II	Type IIIa	Type IIIb
Perforation (endocarditis)	Myxomatous Valve disease	Rheumatic valve	Functional MR:
Mitral annular calcification	Chordal rupture	Radiation	• Ischemic
Mitral annular dilatation	PMs rupture	Drugs	• Nonischemic
Mitral cleft		Inflammatory disease	

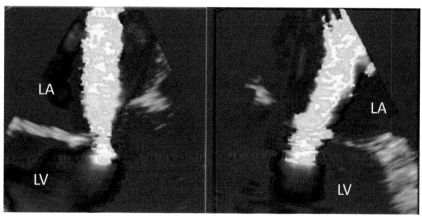

Fig. 1. Three-dimensional TEE echocardiography showing 2D biplane orthogonal views of an MR jet. Note the different shape and size of the flow convergence zone and the vena contracta depending on the view.

an alternative method to evaluate the severity of ischemic mitral regurgitation, although not currently used routinely in clinical practice. The degree of tenting and the annular area in the case of ischemic mitral valve regurgitation may serve as a quantitative measure of severity and serve as a predictor of progression of MR over time.

REFERENCES

1. Enriquez-Sarano M, Akins CW, Vahanian A. Mitral regurgitation. Lancet 2009;373:1382–94.
2. Carpentier A. Cardiac valve surgery—the "French correction". J Thorac Cardiovasc Surg 1983;86:323–37.
3. Gorlin R, Gorlin SG. Hydraulic formula for calculation of the area of the stenotic mitral valve, other cardiac valves, and central circulatory shunts. I. Am Heart J 1951;41·1–29.
4. Levine HJ, Gaasch WH. Vasoactive drugs in chronic regurgitant lesions of the mitral and aortic valves. J Am Coll Cardiol 1996;28:1083–91.
5. Yoran C, Yellin EL, Becker RM, et al. Dynamic aspects of acute mitral regurgitation: effects of ventricular volume, pressure and contractility on the effective regurgitant orifice area. Circulation 1979; 60.170–6.
6. Chaliki HP, Nishimura RA, Enriquez-Sarano M, et al. A simplified, practical approach to assessment of severity of mitral regurgitation by Doppler color flow imaging with proximal convergence: validation with concomitant cardiac catheterization. Mayo Clin Proc 1998;73:929–35.
7. McCully RB, Enriquez-Sarano M, Tajik AJ, et al. Overestimation of severity of ischemic/functional mitral regurgitation by color Doppler jet area. Am J Cardiol 1994;74:790–3.
8. Zoghbi WA, Enriquez-Sarano M, Foster E, et al. Recommendations for evaluation of severity of native valvular regurgitation with two-dimensional and Doppler echocardiography. J Am Soc Echocardiogr 2003;16(7):777–802.
9. Sahn DJ. Instrumentation and physical factors related to visualization of stenotic and regurgitant jets by Doppler color flow mapping. J Am Coll Cardiol 1988;12:1354–65.
10. Hall SA, Brickner ME, Willett DL, et al. Assessment of mitral regurgitation severity by Doppler color flow mapping of the vena contracta. Circulation 1997;95:636–42.
11. Tribouilloy C, Shen WF, Quere JP, et al. Assessment of severity of mitral regurgitation by measuring regurgitant jet width at its origin with transesophageal Doppler color flow imaging. Circulation 1992;85:1248–53.
12. Baumgartner H, Schima H, Kuhn P. Importance of technical variables for quantitative measurements by color Doppler imaging. Am J Cardiol 1991;67:314–5.
13. Lancellotti P, Moura L, Pierard LA, et al. European Association of Echocardiography recommendations for the assessment of valvular regurgitation. Part 2: mitral and tricuspid regurgitation (native valve disease). Eur J Echocardiogr 2010;11(4):307–32.
14. Enriquez-Sarano M, Dujardin KS, Tribouilloy CM, et al. Determinants of pulmonary venous flow reversal in mitral regurgitation and its usefulness in determining the severity of regurgitation. Am J Cardiol 1999;83:535–41.
15. Thomas L, Foster E, Schiller NB. Peak mitral inflow velocity predicts mitral regurgitation severity. J Am Coll Cardiol 1998;31:174–9.
16. Bargiggia GS, Tronconi L, Sahn DJ, et al. A new method for quantitation of mitral regurgitation based

on color flow Doppler imaging of flow convergence proximal to regurgitant orifice. Circulation 1991;84: 1481-9.

17. Enriquez-Sarano M, Miller FA Jr, Hayes SN, et al. Effective mitral regurgitant orifice area: clinical use and pitfalls of the proximal isovelocity surface area method. J Am Coll Cardiol 1995;25:703–9.

18. Vandervoort PM, Thoreau DH, Rivera JM, et al. Automated flow rate calculations based on digital analysis of flow convergence proximal to regurgitant orifices. J Am Coll Cardiol 1993;22:535–41.

19. Schwammenthal E, Chen C, Benning F, et al. Dynamics of mitral regurgitant flow and orifice area. Physiologic application of the proximal flow convergence method: clinical data and experimental testing. Circulation 1994;90:307–22.

20. Hung J, Otsuji Y, Handschumacher MD, et al. Mechanism of dynamic regurgitant orifice area variation in functional mitral regurgitation: physiologic insights from the proximal flow convergence technique. J Am Coll Cardiol 1999;33:538–45.

21. Matsumura Y, Fukuda S, Tran H, et al. Geometry of the proximal isovelocity surface area in mitral regurgitation by 3-dimensional color Doppler echocardiography: difference between functional mitral regurgitation and prolapse regurgitation. Am Heart J 2008;155:231–8.

22. Song JM, Kim MJ, Kim YJ, et al. Three-dimensional characteristics of functional mitral regurgitation in patients with severe left ventricular dysfunction: a real-time three-dimensional colour Doppler echocardiography study. Heart 2008;94:590–6.

23. Kahlert P, Plicht B, Schenk IM, et al. Direct assessment of size and shape of noncircular vena contracta area in functional versus organic mitral regurgitation using real-time three-dimensional echocardiography. J Am Soc Echocardiogr 2008; 21:912–21.

24. Yosefy C, Hung J, Chua S, et al. Direct measurement of vena contracta area by real-time 3-dimensional echocardiography for assessing severity of mitral regurgitation. Am J Cardiol 2009;104:978–83.

25. Pu M, Vandervoort PM, Greenberg NL, et al. Impact of wall constraint on velocity distribution in proximal flow convergence zone. Implications for color Doppler quantification of mitral regurgitation. J Am Coll Cardiol 1996;27:706–13.

26. Matsumura Y, Saracino G, Sugioka K, et al. Determination of regurgitant orifice area with the use of a new three-dimensional flow convergence geometric assumption in functional mitral regurgitation. J Am Soc Echocardiogr 2008;21:1251–6.

27. Cobey FC, McInnis JA, Gelfand BJ, et al. A method for automating 3-dimensional proximal isovelocity surface area measurement. J Cardiothorac Vasc Anesth 2012;26:507–11.

28. Thavendiranathan P, Liu S, Datta S, et al. Quantification of chronic functional mitral regurgitation by automated 3-dimensional peak and integrated proximal isovelocity surface area and stroke volume techniques using real-time 3-dimensional volume color Doppler echocardiography in vitro and clinical validation. Circ Cardiovasc Imaging 2013; 6:125–33.

29. Enriquez-Sarano M, Seward JB, Bailey KR, et al. Effective regurgitant orifice area: a noninvasive Doppler development of an old hemodynamic concept. J Am Coll Cardiol 1994;23:443–51.

How to Grade Mitral Regurgitation
An Integrative Approach

Jorge Solis, MD[a,b,*], Victoria Piro, MD[c],
Gerard Loughlin, MD[a],
Jose Antonio Vazquez de Prada, MD, PhD[d,e]

KEYWORDS

• Mitral valve regurgitation • Mitral regurgitation quantification • Doppler echocardiography
• 3D echocardiography

KEY POINTS

- The American Society of Echocardiography and European Association of Echocardiography recommendations for mitral regurgitation (MR) assessment highlight the importance of an integrated approach.
- Mitral valve anatomy and chamber quantification analysis should always be part of the assessment of MR severity.
- Three-dimensional echocardiography is recommended in complex mitral valve lesions.
  - Distal jet area and vena contracta methods provide semiquantitative methods for assessing MR.
  - With eccentric MR jets, jet area methods may underestimate MR degree due to wall impingement.
  - Quantitate mitral regurgitation by calculating effective regurgitant orifice area or regurgitant volume or fraction using proximal isovelocity surface area or volumetric pulsed Doppler methods when technically possible in moderate or greater degrees of MR.
  - Pulmonary venous Doppler pattern provides supportive evidence of MR severity, particularly the presence of pulmonary venous systolic flow reversal.
- Supportive evidence, such as left atrial and left ventricular (LV) chamber enlargement, LV hypertrophy, elevated right ventricular systolic pressure, and peak mitral E-wave velocity should be included in the overall assessment of MR.

INTRODUCTION

Aside from the clinical examination, an important tool in the diagnosis of mitral regurgitation (MR) is Doppler echocardiography. In particular, the use of color Doppler has allowed for semiquantitative measures of MR. Additionally, the use of pulsed wave and continuous wave Doppler imaging also provides useful qualitative information (based on the intensity, shape, and distribution of the resulting profiles), and allows for the quantification of the degree of MR. Other quantitative measures that are widely used to quantify MR also include the vena contracta (VC) (width or area), regurgitant volume, and regurgitant fraction. Quantification of MR plays a critical role in clinical decision making. Doppler echocardiography has

[a] Department of Cardiology, Hospital General Universitario Gregorio Marañón, Doctor Esquerdo 46, Madrid 28007, Spain; [b] Complutense Medical School, Doctor Esquerdo 46, Madrid 28007, Spain; [c] Division of Cardiology, Massachusetts General Hospital, Blake 2, 55 Fruit Street, Boston, MA 02114, USA; [d] Department of Cardiology, Hospital Universitario Marques de Valdecilla, Avda. de Valdecilla s/n, Santander 39008, Spain; [e] "Marqués de Valdecilla" Research Institute (IFIMAV), Avda. de Valdecilla s/n, Santander 39008, Spain
* Corresponding author. Department of Cardiology, Hospital General Universitario Gregorio Marañón, Doctor Esquerdo 46, Madrid 28007, Spain.
E-mail address: jsolismartin@yahoo.es

Cardiol Clin 31 (2013) 169–175
http://dx.doi.org/10.1016/j.ccl.2013.04.002
0733-8651/13/$ – see front matter © 2013 Elsevier Inc. All rights reserved.

transformed the diagnosis and management of mitral valve disease, providing accurate noninvasive quantification of MR.

As significant MR can impact cardiac structure and function, the evaluation of MR should always include the assessment of atrial and ventricular chamber sizes and function, as these measures influence the decision for intervention and strategy (ie, valve repair or replacement).

This article summarizes recommendations for MR assessment and highlights the importance of an integrated approach, using anatomic information as well as qualitative and quantitative Doppler measures.

MITRAL VALVE QUANTITATION: HEMODYNAMIC BACKGROUND

Understanding the role of the hemodynamic determinants of valvular regurgitation requires an understanding of the Gorlin hydraulic orifice equation. By solving the orifice equation for the regurgitant volume, one can directly derive the hydraulic determinants of regurgitant flow. The Gorlin formula, which also combines the fundamental equation of fluid mechanics (flow = velocity × area), and the Bernoulli equation, which expresses velocity in terms of pressure, is[1] as follows:

$$RV = ROA \times Cd \times \sqrt{LVsm - LAsm} \times Ts$$

Where RV = mitral regurgitant volume, ROA = mitral regurgitant orifice area, Cd = discharge coefficient (contraction of the flow stream as it passes through the anatomic orifice, which depends on fluid viscosity and orifice geometry), $LVsm$ = left ventricular (LV) systolic mean pressure, $LAsm$ = left atrial (LA) systolic mean pressure, and Ts = duration of systole.[2]

As the equation uses the systolic pressure gradient between LV and LA, measuring and recording the patient's blood pressure at the time of the echocardiographic examination is necessary. It is also important to determine the etiology of mitral insufficiency beforehand, as the regurgitant orifice may be dynamic or fixed dependent on the etiology. Furthermore, the regurgitation area is also load dependant. An example of a fixed regurgitant orifice area is severe mitral annular calcification. As opposed to mitral valve prolapse, in which the severity of MR is related to the dynamic variations in orifice area, as a result of dynamic changes in the diameter of the LV throughout the systole.[3]

The duration of MR in systole is also important to consider when grading MR severity, as the duration and pattern of MR can vary depending on mechanism. An example of this variation is when assessing MR severity in myxomatous valves where the MR jet occurs mostly at end systole, as opposed to in dilated cardiomyopathy where MR occurs at the beginning of systole. In the first example, if we were to take into account only late systolic frames, we would run the risk of erroneously considering severe what would in reality be mild or moderate late systolic jets (using the proximal isovelocity surface area method). In such instances, continuous wave Doppler measurements will indicate MR only at late systole.

QUALITATIVE AND SEMIQUANTITATIVE APPROACHES

Qualitative and semiquantitative parameters are useful for identifying the extreme grades of MR severity but not as effective for assessment of the intermediate degrees. These parameters include color flow jet area, VC width, density of the continuous-wave (CW) Doppler profile, pulmonary vein flow pattern, and mitral inflow pattern.[4]

The Color Flow Area

Color flow area is useful for identifying central MR jets and evaluating the spatial orientation of the jet but is not recommended for use in the grading of MR severity of eccentric jets, because this method significantly underestimates the regurgitant volume (up to 40%) when compared with central jets with the same volume.[5]

- <4 cm² or <20% of LA size: mild MR
- >10 cm² or >40% of LA size: severe MR
- Intermediate values: overlap
- Influenced by hemodynamic and technical factors:
  - Low blood pressure, acute MR: underestimate.
  - Eccentric jet: underestimate.
  - Color gain and Nyquist scale optimization.

VC Width

VC width is an easy and quick method that is relatively independent of hemodynamic factors, but is limited by its narrow range. Image optimization is needed: zoom mode with narrow sector and plane perpendicular to the jet is essential to improve spatial and temporal resolution. However, given that the 2-chamber view is parallel to the mitral leaflet coaptation line, even mild degrees of functional regurgitation can appear to show a wide VC; therefore, commissural views are not recommended for VC width measurements.

• <0.3 cm: mild MR	• Can be used in eccentric jet.
• <0.7 cm: severe MR	• Accurate in acute MR.
• Intermediate values: overlap	• Not valid for multiple MR jets.

CW Doppler

Although the use of CW velocities and the density of the CW Doppler profile to evaluate MR severity wave could be considered a qualitative approach to evaluating MR severity, it is a useful adjunct to other quantitative measurements. Adequate alignment of the beam with the MR jet profile is crucial for an accurate representation of the MR severity.

• Soft density, incomplete envelope: mild	• Difficult to obtain in eccentric jet
• Dense signal with triangular shape: severe	

Pulmonary Veins

Pulsed Doppler to evaluate pulmonary vein flow adds additional information to MR severity and should also be used as a complement to other methods. A normal flow pattern is usually associated with mild or mild-to-moderate MR, whereas reversal of the systolic wave is a highly reliable marker of severe or moderate-to-severe regurgitation (Needs a reference here). The presence of blunted systolic waves has less predictive value; hence, should be interpreted with caution.[6]

An additional caveat is that occasionally a nonsignificant MR jet can be selectively directed at a pulmonary vein, causing reversal of flow in that particular vein, and leading to a potential over estimation of MR severity. To overcome this limitation, it is important to asses the flow pattern in 2 or more different pulmonary veins before concluding a positive finding of "blunting" or reversal systolic flow compatible with significant MR.

• Systolic dominance: mild MR	• Influenced by LA pressure and LV relaxation
• Systolic flow reversal: severe MR	• Not accurate if atrial fibrillation

Mitral Inflow Pattern

Mitral inflow pattern is another qualitative and complementary Doppler imaging parameter used in the evaluation of MR severity. A semiquantitative method using the mitral-to-aortic time-velocity integral (TVI) ratio of the pulsed wave Doppler profile of mitral and aortic valves could be used to quantify isolated organic MR. A ratio greater than 1.4 suggests severe MR, whereas values less than 1.0 indicate mild MR.[7]

• A-wave dominant excludes severe MR	• Influenced by LA pressure and LV relaxation
• E-wave >1.5 cm/s indicates severe MR	• Not accurate if atrial fibrillation

QUANTITATIVE APPROACHES

Quantitative approaches to the assessment of MR severity include the regurgitant volume, regurgitant fraction, and effective regurgitant orifice area (EROA). Quantitative measures are particularly useful for defining the intermediate degrees of MR, such as mild-to-moderate and moderate-to-severe regurgitation. The current European recommendations for MR quantitation[8] have taken into account the different characteristics of primary and secondary MR. Different cutoff values have been recommended for the EROA for the diagnosis of severe MR based on the etiology of MR (40 vs 20 mm^2 for primary and secondary MR, respectively). This difference is likely to be related to the underestimation of secondary MR due to the technical limitations rather than to true anatomic differences.

2D Proximal Isovelocity Surface Area

The 2D proximal isovelocity surface area (PISA) method is the current recommended quantitative approach for the assessment of MR severity. Qualitatively, the presence of flow convergence at a Nyquist limit of approximately 50 to 60 cm/s (routine examination) would suggest significant MR. PISA calculations are based on the calculation of the following parameters:

$$EROA = 2\pi r^2 \times Va / PeakMRV \ (CW),$$

where EROA is Effective Regurgitant Orifice Area and Va is aliasing velocity

$$RV \ (cc) = EROA \ (cm^2) \times TVI_{MR}(cm),$$

where RV is regurgitant volume and TVI is MV time-velocity integral.

The PISA method assumes that the ROA is constant throughout systole and is hemispheric in shape. Although the PISA radius tends to be relatively constant in patients with organic rheumatic regurgitation, it frequently increases progressively along the systolic period in patients with mitral valve prolapse. In functional MR, an early peak is followed by a progressive midsystolic decrease, sometimes with another late systolic peak (**Fig. 1**). For this reason, PISA-based methods tend to be more accurate for organic than for functional MR. As previously discussed, in organic, degenerative MR the flow is generally uniform throughout systole as opposed to functional MR, in which a bimodal pattern is more common, with a peak in early and late systole and decreasing during midsystole.

Quantitative Volumetric Measurements

Volumetric methods use pulse-wave Doppler techniques to calculate flow rates and stroke volumes. The stroke volume across a valve annulus can be calculated as follows: TVI across valve annulus multiplied by the cross-sectional area of the annulus. The MR regurgitant volume can be calculated from the flow across cardiac valves. Although many combinations can be used, a common way to derive MR volume is the following:

MR Volume = Mitral inflow minus aortic outflow

Mitral inflow volume is calculated as follows: (TVI of mitral inflow) × (cross-sectional area) of the mitral annulus. The TVI of mitral inflow should be measured at the level of the mitral annular plane, as this is where the cross-sectional area is measured. The cross-sectional area of the mitral annulus is assumed to be circular and calculated as Πr^2, where r is the diameter measured in the in apical 4-chamber view divided by 2.

Anatomically, the mitral annulus is D-shaped and more shaped like an ellipse rather than a circle. However, using a circular assumption for the annulus is reasonable in patients who have developed at least moderate MR, given the annular dilation that occurs with development of moderate or greater MR. Alternatively, the mitral annulus can also be calculated as an ellipse in which the area is Πab, with a and b being the diameters measured in the apical 4-chamber and 2-chamber views divided by 2. Aortic outflow is calculated as TVI of Aortic outflow × Cross-sectional area of LV outflow tract (LVOT). This method assumes that there is no aortic regurgitation; otherwise, pulmonary artery outflow can be used, assuming no significant pulmonary regurgitation. The MR regurgitant volume can also be obtained by calculating LV stroke volume and subtracting aortic outflow volume, assuming no aortic insufficiency is present.

Although straightforward in concept, volumetric methods are time consuming and associated with potential errors that may arise from the multiple measurements required at different views to calculate RV and EROA (**Fig. 2**). For reproducible results, these methods generally require significant training. In addition, as the radius is squared in the area term, small errors in measurement are amplified and accurate resolution of the annulus is important in minimizing measurement errors.

3D ECHOCARDIOGRAPHY

Current 3D echocardiography techniques provide better definition of mitral morphology and pathologic changes, while significantly improving the

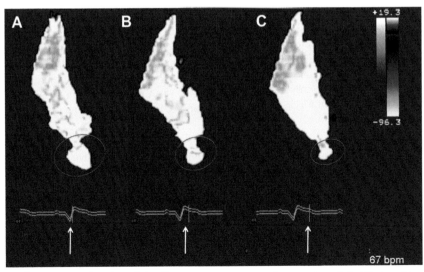

Fig. 1. Functional MR: Decreasing size of the flow convergence area from early systole (*A*), to midsystole (*B*), and end systole (*C*). Note also the changes in shape.

Parameters	view	Approach	example
Mitral annulus (late-Diastole)	Apical 4-Chamber	Hinge point to hinge point	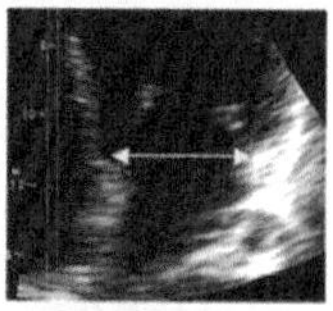
Mitral VTI (Diastole)	Apical 4-Chamber	PW sample at the level of MV annulus	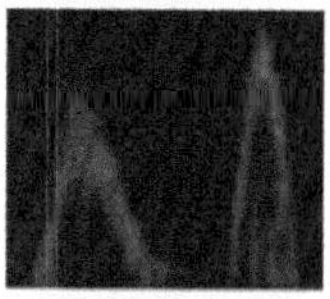
LVOT diameter (mid-Systole)	Parasternal long axis	Zoom at the level of LVOT	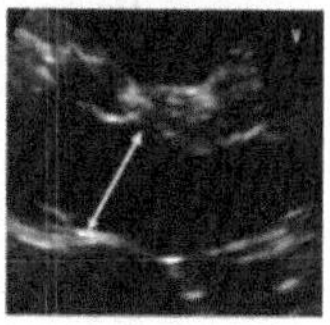
LVOT-VTI (Systole)	Apical 5-Chamber	PW sample at the level of LVOT	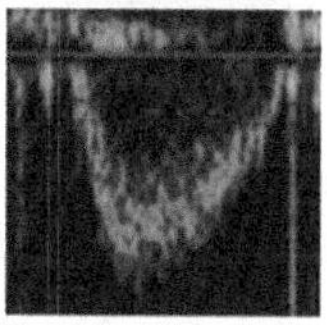

Fig. 2. Parameters needed for MR quantification by quantitative volumetric method. MV, mitral valve; PW, Pulsed wave Doppler.

characterization of mitral regurgitant jets. The unique capability of 3D echocardiography to spatially visualize the shape, size, and orientation of MR jets in real time overcomes some of the limitations of 2D echocardiography, thus enhancing the accuracy of quantification of MR severity.

3D VC Area

Three-dimensional VCA measurements are particularly useful when estimating eccentric or functional regurgitations. In recent years, several studies have validated 3D-guided planimetry of the VCA as a relatively fast, highly feasible, and very precise indicator of MR severity in clinical practice.[9–11]

The VC width can vary dramatically depending on the imaging plane. Traditionally, assessment of VC width in commissural views (2-chamber view) can be inaccurate, as small functional regurgitation can appear to have a wide VC. When using standard 2D imaging, true short-axis imaging, in which the real shape of the VC is visualized, was challenging, as accurate cross-sectional views of the VC was difficult to obtain. Three-dimensional–guided direct planimetry of the VC area (VCA) is able to overcome this problem and accurately establish the real cross-sectional VCA. At this moment, 3D VCA quantitation is possibly the most reproducible and accurate method to establish

the effective regurgitant orifice (as hydrodynamic principles have established the VCA to be just slightly smaller than the real anatomic orifice).[12,13]

The real-time 3D echocardiographic measurement of the VCA has also been validated in the challenging clinical scenario of patients with multiple MR jets.

3D PISA

Direct visualization of the flow convergence area in space by 3D echocardiography color Doppler has confirmed that in most cases the true proximal flow convergence region is rather more hemielliptical than hemispheric. As discussed in the article by Yosefy and colleagues, elsewhere in this issue, the calculation of EROA incorporating the spatial information acquired by 3D can greatly improve the accuracy of 2D-based PISA assessment. Applying the calculations for area for a hemiellipse renders a more accurate and realistic approach when using this quantitative method and underestimation of the overall regurgitation can be significantly corrected.[14–17]

Limitations of Current 3D Color Doppler

Given the large amount of data present in 3D datasets, current technology is limited by a somewhat

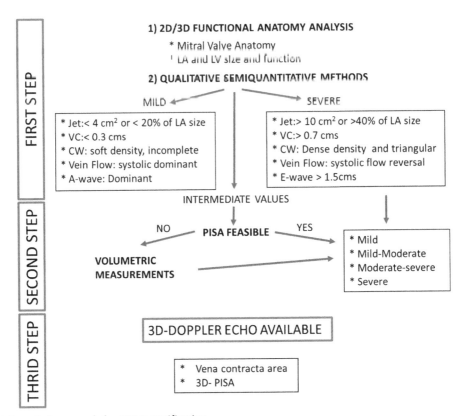

Fig. 3. Integrated approach for MR quantification.

low temporal resolution. This means that even with small angles of view, the "volume" or "voxel" rates in real-time mode is low. Thus, in the presence of high heart rates, limited "volumes" during a systolic period can be obtained. This can be compensated by using multiple-beat full-volume acquisitions, which in turn come with their own limitations, such as stitching artifacts, especially in case of irregular rates or atrial fibrillation.

Also, the accuracy of 3D color Doppler planimetry of the VCA can be affected by factors, such as the color Doppler gain. Gain settings can have a significant effect on the size of the visible VCA, but should technically have no effect on the true VCA. The VCA should be measured at aliased velocities to avoid the possibility of "color bleeding" that may occur at lower nonaliased velocities.

Finally, the dynamic variation in ROA during systole has to be considered. Theoretically, the instantaneous ROA should be integrated throughout the cardiac cycle, but this is not practical in the clinical setting unless automated analysis methods are implemented. However, this is not a limitation of 3D echocardiography but something inherent to any ultrasound Doppler technology. Practice guidelines support the use of a single ROA

measurement, usually at midsystole, for quantification of MR.

In spite of these limitations, the integration of all the previously described 3D echocardiography information will help to achieve a more accurate grading of MR severity.

DOPPLER INTEGRATED APPROACH

The American Society of Echocardiography and European Association of Echocardiography recommendations establish that the approach to MR evaluation should integrate multiple methods to minimize the effects of technical or measurement errors. **Fig. 3** shows an algorithm based on this principle and distinguishes 3 steps that can be applied in daily clinical practice. Step 1 consists of identifying the extreme grades of MR severity, step 2 is centered on defining the intermediate grades, and step 3, if available, the use of 3D echocardiographic methods to further refine the estimation of MR.

SUMMARY

Evaluation of MR severity remains complex and challenging. An integrative approach to grading

MR is recommended. The use of multiple Doppler methods should be used to help discriminate between grades of severity. Importantly, MR severity should always be considered in the context of clinical data. The emerging inclusion of 3D echocardiography may provide complementary data for MR quantification and better anatomic and pathophysiological detail of the mitral valve.

REFERENCES

1. Gorlin R, Gorlin SG. Hydraulic formula for calculation of the area of the stenotic mitral valve, other cardiac valves, and central circulatory shunts. Am Heart J 1951;41:1–29.
2. Levine HJ, Gaasch WH. Vasoactive drugs in chronic regurgitant lesions of the mitral and aortic valves. J Am Coll Cardiol 1996;28:1083–91.
3. Yoran C, Yellin EL, Becker RM, et al. Dynamic aspects of acute mitral regurgitation: effects of ventricular volume, pressure and contractility on the effective regurgitant orifice area. Circulation 1979;60:170–6.
4. Zoghbi WA, Enriquez-Sarano M, Foster E, et al. Recommendations for evaluation of severity of native valvular regurgitation with two-dimensional and Doppler Echocardiography. J Am Soc Echocardiogr 2003;16(7):777–802.
5. Yoshida K, Yoshikawa J, Shakudo M, et al. Color Doppler evaluation of valvular regurgitation in normal subjects. Circulation 1988;78(4):840–7.
6. Pu M, Griffin BP, Vandervoort PM, et al. The value of assessing pulmonary venous flow velocity for predicting severity of mitral regurgitation: A quantitative assessment integrating left ventricular function. J Am Soc Echocardiogr 1999;12(9):736–43.
7. Tribouilloy C, Shen WF, Rey JL, et al. Mitral to aortic velocity-time integral ratio. A non-geometric pulsed-Doppler regurgitant index in isolated pure mitral regurgitation. Eur Heart J 1994;15(10):1335–9.
8. Vahanian A, Alfieri O, Andreotti F, et al. Guidelines on the management of valvular heart disease (version 2012): the Joint Task Force on the Management of Valvular Heart Disease of the European Society of Cardiology (ESC) and the European Association for Cardio-Thoracic Surgery (EACTS). Eur J Cardiothorac Surg 2012;42(4):S1–44.
9. Kahlert P, Plicht B, Schenk IM, et al. Direct assessment of size and shape of noncircular vena contracta area in functional versus organic mitral regurgitation using real-time three-dimensional echocardiography. J Am Soc Echocardiogr 2008;21(8):912–21.
10. Little SH, Pirat B, Kumar R, et al. Three-dimensional color Doppler echocardiography for direct measurement of vena contracta area in mitral regurgitation: in vitro validation and clinical experience. JACC Cardiovasc Imaging 2008;1(6):695–704.
11. Zeng X, Levine RA, Hua L, et al. Diagnostic value of vena contracta area in the quantification of mitral regurgitation severity by color Doppler 3D echocardiography. Circ Cardiovasc Imaging 2011;4(5):506–13.
12. Grayburn PA, Weissman NJ, Zamorano JL. Quantitation of mitral regurgitation. Circulation 2012;126(16):2005–17.
13. Thavendiranathan P, Phelan D, Thomas JD, et al. Quantitative assessment of mitral regurgitation: validation of new methods. J Am Coll Cardiol 2012;60(16):1470–83.
14. Cobey FC, McInnis JA, Gelfand BJ, et al. A method for automating 3-dimensional proximal isovelocity surface area measurement. J Cardiothorac Vasc Anesth 2012;26(3):507–11.
15. Thavendiranathan P, Liu S, Datta S, et al. Quantification of Chronic Functional Mitral Regurgitation by Automated 3-Dimensional Peak and Integrated proximal Isovelocity Surface Area and Stroke Volume Techniques Using Real-Time 3-Dimensional Volume Color Doppler Echocardiography In Vitro and Clinical Validation. Circ Cardiovasc Imaging 2013;6:125–33.
16. Matsumura Y, Saracino G, Sugioka K, et al. Determination of regurgitant orifice area with the use of a new three-dimensional flow convergence geometric assumption in functional mitral regurgitation. J Am Soc Echocardiogr 2008;21(11):1251–6.
17. Lancellotti P, Cosyns B, Zacharakis D, et al. Importance of left ventricular longitudinal function and functional reserve in patients with degenerative mitral regurgitation: assessment by two-dimensional speckle tracking. J Am Soc Echocardiogr 2008;21(12):1331–6.

.

Echocardiographic Assessment of Mitral Stenosis
Echocardiographic Features of Rheumatic Mitral Stenosis

Sonia Jain, MBBS, Sunil V. Mankad, MD*

KEYWORDS

- Echocardiography • Mitral stenosis • Rheumatic heart disease • Balloon valvuloplasty

KEY POINTS

- Echocardiography is the primary imaging modality in rheumatic mitral stenosis.
- It is essential for diagnosis, serial follow up, therapeutic procedural guidance and prognostication.
- In middle- and low-income countries, portable echocardiography devices are a useful tool in large-scale population screening for early identification of rheumatic heart disease, and prevention of chronic sequelae.
- Salient echocardiographic data include mitral valvular morphology, valve area, transmitral gradient, pulmonary hypertension, and concomitant valvular disease.
- Echocardiography aids assessment of patient candidacy for percutaneous balloon valvuloplasty versus surgery.
- Baseline echocardiographic features are strong independent predictors of procedural success and long-term outcome.

 Videos of a patient with mitral stenosis and the mitral valve directly viewed en face from the left ventricular perspective accompany this article at http://www.cardiology.theclinics.com/

INTRODUCTION

Mitral stenosis (MS) is characterized by pathologic thickening and narrowing of the valve, resulting in a reduction in the valve orifice area. This process results in obstruction to transmitral flow in diastole, an increase in upstream pressures, pulmonary hypertension, and eventually a decrease in cardiac output.

ETIOLOGY

Globally, rheumatic heart disease (RHD) is the most common cause of MS. Other less frequent causes include congenital MS, inflammatory diseases such as systemic lupus erythematosus,[1] drug-induced valvulopathy, mitral annular calcification or nonvalvular obstruction secondary to left atrial myxoma, large thrombus, or congenital cor triatriatum.

GLOBAL DISEASE BURDEN AND TRENDS

Over the last century there has been a dramatic decline in the incidence and severity of RHD in the United States and Western Europe, currently estimated to be up to 10 per 100,000 per year.[2]

Division of Cardiovascular Diseases, Department of Medicine, Mayo Clinic College of Medicine, 200 First Street Southwest, Rochester, MN 55905, USA
* Corresponding author.
E-mail address: mankad.sunil@mayo.edu

Cardiol Clin 31 (2013) 177–191
http://dx.doi.org/10.1016/j.ccl.2013.03.006
0733-8651/13/$ – see front matter © 2013 Elsevier Inc. All rights reserved.

Although not definitively established, proposed reasons for this decline include a combination of improved socioeconomic conditions, robust public health measures, prompt antibiotic therapy,[3] and alteration in virulence of streptococcal strains.[4] In the mid- to late 1980s, there were focal resurgences of RHD in the United States that were effectively treated with antibiotic therapy.[4–6] However, RHD continues to pose a huge disease burden in the developing world.[7,8] Ninety-seven percent of all cases of RHD occur in low-income and middle-income countries,[9] where it remains the most common cardiovascular disease in school-age children and young adults. Furthermore, it continues to be the most common cardiac cause of mortality and morbidity in pregnant women. In Africa, it is estimated that RHD is responsible for approximately 90% of cardiac disease in pregnancy and a third of maternal deaths.[10–12] In addition, there are significant differences in epidemiologic patterns, with earlier age of onset, susceptibility to repeated infections, and greater severity of symptoms and sequelae in low-income and middle-income countries. Socioeconomic constraints that limit public health measures for effective prophylaxis, and limited treatment options are largely responsible for this huge global disparity in RHD.

PREVALENCE

Reliable disease prevalence is difficult to ascertain because of geographic diversity, and variability in screening methods, data collection, and reporting.[13] A meta-analysis by Carapetis and colleagues[14] estimated that worldwide, 15.6 to 19.6 million have RHD, of whom 2.4 million are children aged 5 to 14 years. Annually about 233,000 deaths in developing countries are due to RHD. There is an apparent female predominance.[13,15,16] More cases are observed in urban slums than in rural areas,[16,17] most likely because of overcrowding. There is extensive geographic variation, with the highest all age prevalence in sub-Saharan Africa (5.7 cases per 1000), followed by the indigenous populations of the Pacific Islands, New Zealand, and Australia (3.5 per 1000), and Southeast Asia (2.2 per 1000).[9,14] Economically developed countries have the lowest incidence of 0.3 per 1000.

ROLE OF ECHOCARDIOGRAPHY IN DISEASE SCREENING

Historically, most of the prevalence data were obtained from epidemiologic studies that used auscultation school surveys of children aged 5 to 15 years. Marijon and colleagues[15] demonstrated a prevalence of 2.3 cases per 1000 by auscultation alone, and a 10-fold higher prevalence of 30.4 cases per 1000 by echocardiographic screening of school-age children in Cambodia and Mozambique (**Table 1**). Multiple other studies have reiterated a higher prevalence by echocardiographic screening in endemic regions such as Tonga,[20] India,[22] Nicaragua,[16] Fiji,[19] and New Zealand.[21] The single most effective strategy to prevent chronic debilitating sequelae is early case detection and penicillin prophylaxis for initial and subsequent episodes of acute rheumatic fever (ARF).[23–25] As many as 54% of patients with echocardiographic features of RHD can be missed by auscultation alone.[20] A strategy using auscultation of a murmur leading to echocardiographic assessment will underdiagnose subclinical cases, thereby denying a valuable opportunity for early penicillin therapy for initial and subsequent episodes of ARF.

Several studies have successfully demonstrated the feasibility of implementing screening programs in endemic countries using portable echocardiography. Using a focused screening protocol to assess the mitral and aortic valves in the parasternal long-axis and apical 4-chamber views, each study can be completed in 5 to 10 minutes,[20] with an estimated cost of approximately US $40.0 per patient detected. The price

Table 1
Prevalence data

	Region	Prevalence by Clinical Auscultation (per 1000)	Prevalence by Echo Screening (per 1000)
Anabwani et al,[18] 1996	Kenya		27
Marijon et al,[15] 2007	Cambodia, Mozambique	2.3	30.4
Carapetis et al,[20] 2008	Tonga		33.2
Bhaya et al,[22] 2010	India		51.0
Parr et al,[16] 2010	Nicaragua		48.0
Reeves at al,[19] 2011	Fiji	11	55.2
Webb et al,[21] 2011	New Zealand		26.0

of training personnel is offset by the significant downstream costs incurred in the treatment of chronic sequelae. Although there have been concerns about overdiagnosis, echocardiography is highly specific for RHD, with a positive predictive value of 94%.[26] In one study, only 2.6% of children who had physiologic regurgitation or minor congenital mitral valvular abnormalities were misidentified as having features of RHD. Echocardiography is a highly sensitive, specific, portable, cost-effective, and evidence based screening test that can decrease the global burden of RHD.

Since 2005, the World Health Organization (WHO) and National Institutes of Health (NIH) have recommended echocardiographic screening of endemic populations. The most recent guidelines are the 2012 World Heart Federation (WHF) criteria for echocardiographic diagnosis of RHD.[27] American College of Cardiology (ACC)/American Heart Association (AHA) guidelines for indications of echocardiography in MS are available online at: http://content.onlinejacc.org/article.aspx?articleid=1139137.

GROUP A STREPTOCOCCAL INFECTIONS AND RHEUMATIC HEART DISEASE

For a comprehensive understanding of the fascinating pathophysiology of RHD, a review of streptococcal immunology is essential. Group A streptococcal infections are a common cause of childhood infections. ARF occurs in 3% to 5% of patients, typically following a group A streptococcal throat infection. It has been recently suggested that streptococcal skin infections maybe associated with ARF, but this has not been conclusively demonstrated.[28,29] In 1928, Lancefield[30,31] identified the streptococcal M protein antigen, which is the major virulence factor responsible for tissue adherence and resistance from phagocytosis.[32] In the 1960s, an immunologic cross-reactivity between streptococcal antigens and glycoproteins of the cardiac valves was demonstrated.[33–35] In the 1980s, similar cross-reactivity with cardiac myosin was noted.[36–39]

Based on M serotyping, more than 80 bacterial strains have been identified. Hence, a single person can have repeated episodes of ARF with different rheumatogenic strains.[40,41] In addition, studies from India, Brazil, South Africa, and Australia have demonstrated antigenic diversity, making the possibility of a vaccine elusive.

CLINICAL MANIFESTATIONS OF ARF

The manifestations of ARF include arthritis, carditis, skin manifestations (erythema marginatum, subcutaneous nodules), and chorea. Curiously, arthritis and carditis rarely coexist in the same patient. Cardiac involvement is said to occur in one-third of patients with ARF. The manifestations include carditis, pericarditis, valvulitis in the form of mitral regurgitation, and congestive heart failure. Recurrences mimic the initial attack and increase the extent of valve disease; that is, carditis begets carditis.[42] The spectrum of RHD may have different clinical manifestations and severity in middle-income and low-income countries,[43] thought to be secondary to recurrent streptococcal infections.

PATHOPHYSIOLOGY

The mitral valve apparatus is an architecturally complex structure consisting of the anterior and posterior mitral valve leaflets, mitral annulus, commissures, papillary muscles, and chordae tendineae. The anterior leaflet comprises one-third and the posterior leaflet two-thirds of the annulus. The normal leaflets are thin, translucent, and briskly mobile structures. In rheumatic MS there is leaflet thickening, fibrosis and calcification, chordal shortening, and commissural fusion and calcification, resulting in progressive narrowing of the mitral valve orifice.

ECHOCARDIOGRAPHY IN RHEUMATIC MITRAL STENOSIS

Ever since Edler and Hertz[44] pioneered ultrasound technology to assess heart motion in 1954, echocardiography has played a pivotal role in the diagnosis and management of rheumatic MS. Today, echocardiography is the primary imaging modality for the diagnosis, quantification, and detection of concomitant valvular involvement, assessment of morphologic suitability for intervention, and serial follow-up of MS.[45–47] The main echocardiographic variables to quantify severity include transmitral gradient, valve area, and pulmonary hypertension.

M MODE

Two-dimensional (2D) guided M-mode assessment of the mitral valve is typically performed in the parasternal long-axis and short-axis views. Because of the high temporal resolution, M mode beautifully illustrates leaflet motion. The movement of the normal anterior mitral valve leaflet has 4 distinct phases, giving it the characteristic M shape during diastole.

1. Early diastole: a brisk rapid opening or anterior excursion (E wave) at the onset of diastole, resulting in early rapid filling of the left ventricle

2. Mid diastole or diastasis: near closure during passive filling of the left ventricle

3. Late diastole: a smaller anterior excursion caused by left atrial contraction (A wave)

4. Early systole/isovolumic contraction: valve closure

The posterior leaflet has a similar but less exaggerated independent pattern of motion, with a W shape.

In rheumatic MS, there is a distinct and easily recognizable distortion of this M-mode pattern.[48–50] There is thickening of the leaflets, a delay in amplitude and slope of the E wave (delayed valve opening), a slow descent or flattening of the E-F slope (increase in left ventricular filling pressures), and decrease in amplitude of the A wave (decreased contribution from atrial contraction). The slower and flatter the slope of the E wave, the more severe the MS. A slow slope of 10 to 30 cm/s and an E-wave height of 20 mm indicate severe MS with a valve area of less than 1.0 cm^2.[51] The flattening of the E-F slope of the anterior mitral valve leaflet indicates an increase in left ventricular filling pressures, and may also be seen in conditions of poor left ventricular compliance and pulmonary hypertension.[52,53] The posterior mitral valve leaflet moves anteriorly and in parallel with the anterior leaflet, rather than in the usual posterior direction. This cardinal finding is highly specific to MS. The A wave is absent in the presence of atrial fibrillation. M-mode examples of a normal mitral valve and MS are shown in **Fig. 1**.

TWO-DIMENSIONAL ECHOCARDIOGRAPHY

With the introduction of real-time 2D echocardiography in the early 1970s came the unique ability to visualize the morphology and motion of the mitral valve apparatus. The normal mitral valve leaflets are thin (<4 mm), translucent, and highly mobile structures, with the anterior mitral leaflet exhibiting the greater mobility. The maximum mobility is seen in the leaflet tips.

In rheumatic MS the leaflet thickening is most pronounced at the tips, with relative sparing of the mid portion, giving the characteristic "bent-knee" or "hockey-stick" appearance. The leaflets open and close suddenly, with the appearance of convexity into the left ventricle in diastole (doming), and convexity into the left atrium during systole. In some patients, this may have the appearance of mitral valve prolapse. The posterior leaflet is also thickened and restricted, and is paradoxically "pulled forward" by the anterior leaflet, rather than the normal posterior movement in diastole. Between leaflet opening and closing, there is very little motion of the leaflets. An example of the typical 2D appearance of MS is shown in **Fig. 2** and Video 1.

ASSESSMENT OF SEVERITY OF MITRAL STENOSIS

Severity is quantified by Doppler transmitral pressure gradient, pulmonary hypertension, and mitral valve area (MVA) (**Table 2**).

DOPPLER EVALUATION
Transmitral Pressure Gradient

The mean transmitral gradient is extremely important for grading the severity of MS (<5 mm Hg, mild; 5–10 mm Hg, moderate; >10 mm Hg, severe). The gradient is obtained by application of the simplified Bernoulli equation $\Delta Pressure = 4v^2$, where v is the transmitral velocity obtained from continuous-wave Doppler (CWD) interrogation of mitral flow in the apical 4-chamber view. The peak gradient is obtained using the peak Doppler velocity, and the mean gradient is the average of digitized instantaneous gradients enveloped in the CWD signal. Integrated software automatically calculates and displays the peak and mean gradients. In general, severity classification is based on the mean, not peak, transmitral gradient. Doppler-derived mean transmitral gradient correlates well with invasive measurements, and is easily reproducible.[54–56] If the Doppler beam is not in parallel alignment with the direction of flow, as in very eccentric jets, the gradient will be underestimated. The mean transmitral gradient is highly sensitive to alterations in mitral flow, atrioventricular compliance, and heart rate. With tachycardia there is a decrease in diastolic filling, resulting in elevation of the mean gradient. In the presence of atrial fibrillation, at least 5 and usually 10 cycles have to be averaged to obtain an accurate mean gradient.

Estimation of Pulmonary Artery Pressure

The obstruction of flow at the mitral orifice results in pulmonary hypertension and increased pulmonary vascular resistance. The degree of pulmonary hypertension is a measure of the hemodynamic burden. Even patients with unremarkable pulmonary hypertension at rest can have impressive elevations of pressure during exercise. Pulmonary artery systolic pressure (PAP) is incorporated in grading severity of MS (<30 mm Hg, mild; 30–50 mm Hg, moderate; >50 mm Hg, severe).[45,46]

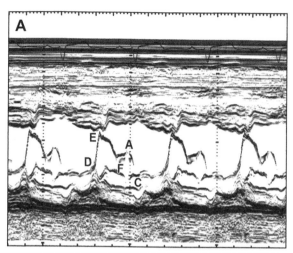

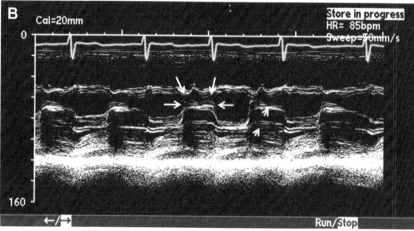

Fig. 1. (*A*) M mode of normal mitral valve. Shown is the M-mode echocardiogram of a normal mitral valve obtained from a parasternal long-axis view. During diastole, the mitral leaflets separate widely with the anterior leaflet approaching the interventricular septum and the posterior leaflet moving toward the posterior wall of the left ventricle. The anterior mitral leaflet produces an M-shaped configuration while the posterior leaflet, which moves in the opposite direction of the anterior leaflet, produces a W-shaped configuration. The D point marks the position of the mitral valve leaflets at the onset of diastole; the E point is the point of maximal opening of the mitral valve and correlates with early, rapid filling of the left ventricle, the F point represents the most posterior position of the anterior leaflet following the E point; the E-F slope represents the initial diastolic motion of the anterior leaflet and is an indication of the rate of left atrial emptying (normally this is quite steep); the A point represents reopening of the mitral valve leaflets with atrial contraction; and the C point denotes the final position of the mitral valve leaflets immediately before ventricular systole. (*B*) M mode of mitral valve with mitral stenosis. Shown is the typical M mode obtained from a parasternal long-axis view of mitral stenosis. Note the marked thickening of the anterior mitral leaflet (*white arrows*). The mitral leaflets are bright (calcified) and thickened. The E-F slope is markedly decreased, and instead of moving in opposite directions during systole, the mitral anterior and posterior leaflets move in the same direction (anteriorly), demonstrated by the yellow arrows.

In the absence of pulmonic stenosis, echocardiographically estimated right ventricular systolic pressure (RVSP) is used as a surrogate for PAP. The gradient across the tricuspid valve is ΔPressure $= 4v^2$, where v is the maximum CWD tricuspid velocity. The right atrial pressure (RAP) is estimated from size of the inferior vena cava and respiratory collapsibility.[47]

$$RVSP \text{ (mm Hg)} = \text{Transtricuspid gradient} + RAP$$

Mitral Valve Area

The normal MVA is 4.0 to 5.0 cm². Typically, patients with MS do not experience symptoms until the valve area is less than 2.5 cm². Based on valve

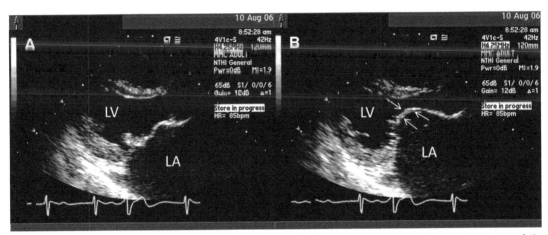

Fig. 2. Two-dimensional (2D) echo features of mitral stenosis. Shown are parasternal long-axis images of the mitral valve during end-systole (*A*) and end-diastole (*B*). Note the markedly enlarged left atrium (LA), and the thickening and doming or "hockey-stick" appearance of the anterior mitral leaflet during systole (*white arrows*). LV, left ventricle. The corresponding 2D echocardiographic movie of a parasternal long-axis image of a patient with mitral stenosis is shown in Video 1.

area, stenosis is classified as mild (>1.5 cm²), moderate (1.0–1.5 cm²), or severe (<1.0 cm²). Echocardiographically there are 5 common methods to estimate MVA: (1) 2D planimetry, (2) pressure half-time (PHT), (3) continuity method, (4) proximal isovelocity surface area (PISA) method, and (5) 3D planimetry. In addition, the color Doppler method, which assumes an elliptical orifice, has also been used.[57] Although this method has the advantage of not being influenced by the presence of coexistent mitral regurgitation, atrial fibrillation, left ventricular dysfunction, or aortic regurgitation, it is not commonly used and is not discussed further in this review. Valve area indexed to body surface area has not been validated. Planimetry and the PHT methods are the most widely used and easily applicable. Planimetry is considered the reference method. Although individually all 5 aforementioned techniques have been shown to have good correlation with invasively derived area and surgical anatomic sizing,[58] there are inherent limitations.

No single method should be solely relied on, and data from multiple methods should be interpreted in the appropriate clinical setting.

Mitral valve area by direct 2D planimetry

Planimetry is based on direct visualization of the mitral valve orifice, and is not limited by hemodynamic loading conditions. Multiple studies have confirmed that mitral orifice area measured by 2D echocardiographic planimetry has an excellent correlation with direct sizing at surgery ($r = 0.92$),[59] and invasively derived area using the Gorlin hydraulic formula[60] ($r = 0.95$).[61]

Because of the typical pattern of leaflet fibrosis, the mitral inflow is funnel shaped, with the narrowest orifice at the level of the leaflet tips. Therefore, if the orifice is traced at a level below the leaflet tips, the area can be overestimated. To perform a satisfactory planimetry the 2D image of the mitral valve in the parasternal short-axis view is optimized, and meticulously scanned to obtain the frame with the smallest orifice. The inner rim of the orifice, including opened commissures, is traced in mid-diastole to calculate the MVA. Several measurements should be averaged in patients with heart-rate variability and atrial fibrillation. Guidelines emphasize planimetry as the reference measurement.[47] However, it may be challenging to achieve in the setting of poor image quality, and heavily calcified or distorted valves. An example of 2D planimetry is shown in **Fig. 3**.

Mitral valve area by pressure half-time method

In 1979, Hatle and colleagues[62] explored the concept of PHT as a relatively flow-independent

Table 2
Grading severity of mitral stenosis

	Mild	Moderate	Severe
Mean gradient (mm Hg)	<5	5–10	>10
Pulmonary artery systolic pressure (mm Hg)	<30	30–50	>50
Valve area (cm²)	>1.5	1.0–1.5	<1.0

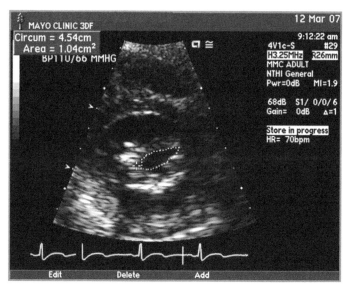

Fig. 3. 2D planimetry–derived measurement of mitral valve area. Shown is the zoomed-in parasternal short-axis image of the mitral valve in a patient with mitral stenosis during diastole. The image is frozen, and direct area measurement at the tips of the mitral valve is made to determine mitral valve area. Note the echo-bright or calcified portions of the mitral valve, which can sometimes make accurate planimetric measurements difficult. In this case, the mitral valve area of 1.04 cm^2 is consistent with severe mitral stenosis.

assessment of MS severity. The maximum transmitral pressure gradient is obtained from the Bernoulli equation $4v^2$ (where v is the peak velocity across the mitral valve in diastole). The PHT is the time taken for the transmitral pressure gradient to decay to half the value at the onset of diastole. Mathematically, it approximates the time required for the peak velocity to decrease to v/square root of 2 or 1.4. In stenotic mitral valves, there is a linear and inverse relationship between MVA and PHT: the more severe the MS, the longer the PHT. The PHT across isolated MS can be between 90 and 383 milliseconds.[62] Hatle and colleagues proposed a derivation of MVA by using the empirical formula MVA = 220/PHT, relating an inverse relationship between PHT and the anatomic MVA. The correlation coefficient with area determined by cardiac catheterization was excellent ($r = 0.92$). The PHT can also be calculated by multiplying the deceleration time (time required for the peak velocity to decrease to the zero baseline) by 0.29.

There are important caveats to the blanket use of the PHT method. PHT measurements can be unreliable in the presence of tachycardia and atrial fibrillation. PHT is directly proportional to left atrial and ventricular chamber compliance and the square root of the initial peak gradient. In the acute postvalvotomy period, there are abrupt changes in the atrioventricular pressure-compliance relationships[63] and transmitral gradient, rendering PHT-derived aortic valve area unreliable and inaccurate.[64,65] In conditions of increased left ventricular stiffness, such as aortic valve disease or coronary artery disease, the PHT is shortened and may overestimate MVA even in the presence of significant MS.[66] Similarly, concomitant aortic regurgitation causes a shortening of PHT and overestimation of the MVA.[67]

Mitral valve area by continuity method

The continuity method is based on the principle of conservation of mass. In other words, the stroke volumes proximal and distal to the stenotic mitral valve must be equal. The proximal (or transmitral) stroke volume (SV) can be obtained from the right ventricular or left ventricular outflow tract (LVOT), as long as there is no significant aortic or pulmonic valve regurgitation, respectively.

$$SV = \text{Valve area} \times VTI$$

$$MVA = LVOT\ SV/VTI_{MS}$$

where VTI is velocity-time integral.

Mitral valve area by PISA method

The principle of flow convergence or PISA states that as flow accelerates toward an orifice, it forms multiple hemispheric shells of increasing velocity and decreasing radius. All blood cells at a particular hemisphere must have the same velocity and radius. To conserve mass, the flow rate at a given hemispheric shell must be equal to the flow rate across the stenotic mitral valve.

Diastolic flow rate at stenotic mitral valve = Flow rate at PISA

Flow rate = Area × Velocity

$$Area = 2 \pi (r)^2 = 6.28 \times (r)^2$$

$$MVA = 6.28 (r)^2 \times Alias_{vel}/Peak_{MS\ velocity} \times \alpha°/180°$$

PISA measurements are made by color flow Doppler assessment of the mitral inflow in the apical 4-chamber window. The color Doppler baseline is shifted upwards toward the left ventricle (ie, the direction of the jet of interest), and optimized to visualize a red-blue boundary and hemispheric contour. The velocity at the shell is the aliasing velocity (V_{alias}), which is typically 25 to 40 cm/s. The peak mitral velocity is obtained by CWD. The hemispheric radius (r) is measured from the level of the stenotic orifice to the center of the shell. Because of the typical rheumatic leaflet doming and funnel-shaped inflow, only a fraction of a given hemisphere crosses the orifice, necessitating an angle correction factor $\alpha/180$, which is the angle between the 2 mitral leaflets at the atrial side. Some investigators have proposed simplifying the equation using a fixed α of 100 for all patients.[68] The PISA method has been shown to have a good correlation with other methods of MVA estimation.[69] In the presence of atrial fibrillation, the correlation is decreased but reasonable.[70] An example of the PISA method for calculating mitral valve area in MS is shown in **Fig. 4**.

THREE-DIMENSIONAL ECHOCARDIOGRAPHY

In the last 2 decades, real-time 3-dimensional echocardiography (RT3DE) using phased, matrix-array transducer probes has evolved as an exciting technology with which to visualize the mitral valve en face. RT3DE can be performed via both transthoracic and transesophageal approaches. A volumetric pyramid is scanned, and images are displayed as intersecting orthogonal views. The data can be analyzed in real time (live 3D or "zoom" modes) or stored and analyzed off-line (full volume). Irrespective of the window of acquisition, the volumetric pyramid can be steered and rotated to visualize the mitral valve from the left atrial or ventricular aspects, and at any angle or cross-sectional plane. Hence, the smallest diastolic orifice area can be accurately planimetered. Whereas 2D planimetry requires a satisfactory parasternal window, 3D echocardiography can be performed via a parasternal or apical window.

MVA by 3D planimetry has been shown to be a feasible and reproducible measurement that correlates well with 2D planimetry ($r = 0.93$) and PHT ($r = 0.87$).[71] When compared with the various 2D methods (planimetry, PHT, and PISA), 3D planimetry has the closest agreement with invasive Gorlin-derived MVA.[72] In patients undergoing percutaneous mitral commissurotomy, RT3DE provides superior assessment of commissural

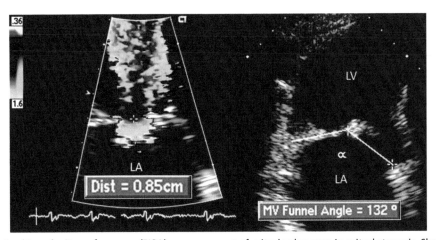

Fig. 4. Proximal isovelocity surface area (PISA) measurement of mitral valve area in mitral stenosis. Shown on the left panel is color Doppler measurement of flow from the left atrium (LA) across the mitral valve in a patient with mitral stenosis. The color baseline is shifted toward the left ventricle (aliasing velocity 0.36 m), which allows for blooming of the hemispheric shell as flow accelerates through the stenotic mitral orifice. The image is frozen, and direct measurement of the radius of the hemisphere is measured (0.85 cm in the example shown). Because of the funnel shape of the mitral valve, calculation of mitral valve area has to be corrected for the angle of the leaflets. In the case shown (*right panel*), the mitral valve leaflet angle is 132°. The formula for calculation of the mitral valve area is described in the text. LV, left ventricle.

anatomy,[73] and accurate valve area immediately after valvuloplasty when 2D methods may be unreliable.[74] An example of 3D-guided 2D planimetry measured from the left ventricular perspective is shown in **Fig. 5** and Video 2.

STRESS ECHOCARDIOGRAPHY

The ACC/AHA guidelines endorse a Class 1 indication for exercise echocardiography in patients with discordant clinical features and stenosis severity by resting echo.[45] Intervention may be considered in patients with a mean gradient greater than 15 mm Hg or PAP greater than 60 mm Hg with exercise.[45] Exercise testing recapitulates symptoms and provides an objective assessment of mitral flow hemodynamics, left ventricular function, PAP, and exercise capacity. As early as 1951, Gorlin and colleagues[75] demonstrated that patients with MS experience a significant increase in heart rate, left atrial pressure, and PAP during supine bike exercise. In addition, a subset of patients with very poor left atrial compliance can have substantial elevations in PAP during exercise.[76] Studies comparing invasive and Doppler-derived estimation of exercise valve gradients and PAP have shown an excellent correlation.[77,78]

Both exercise and dobutamine stress echocardiography (DSE) have been studied. Supine bike exercise is preferred to dobutamine. Exercise is a more physiologic stressor, and results in greater elevations of heart rate, left ventricular filling pressures, and PAP.[79] In patients who are unable to exercise, DSE may be performed.

Planimetered valve area and Doppler quantification of mean transmitral gradient and PAP is performed at rest and during exercise, or following intravenous dobutamine infusions, at a rate of 10 to 40 µg/kg/min. DSE has few complications, and provides incremental prognostic data for patients with moderate MS with an MVA of 1.0 to 1.5 cm². A DSE mean gradient of 18 mm Hg or more identifies patients with a high risk of future clinical events.[80] Stress echocardiography can demonstrate an improvement in mitral flow hemodynamics as early as 5 days after percutaneous transvenous mitral commissurotomy[81] and after mitral valve replacement.[82]

ROLE OF ECHOCARDIOGRAPHY IN MITRAL BALLOON VALVULOPLASTY

Percutaneous balloon mitral valvuloplasty (PBMV) is indicated (1) in patients with symptomatic severe MS, and amenable anatomy, (2) in high-risk patients with contraindications to surgery, or (3) as a bridge to surgery. Patient candidacy for the procedure is determined by echocardiographic assessment of mitral valve morphology. The mechanism of improvement in transmitral gradient and valve area is commissural splitting.[83] Assessment of commissural morphology is extremely

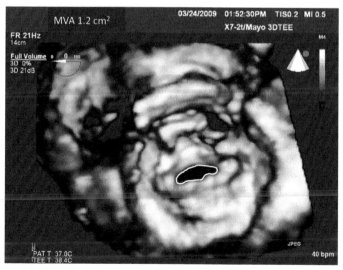

Fig. 5. Three-dimensional (3D) guided planimetry measurement of mitral valve area. Shown is the mitral valve orifice by 3D transesophageal echocardiography from the left ventricular perspective. Using 3D echocardiography, the leaflet tips can be confidently identified using multiple planes, to be certain the mitral orifice is viewed at the appropriate angle and en face. The image can be frozen and a direct 3D-guided 2D planimetry tracing performed of the mitral valve area. In the case shown, the orifice measured 1.2 cm² and is consistent with moderate mitral stenosis. The corresponding movie illustrating the mitral valve directly viewed en face from the left ventricular perspective is shown in Video 2.

important.[84] The widely recognized 2D echocardiographic Wilkins score[85] describes 4 morphologic characteristics: leaflet mobility, thickening, calcification, and subvalvar thickening. Each characteristic is ascribed a score of 0 to 4 (with increasing severity) (**Table 3**). A Wilkins score of less than 8 predicts improved survival. The echocardiographic visualization of commissural calcium alone can identify patients with poor survival on follow-up.[86] 3D echocardiography (3DE) enables superior visualization of the mitral valve morphology. More recently, a 3DE score has been proposed.[87]

Once patients have been identified as suitable for PBMV, TEE is recommended to rule out left atrial thrombus and/or further assessment of significant mitral regurgitation, which are contraindications to proceed.

Postprocedure transthoracic echocardiography (TTE) is necessary for assessment of valve area determined by 2D or 3D planimetry, Doppler transmitral gradient, degree of commissural separation, and worsening or new mitral regurgitation. As already described, MVA by the PHT method is unreliable up to 72 hours following valvuloplasty, owing to abrupt changes in chamber compliance and gradient.[88] However, a PHT of less than 130 milliseconds has been shown to be associated with good valve opening.[65] Mitral regurgitation can occur or worsen in 2% to 10% of patients.

The baseline echocardiographic score is the strongest independent predictor of both immediate procedural success and long-term clinical outcomes including restenosis and mortality.[90,91] Other independent echocardiographic predictors include postvalvuloplasty area, transmitral gradient (mean and peak),[85,89,91] degree of commissural opening,[83] and presence of commissural mitral regurgitation.[92] These conclusions have been reiterated by a recent publication of the largest study to date.[93]

TRANSESOPHAGEAL ECHOCARDIOGRAPHY

TEE is useful for the assessment of MS in selected patients with suboptimal imaging windows. Where satisfactory TTE data are available, TEE is not routinely indicated. The primary indication for TEE is to rule out left atrial thrombus, and confirm the degree of mitral regurgitation in patients undergoing PBMV (Class 1 recommendation).[45,46] Patients with rheumatic MS are at high risk of atrial fibrillation, left atrial thrombi, and thromboembolism, despite systemic anticoagulation.[94] The presence of thrombus is a contraindication for PBMV. Compared with TEE, TTE has limited sensitivity for detecting clots in the left atrium, particularly the appendage.[94,95] The majority of patients with rheumatic MS, up to two-thirds, have spontaneous left atrial contrast on TEE. Atrial fibrillation, spontaneous echo contrast, and an enlarged left

Table 3
Wilkins score to assess suitability for percutaneous mitral balloon valvuloplasty

Grade	Mobility	Subvalvular Thickening	Thickening	Calcification
1	Highly mobile valve with only leaflet tips restricted	Minimal thickening just below the mitral leaflets	Leaflets near normal in thickness (4–5 mm)	A single area of increased echo brightness
2	Leaflet mid and base portions have normal mobility	Thickening of chordal structures extending up to one-third of the chordal length	Midleaflets normal, considerable thickening of margins (5–8 mm)	Scattered areas of brightness confined to leaflet margins
3	Valve continues to move forward in diastole, mainly from the base	Thickening extending to the distal third of the chords	Thickening extending through the entire leaflet (5–8 mm)	Brightness extending into the midportion of the leaflets
4	No or minimal forward movement of the leaflets in diastole	Extensive thickening and shortening of all chordal structures extending down to the papillary muscles	Considerable thickening of all leaflet tissue (greater than 8–10 mm)	Extensive brightness throughout much of the leaflet tissue

Reprinted from Wilkins GT, Weyman AE, Abascal VM, et al. Percutaneous balloon dilatation of the mitral valve: an analysis of echocardiographic variables related to outcome and the mechanism of dilatation. Br Heart J 1988;60:299–308 (PMCID: PMC1216577); with permission.

atrium are associated with high thromboembolic risk.[96,97] During the PBMV, 2D and 3D TEE can provide navigational guidance for transseptal puncture and balloon placement, and evaluate for procedural success and complications such as new or worsening mitral regurgitation, interatrial shunting, or, rarely, pericardial effusion.[98–100] It can be done expeditiously, reliably, and with minimal complications.

ROLE OF ECHOCARDIOGRAPHY IN FOLLOW-UP

As per current guidelines,[45,46] echocardiography should be performed every year in asymptomatic patients with severe MS, and every 2 to 3 years in patients with less severe MS. Patients who have undergone PBMV should undergo similar surveillance.

SUMMARY

Echocardiography is the primary imaging modality in rheumatic MS. It is readily available, noninvasive, and reproducible, and has a robust evidence base. It has played an important role in describing the natural history of the disease. In middle-income and low-income countries, portable echocardiography devices are a useful tool in large-scale population screening for the early identification and treatment of RHD, and prevention of chronic sequelae. The salient echocardiographic data are mitral valvular morphology, valve area, transmitral gradient, pulmonary hypertension, and concomitant valvular disease. From a clinician's perspective, it is important to appreciate the applicability and pitfalls of the various echocardiographic techniques used in MS. Apart from its diagnostic role, echocardiography aids assessment of patient candidacy for PBMV versus surgery. Baseline echocardiographic features are strong independent predictors of procedural success and long-term outcome. Consistent reproducibility lends itself to disease surveillance. Evolving technology such as 3D echocardiography has the exciting potential to improve our understanding and management of this globally relevant disease entity.

SUPPLEMENTARY DATA

Supplementary data related to this article can be found online at http://dx.doi.org/10.1016/j.ccl. 2013.03.006.

REFERENCES

1. Galve E, Candell-Riera J, Pigrau C, et al. Prevalence, morphologic types, and evolution of cardiac valvular disease in systemic lupus erythematosus. N Engl J Med 1988;319:817–23.
2. Tibazarwa KB, Volmink JA, Mayosi BM. Incidence of acute rheumatic fever in the world: a systematic review of population-based studies. Heart 2008;94: 1534–40.
3. Massell BF, Chute CG, Walker AM, et al. Penicillin and the marked decrease in morbidity and mortality from rheumatic fever in the united states. N Engl J Med 1988;318:280–6.
4. Bisno AL. Group a streptococcal infections and acute rheumatic fever. N Engl J Med 1991;325: 783–93.
5. Veasy LG, Wiedmeier SE, Orsmond GS, et al. Resurgence of acute rheumatic fever in the intermountain area of the united states. N Engl J Med 1987;316:421–7.
6. Bisno AL. The resurgence of acute rheumatic fever in the United States. Annu Rev Med 1990;41: 319–29.
7. Padmavati S. Rheumatic fever and rheumatic heart disease in developing countries. Bull World Health Organ 1978;56:543–50.
8. Agarwal BL. Rheumatic heart disease unabated in developing countries. Lancet 1981;2:910–1.
9. White H, Walsh W, Brown A, et al. Rheumatic heart disease in indigenous populations. Heart Lung Circ 2010;19:273–81.
10. Abdel-Hady ES, El-Shamy M, El-Rifai AA, et al. Maternal and perinatal outcome of pregnancies complicated by cardiac disease. Int J Gynaecol Obstet 2005;90:21–5.
11. Cole TO, Adeleye JA. Rheumatic heart disease and pregnancy in Nigerian women. Clin Cardiol 1982;5:280 6.
12. Nkomo VT. Epidemiology and prevention of valvular heart diseases and infective endocarditis in Africa. Heart 2007;93:1510–9.
13. Padmavati S. Rheumatic heart disease: prevalence and preventive measures in the Indian subcontinent. Heart 2001;86:127.
14. Carapetis JR, Steer AC, Mulholland EK, et al. The global burden of group a streptococcal diseases. Lancet Infect Dis 2005;5:685–94.
15. Marijon E, Ou P, Celermajer DS, et al. Prevalence of rheumatic heart disease detected by echocardiographic screening. N Engl J Med 2007;357:470–6.
16. Paar JA, Berrios NM, Rose JD, et al. Prevalence of rheumatic heart disease in children and young adults in Nicaragua. Am J Cardiol 2010;105: 1809–14.
17. Longo-Mbenza B, Bayekula M, Ngiyulu R, et al. Survey of rheumatic heart disease in school

children of Kinshasa town. Int J Cardiol 1998;63:
287–94.

18. Anabwani GM, Bonhoeffer P. Prevalence of heart
disease in school children in rural Kenya using
colour-flow echocardiography. East Afr Med J
1996;73:215–7.

19. Reeves BM, Kado J, Brook M. High prevalence of
rheumatic heart disease in Fiji detected by echocardiography screening. J Paediatr Child Health
2011;47:473–8.

20. Carapetis JR, Hardy M, Fakakovikaetau T, et al.
Evaluation of a screening protocol using auscultation and portable echocardiography to detect
asymptomatic rheumatic heart disease in Tongan
schoolchildren. Nat Clin Pract Cardiovasc Med
2008;5:411–7.

21. Webb RH, Wilson NJ, Lennon DR, et al. Optimising
echocardiographic screening for rheumatic heart
disease in New Zealand: not all valve disease is
rheumatic. Cardiol Young 2011;21:436–43.

22. Bhaya M, Panwar S, Beniwal R, et al. High prevalence of rheumatic heart disease detected by
echocardiography in school children. Echocardiography 2010;27:448–53.

23. Feinstein AR. Prophylaxis of rheumatic fever. Am
Heart J 1964;67:278–9.

24. Steer A, Colquhoun S, Noonan S, et al. Control of
rheumatic heart disease in the Pacific region. Pac
Health Dialog 2006;13:49–55.

25. Marijon E, Jouven X. Early detection of rheumatic
heart disease and prevention of heart failure in
Sub-Saharan Africa. J Am Coll Cardiol 2008;51:
1125–6 [author reply: 1126].

26. Minich LL, Tani LY, Pagotto LT, et al. Doppler echocardiography distinguishes between physiologic and
pathologic "silent" mitral regurgitation in patients
with rheumatic fever. Clin Cardiol 1997;20:924–6.

27. Remenyi B, Wilson N, Steer A, et al. World Heart
Federation criteria for echocardiographic diagnosis of rheumatic heart disease—an evidence-
based guideline. Nat Rev Cardiol 2012;9:297–309.

28. McDonald MI, Towers RJ, Andrews RM, et al. Low
rates of streptococcal pharyngitis and high rates
of pyoderma in Australian Aboriginal communities
where acute rheumatic fever is hyperendemic.
Clin Infect Dis 2006;43:683–9.

29. Steer AC, Carapetis JR. Prevention and treatment
of rheumatic heart disease in the developing world.
Nat Rev Cardiol 2009;6:689–98.

30. Lancefield RC. The antigenic complex of Streptococcus haemolyticus: I. Demonstration of a type-
specific substance in extracts of Streptococcus
haemolyticus. J Exp Med 1928;47:91–103.

31. Lancefield RC. The antigenic complex of Streptococcus haemolyticus: II. Chemical and immunological properties of the protein fractions. J Exp Med
1928;47:469–80.

32. Manjula BN. Molecular aspects of the phagocytosis resistance of group A streptococci. Eur J Epi-
demiol 1988;4:289–300.

33. Kaplan MH, Meyeserian M. An immunological
cross-reaction between group-A streptococcal
cells and human heart tissue. Lancet 1962;1:
706–10.

34. Kaplan MH. Immunologic relation of streptococcal
and tissue antigens. I. Properties of an antigen in
certain strains of group A streptococci exhibiting
an immunologic cross-reaction with human heart
tissue. J Immunol 1963;90:595–606.

35. Goldstein I, Rebeyrotte P, Parlebas J, et al. Isolation from heart valves of glycopeptides which share
immunological properties with Streptococcus haemolyticus group A polysaccharides. Nature 1968;
219:866–8.

36. Dale JB, Beachey EH. Sequence of myosin-
crossreactive epitopes of streptococcal M protein.
J Exp Med 1986;164:1785–90.

37. Cunningham MW, Hall NK, Krisher KK, et al.
A study of anti-group A streptococcal monoclonal
antibodies cross-reactive with myosin. J Immunol
1986;136:293–8.

38. Bronze MS, Beachey EH, Dale JB. Protective and
heart-crossreactive epitopes located within the
NH2 terminus of type 19 streptococcal M protein.
J Exp Med 1988;167:1849–59.

39. Fenderson PG, Fischetti VA, Cunningham MW.
Tropomyosin shares immunologic epitopes with
group A streptococcal M proteins. J Immunol
1989;142:2475–81.

40. Fox EN. M proteins of group A streptococci. Bac-
teriol Rev 1974;38:57–86.

41. Fischetti VA. Streptococcal M protein: molecular
design and biological behavior. Clin Microbiol
Rev 1989;2:285–314.

42. Sanyal SK, Berry AM, Duggal S, et al. Sequelae of
the initial attack of acute rheumatic fever in children
from North India. A prospective 5-year follow-up
study. Circulation 1982;65:375–9.

43. Marcus RH, Sareli P, Pocock WA, et al. The spectrum of severe rheumatic mitral valve disease in a
developing country. Correlations among clinical
presentation, surgical pathologic findings, and hemodynamic sequelae. Ann Intern Med 1994;120:
177–83.

44. Edler I, Hertz CH. The use of ultrasonic reflecto-
scope for the continuous recording of the move-
ments of heart walls. 1954. Clin Physiol Funct
Imaging 2004;24:118–36.

45. Bonow RO, Carabello BA, Chatterjee K, et al. 2008
focused update incorporated into the ACC/AHA
2006 guidelines for the management of patients
with valvular heart disease: a report of the American College of Cardiology/American Heart Association Task Force on Practice Guidelines (Writing

Committee to revise the 1998 guidelines for the management of patients with valvular heart disease): endorsed by the Society of Cardiovascular Anesthesiologists, Society for Cardiovascular Angiography and Interventions, and Society of Thoracic Surgeons. Circulation 2008;118:e523–661.

46. Vahanian A, Alfieri O, Andreotti F, et al. Guidelines on the management of valvular heart disease (version 2012): the Joint Task Force on the Management of Valvular Heart Disease of the European Society Of Cardiology (ESC) and the European Association for Cardio-Thoracic Surgery (EACTS). Eur J Cardiothorac Surg 2012;42:S1–44.

47. Baumgartner H, Hung J, Bermejo J, et al. Echocardiographic assessment of valve stenosis: EAE/ASE recommendations for clinical practice. Eur J Echocardiogr 2009;10:1–25.

48. Edler I, Gustafson A. Ultrasonic cardiogram in mitral stenosis; preliminary communication. Acta Med Scand 1957;159:85–90.

49. Effert S. Pre- and postoperative evaluation of mitral stenosis by ultrasound. Am J Cardiol 1967;19:59–65.

50. Joyner CR Jr, Reid JM, Bond JP. Reflected ultrasound in the assessment of mitral valve disease. Circulation 1963;27:503–11.

51. Segal BL, Likoff W, Kingsley B. Echocardiography. Clinical application in mitral stenosis. JAMA 1966; 195:161–6.

52. McLaurin LP, Gibson TC, Waider W, et al. An appraisal of mitral valve echocardiograms mimicking mitral stenosis in conditions with right ventricular pressure overload. Circulation 1973; 48:801–9.

53. Goodman DJ, Harrison DC, Popp RL. Echocardiographic features of primary pulmonary hypertension. Am J Cardiol 1974;33:438–43.

54. Holen J, Aaslid R, Landmark K, et al. Determination of pressure gradient in mitral stenosis with a non-invasive ultrasound Doppler technique. Acta Med Scand 1976;199:455–60.

55. Hatle L, Brubakk A, Tromsdal A, et al. Noninvasive assessment of pressure drop in mitral stenosis by Doppler ultrasound. Br Heart J 1978;40:131–40.

56. Nishimura RA, Rihal CS, Tajik AJ, et al. Accurate measurement of the transmitral gradient in patients with mitral stenosis: a simultaneous catheterization and Doppler echocardiographic study. J Am Coll Cardiol 1994;24:152–8.

57. Kawahara T, Yamagishi M, Seo H, et al. Application of Doppler color flow imaging to determine valve area in mitral stenosis. J Am Coll Cardiol 1991;18: 85–92.

58. Faletra F, Pezzano A Jr, Fusco R, et al. Measurement of mitral valve area in mitral stenosis: four echocardiographic methods compared with direct measurement of anatomic orifices. J Am Coll Cardiol 1996;28:1190–7.

59. Henry WL, Griffith JM, Michaelis LL, et al. Measurement of mitral orifice area in patients with mitral valve disease by real-time, two-dimensional echocardiography. Circulation 1975;51:827–31.

60. Gorlin R, Gorlin SG. Hydraulic formula for calculation of the area of the stenotic mitral valve, other cardiac valves, and central circulatory shunts. I. Am Heart J 1951;41:1–29.

61. Nichol PM, Gilbert BW, Kisslo JA. Two-dimensional echocardiographic assessment of mitral stenosis. Circulation 1977;55:120–8.

62. Hatle L, Angelsen B, Tromsdal A. Noninvasive assessment of atrioventricular pressure half-time by Doppler ultrasound. Circulation 1979;60:1096–104.

63. Stefanadis C, Dernellis J, Stratos C, et al. Effects of balloon mitral valvuloplasty on left atrial function in mitral stenosis as assessed by pressure-area relation. J Am Coll Cardiol 1998;32:159–68.

64. Thomas JD, Wilkins GT, Choong CY, et al. Inaccuracy of mitral pressure half-time immediately after percutaneous mitral valvotomy. Dependence on transmitral gradient and left atrial and ventricular compliance. Circulation 1988;78:980–93.

65. Messika-Zeitoun D, Meizels A, Cachier A, et al. Echocardiographic evaluation of the mitral valve area before and after percutaneous mitral commissurotomy: the pressure half-time method revisited. J Am Soc Echocardiogr 2005;18:1409–14.

66. Karp K, Teien D, Bjerle P, et al. Reassessment of valve area determinations in mitral stenosis by the pressure half-time method: impact of left ventricular stiffness and peak diastolic pressure difference. J Am Coll Cardiol 1989;13:594–9.

67. Flachskampf FA, Weyman AE, Gillam L, et al. Aortic regurgitation shortens Doppler pressure half-time in mitral stenosis: clinical evidence, in vitro simulation and theoretic analysis. J Am Coll Cardiol 1990; 16:396–404.

68. Messika-Zeitoun D, Cachier A, Brochet E, et al. Evaluation of mitral valve area by the proximal isovelocity surface area method in mitral stenosis: could it be simplified? Eur J Echocardiogr 2007;8: 116–21.

69. Rodriguez L, Thomas JD, Monterroso V, et al. Validation of the proximal flow convergence method. Calculation of orifice area in patients with mitral stenosis. Circulation 1993;88:1157–65.

70. Rifkin RD, Harper K, Tighe D. Comparison of proximal isovelocity surface area method with pressure half-time and planimetry in evaluation of mitral stenosis. J Am Coll Cardiol 1995;26:458–65.

71. Binder TM, Rosenhek R, Porenta G, et al. Improved assessment of mitral valve stenosis by volumetric real-time three-dimensional echocardiography. J Am Coll Cardiol 2000;36:1355–61.

72. Zamorano J, Cordeiro P, Sugeng L, et al. Real-time three-dimensional echocardiography for rheumatic

mitral valve stenosis evaluation: an accurate and novel approach. J Am Coll Cardiol 2004;43: 2091–0

73. Messika-Zeitoun D, Brochet E, Holmin C, et al. Three-dimensional evaluation of the mitral valve area and commissural opening before and after percutaneous mitral commissurotomy in patients with mitral stenosis. Eur Heart J 2007;28:72–9.

74. Zamorano J, Perez de Isla L, Sugeng L, et al. Non-invasive assessment of mitral valve area during percutaneous balloon mitral valvuloplasty: role of real-time 3D echocardiography. Eur Heart J 2004; 25:2086–91.

75. Gorlin R, Sawyer CG, Haynes FW, et al. Effects of exercise on circulatory dynamics in mitral stenosis. III. Am Heart J 1951;41:192–203.

76. Schwammenthal E, Vered Z, Agranat O, et al. Impact of atrioventricular compliance on pulmonary artery pressure in mitral stenosis: an exercise echocardiographic study. Circulation 2000;102: 2378–84.

77. Gonzalez MA, Child JS, Krivokapich J. Comparison of two-dimensional and Doppler echocardiography and intracardiac hemodynamics for quantification of mitral stenosis. Am J Cardiol 1987;60:327–32.

78. Yock PG, Popp RL. Noninvasive estimation of right ventricular systolic pressure by Doppler ultrasound in patients with tricuspid regurgitation. Circulation 1984;70:657–62.

79. Hwang MH, Pacold I, Piao ZE, et al. The usefulness of dobutamine in the assessment of the severity of mitral stenosis. Am Heart J 1986;111:312–6.

80. Reis G, Motta MS, Barbosa MM, et al. Dobutamine stress echocardiography for noninvasive assessment and risk stratification of patients with rheumatic mitral stenosis. J Am Coll Cardiol 2004;43: 393–401.

81. Tamai J, Nagata S, Akaike M, et al. Improvement in mitral flow dynamics during exercise after percutaneous transvenous mitral commissurotomy. Noninvasive evaluation using continuous wave Doppler technique. Circulation 1990;81:46–51.

82. Leavitt JI, Coats MH, Falk RH. Effects of exercise on transmitral gradient and pulmonary artery pressure in patients with mitral stenosis or a prosthetic mitral valve: a Doppler echocardiographic study. J Am Coll Cardiol 1991;17:1520–6.

83. Messika-Zeitoun D, Blanc J, Iung B, et al. Impact of degree of commissural opening after percutaneous mitral commissurotomy on long-term outcome. JACC Cardiovasc Imaging 2009;2:1–7.

84. Fatkin D, Roy P, Morgan JJ, et al. Percutaneous balloon mitral valvotomy with the Inoue single-balloon catheter: commissural morphology as a determinant of outcome. J Am Coll Cardiol 1993; 21:390–7.

85. Abascal VM, Wilkins GT, Choong CY, et al. Echocardiographic evaluation of mitral valve structure and function in patients followed for at least 6 months after percutaneous balloon mitral valvuloplasty. J Am Coll Cardiol 1988;12:606–15.

86. Cannan CR, Nishimura RA, Reeder GS, et al. Echocardiographic assessment of commissural calcium: a simple predictor of outcome after percutaneous mitral balloon valvotomy. J Am Coll Cardiol 1997;29:175–80.

87. Anwar AM, Attia WM, Nosir YF, et al. Validation of a new score for the assessment of mitral stenosis using real-time three-dimensional echocardiography. J Am Soc Echocardiogr 2010;23:13–22.

88. Chen CG, Wang YP, Guo BL, et al. Reliability of the Doppler pressure half-time method for assessing effects of percutaneous mitral balloon valvuloplasty. J Am Coll Cardiol 1989;13:1309–13.

89. Cohen DJ, Kuntz RE, Gordon SP, et al. Predictors of long-term outcome after percutaneous balloon mitral valvuloplasty. N Engl J Med 1992;327: 1329–35.

90. Fawzy ME, Shoukri M, Al Buraiki J, et al. Seventeen years' clinical and echocardiographic follow up of mitral balloon valvuloplasty in 520 patients, and predictors of long-term outcome. J Heart Valve Dis 2007;16:454–60.

91. Langerveld J, Thijs Plokker HW, Ernst SM, et al. Predictors of clinical events or restenosis during follow-up after percutaneous mitral balloon valvotomy. Eur Heart J 1999;20:519–26.

92. Kim MJ, Song JK, Song JM, et al. Long-term outcomes of significant mitral regurgitation after percutaneous mitral valvuloplasty. Circulation 2006;114:2815–22.

93. Bouleti C, Iung B, Laouenan C, et al. Late results of percutaneous mitral commissurotomy up to 20 years: development and validation of a risk score predicting late functional results from a series of 912 patients. Circulation 2012;125:2119–27.

94. Manning WJ, Reis GJ, Douglas PS. Use of transoesophageal echocardiography to detect left atrial thrombi before percutaneous balloon dilatation of the mitral valve: a prospective study. Br Heart J 1992;67:170–3.

95. Kronzon I, Tunick PA, Glassman E, et al. Transesophageal echocardiography to detect atrial clots in candidates for percutaneous transseptal mitral balloon valvuloplasty. J Am Coll Cardiol 1990;16: 1320–2.

96. Daniel WG, Nellessen U, Schroder E, et al. Left atrial spontaneous echo contrast in mitral valve disease: an indicator for an increased thromboembolic risk. J Am Coll Cardiol 1988;11: 1204–11.

97. Goswami KC, Yadav R, Rao MB, et al. Clinical and echocardiographic predictors of left atrial

clot and spontaneous echo contrast in patients with severe rheumatic mitral stenosis: a prospective study in 200 patients by transesophageal echocardiography. Int J Cardiol 2000;73: 273–9.
98. Jaarsma W, Visser CA, Suttorp MJ, et al. Transesophageal echocardiography during percutaneous balloon mitral valvuloplasty. J Am Soc Echocardiogr 1990;3:384–91.

99. Rittoo D, Sutherland GR, Currie P, et al. The comparative value of transesophageal and transthoracic echocardiography before and after percutaneous mitral balloon valvotomy: a prospective study. Am Heart J 1993;125:1094–105.
100. Goldstein SA, Campbell AN. Mitral stenosis. Evaluation and guidance of valvuloplasty by transesophageal echocardiography. Cardiol Clin 1993;11: 409–25.

Calcific Mitral Stenosis

Laila A. Payvandi, MD, Vera H. Rigolin, MD*

KEYWORDS

- Calcific mitral stenosis • Mitral annular calcification • Mitral stenosis • Mitral valve
- Echocardiography

KEY POINTS

- Key risk factors for mitral annular calcification (MAC) include advanced age, female gender, and end-stage renal disease.
- MAC is associated with an increased risk of atrial fibrillation, coronary artery disease, stroke, and cardiovascular morbidity and mortality.
- Severe MAC can extend onto the base of the mitral valve leaflets, particularly the posterior leaflet, and cause a calcific, degenerative form of mitral stenosis (MS).
- The morphologic features of calcific versus rheumatic MS are different. Therefore, the echo approach to quantifying MS severity is different for these two disease entities.
- 3-dimensional transthoracic and transesophageal echo are valuable adjunctive methods for evaluating calcific MS and determining stenosis severity.

INTRODUCTION

The mitral valve annulus is a complex structure that forms an integral part of the mitral valve apparatus. The saddle-shaped annulus plays an active role in mitral valve leaflet coaptation and in left atrial and left ventricular (LV) systole and diastole.[1] Situated in continuity with the aortomitral curtain anteriorly and the posterior mitral valve leaflet posteriorly, the annulus is susceptible to disease processes that are distinct from those that affect the mitral valve leaflets. In addition, advanced annular calcification may extend onto the mitral valve leaflets, particularly the posterior leaflet, thereby by causing increased diastolic gradients across the mitral valve. This form of mitral stenosis (MS) is often referred to as calcific, or degenerative, MS and must be distinguished from the disease process and valve morphology inherent to rheumatic MS. The following review highlights risk factors for mitral annular calcification (MAC), features of calcific MS, and the echo approach to this unique form of valvular heart disease.

MITRAL ANNULAR CALCIFICATION
Description

Annular calcification, one of the most common cardiac findings at autopsy, occurs when calcium is deposited in the region between the posterior LV wall and the posterior mitral valve leaflet.[2] Surgical and autopsy studies suggest that calcium may also extend into the LV myocardium and beneath the endocardial surface of the posterior leaflet.[1] MAC is typically appreciated by transthoracic echo (TTE) in the parasternal long-axis and short-axis views as an echogenic structure in this region (**Fig. 1**). Anterior involvement is less common but may occur in advanced cases. Calcification of the aortic valve, papillary muscles, and chordae tendinae frequently coexist with MAC and, if present, will also be appreciated by echo.[1]

Caseous calcification of the mitral annulus (CCMA) is a rare variant of MAC that may be misinterpreted as tumor, abscess, or thrombus on echo. This finding is sometimes described as soft annular calcification that consists of a combination

Division of Cardiology, Department of Medicine, Bluhm Cardiovascular Institute, Northwestern University Feinberg School of Medicine, 676 North Saint Clair Street, Suite 600, Chicago, IL 60611, USA
* Corresponding author.
E-mail address: v-rigolin@northwestern.edu

Cardiol Clin 31 (2013) 193–202
http://dx.doi.org/10.1016/j.ccl.2013.03.007
0733-8651/13/$ – see front matter © 2013 Elsevier Inc. All rights reserved.

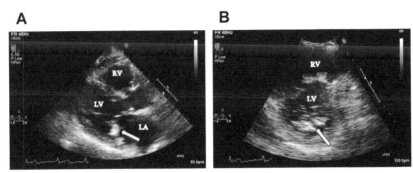

Fig. 1. MAC. MAC is best appreciated in the parasternal long axis (A) and short axis (B) views as a bright echo-density along the posterior mitral annular plane (arrow). LA, left atrium; LV, left ventricle; RV, right ventricle.

of calcium, fatty acids, and cholesterol.[2,3] These components, which form a white, caseous, tooth-pastelike material, are surrounded by a calcified shell.[2,3] Microscopic analysis of the caseous material demonstrates amorphous eosinophils, macrophages, and lymphocytes with scattered areas of calcification and necrosis.[2] By TTE, CCMA appears as a round, echo-dense mass with smooth borders that is typically located in the posterior periannular region. A central area of echolucency, which represents liquification necrosis, and the absence of acoustic shadowing help distinguish this entity from true MAC.[2]

The cause of CCMA is unknown, and serial echo studies may demonstrate progression or spontaneous resolution, reflecting the dynamic nature of this entity.[1,3] No clinical differences have been show to exist between patients with MAC and those with CCMA; thus, appropriate diagnosis rests on a detailed echo evaluation. Although the clinical course is typically benign, CCMA has, in rare cases, been reported to cause MS or regurgitation by mass effect, erosion into the left atrium, and erosion into the left circumflex artery.[1]

CCMA may also be misinterpreted by echo as tumor, abscess, or even thrombus. Appropriate diagnosis is critical becauasae misdiagnosis in this context may lead to unnecessary and invasive management strategies. Clinical correlation with features that support malignancy, infection, or hypercoaguability will distinguish these entities from CCMA and additional imaging modalities, such as transesophageal echo (TEE) and cardiac magnetic resonance imaging, may be required.

Demographics

MAC is associated with female gender, advanced age, diabetes, hypertension, and coronary artery disease (CAD).[4] MAC has also been found in patients with mitral valve prolapse. In this disorder, dystrophic calcification at sites of annular trauma is thought to result from excess tension exerted

by the redundant leaflets.[1] It is estimated that MAC is present in approximately 9% of women and 3% of men who are more than 60 years of age.[1] Annular calcification is also common among patients with chronic renal disease, particularly those with end-stage renal disease (ESRD) requiring dialysis (**Fig. 2**). Prior studies suggest MAC is present in greater than 40% of patients with ESRD and that it tends to develop in younger patients and at a more rapid rate compared with patients without advanced renal disease.[5,6] Studies also show that even mild forms of chronic kidney disease (CKD) confer an increased risk for MAC. A subgroup analysis from the Framingham Heart Study, for example, demonstrated that individuals with chronic kidney disease (defined as a glomerular filtration rate <60 mL/min per 1.73 m^2) were 1.9 times more likely to have MAC compared to those without chronic kidney disease even after adjusting for age and gender.[7]

The major contributor to MAC in patients with renal disease is deranged calcium and phosphorus metabolism caused by secondary hyperparathyroidism. This condition results in a high systemic burden of calcium-phosphorus products, with subsequent calcification of soft tissue structures like the annulus. The presence of MAC in this population bears relevance to the increased cardiovascular risk associated with CKD because MAC is a marker for atherosclerotic burden and is associated with an increased risk of atrial arrhythmias, stroke, and cardiovascular morbidity and mortality.[7]

Clinical Manifestations

MAC is associated with an increased risk of atrial fibrillation, CAD, stroke, and cardiovascular mortality in patients with and without renal disease. Studies have demonstrated the association between MAC and the presence of CAD in younger (<65 years old) and older patients.[8,9] The association between MAC and the risk of cardiovascular

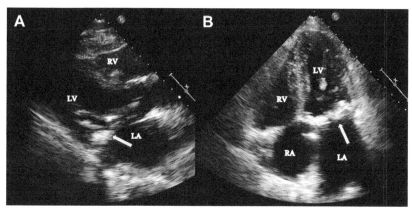

Fig. 2. MAC in ESRD. This Fig. highlights severe MAC, involving both the anterior and posterior aspects of the annulus (*arrow*) in a patient with ESRD. The parasternal long-axis (*A*) and 4-chamber (*B*) views are shown. Abnormal calcium and phosphate metabolism is believed to be the cause of accelerated MAC in this patient population. LA, left atrium; LV, left ventricle; RA, right atrium; RV, right ventricle.

outcomes has been shown in a large cohort (1197 patients) of the Framingham group. After an average of 16 years of follow-up, individuals with MAC had a higher risk for cardiovascular disease, cardiovascular death, and all-cause death. For each 1-mm increase in the size of the MAC, the event rate increased by approximately 10%.[10] Others have also demonstrated the association between MAC, CAD, and cardiovascular death.[11]

The relationship between MAC and increased cardiovascular risk can be explained in several ways. First, there is the burden of shared risk factors, including age, hypertension, hyperlipidemia, diabetes, and obesity. Second, MAC may reflect the long-term exposure of the cardiovascular system to such risk factors. Third, MAC may be a marker for the burden of atherosclerosis. Fourth, other metabolic, inflammatory, and hemostatic factors may be responsible for this relationship.[10] It has also been suggested that vascular and valvular calcification may arise from the same precursor cells suggesting that both entities may be involved in the atherosclerotic process.[8] Finally, cardiovascular effects independent of atherosclerosis, such as mitral valve dysfunction, conduction disease, and increased left atrial size, may also contribute to cardiovascular death.

Aside from cardiac disease, several studies have also demonstrated an increased risk of stroke in individuals with MAC.[12–15] This risk can be explained by the presence of associated risk factors similar to those seen in patients with CAD. In addition, a higher burden of aortic atherosclerosis has been shown in individuals with MAC.[12,16] Less commonly, calcific or thrombotic emboli originating from the MAC may directly cause stroke.[5]

MITRAL VALVULAR DYSFUNCTION
Mitral Regurgitation

The most common form of valvular dysfunction from MAC is mitral regurgitation (MR) (**Fig. 3**). In the normal heart, the base of LV contracts like a sphincter. The posterior aspect of the annulus is included in the base of the LV. During systole, the circumference of the annulus decreases and acts like a sphincter. When the annulus becomes calcified, this sphincterlike contraction does not occur. Because the size of the annulus is not decreased, MR then results.[17] MR may also result from calcium deposition at the base of the posterior leaflet that causes leaflet elevation. As a result, there is less surface area for coaptation with the anterior leaflet and increased risk of chordal elongation and rupture, all of which increase the risk of MR.[1]

Mitral Stenosis

Less commonly, MAC may cause increased diastolic gradients across the mitral valve. This process occurs when the burden of annular calcification is heavy and extends onto the mitral valve leaflets. The resulting decrease in anatomic orifice area leads to calcific, or degenerative, MS.[4] This form of MS is markedly different from rheumatic MS. Rheumatic MS is defined by commissural fusion, leaflet tip restriction, and chordal shortening with relative pathologic sparing of the annulus and base of the mitral leaflets (**Fig. 4**). The limiting orifice area is at the rheumatic leaflet tips (**Fig. 5**), whereas in calcific MS, the limiting orifice area is at the base of the mitral leaflets (**Fig. 6**). These differences are well appreciated by transthoracic real-time 3-dimensional echo (RT3DE). This modality highlights the leaflet doming and funnel-shaped geometry of a rheumatic mitral valve, in contrast to

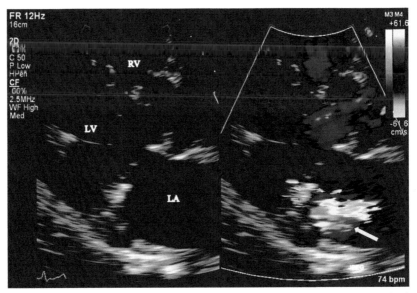

Fig. 3. MR caused by MAC. MR (*arrow*) is the most common valve lesion associated with MAC. This lesion is caused by a combination of factors, including dysfunctional annular contraction and posterior leaflet elevation caused by calcium deposition under the leaflet base. LA, left atrium; LV, left ventricle; RV, right ventricle.

the long, tubular geometry of a mitral orifice affected by calcific stenosis.[18]

Echo Features of Calcific MS and Methods of Quantifying Severity

In addition to structural difference between rheumatic and calcific forms of MS, the respective

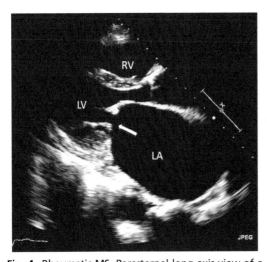

Fig. 4. Rheumatic MS. Parasternal long-axis view of a patient with rheumatic MS is shown. Leaflet tip fusion (*arrow*), commissural fusion, and chordal thickening and shortening are the key morphologic features of rheumatic MS. The annulus and base of the leaflets are normally spared. LA, left atrium; LV, left ventricle; RV, right ventricle.

methods for evaluating stenosis severity are also different. The severity of rheumatic MS is typically evaluated by a combination of 2-dimensional and Doppler-derived techniques, some of which cannot be reliably applied to calcific MS because of the pattern of valve deformation and coexisting hemodynamic abnormalities.

Commissural and leaflet tip fusion, the structural hallmarks of rheumatic MS, lend themselves to planimetry of the mitral orifice area, which may be performed independent of assumptions regarding flow conditions, LV compliance, or associated valvular lesions.[19] This assessment of mitral valve area (MVA), which correlates well with the anatomic area of explanted valves, cannot be reliably applied in the context of calcific MS. In calcific MS, stenosis originates from heavy annular calcification that subsequently extends to the leaflets starting at the base. As such, the limiting orifice in calcific MS cannot be readily appreciated in short axis by 2-dimensional echo; planimetry should, therefore, be avoided.[4,19]

In terms of spectral Doppler, rheumatic MS assessment is based on mean diastolic gradient and MVA derived from the pressure half-time (PHT) method (MVA = 220/PHT). Both of these techniques involve continuous wave Doppler and are described in the American Society of Echocardiography's guidelines on valve stenosis[19] (**Fig. 7**). Mean diastolic gradient may also be used in the context of calcific MS; but this method, in general, becomes unreliable in the presence tachycardia, atrial fibrillation, increased

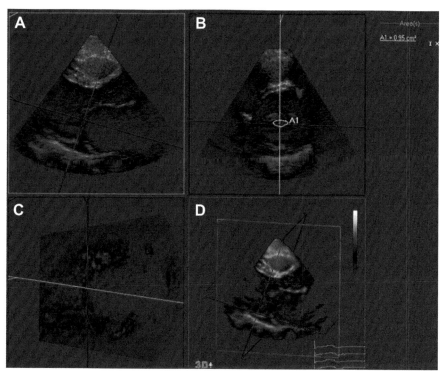

Fig. 5. Three-dimensional assessment of rheumatic MS. Transthoracic full-volume 3-dimensional imaging allows precise evaluation of the stenotic mitral valve orifice. By aligning perpendicular planes in (A) and (C), a short-axis view of the mitral valve is obtained at the level of the leaflet tips (B). In this example, planimetry at this level resulted in a mitral valve area of 0.95 cm², consistent with severe MS. Full 3D volume of the heart demonstrating all 3 cropping planes simultaneously (D). A1, mitral valve area.

cardiac output, and/or MR.[4,19] On the other hand, area measurements derived from the PHT method should be avoided in calcific MS. This measurement is significantly affected by LV compliance,

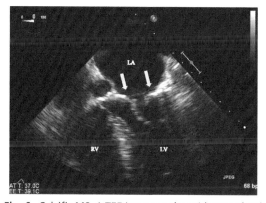

Fig. 6. Calcific MS. A TEE image at the midesopagheal 0° plane from a patient with ESRD disease is shown. In calcific MS, calcium extends from the annulus onto the mitral valve leaflets, resulting in a decreased orifice area in diastole. Unlike rheumatic MS, the limiting orifice occurs at the base of the leaflets (arrows). The leaflet tips are unaffected. LA, left atrium; LV, left ventricle; RV, right ventricle.

which is decreased in patients with advanced age, hypertension, diabetes mellitus, and aortic stenosis—comorbidities that commonly coexist with MAC and calcific MS. Decreased LV compliance results in more rapid equilibration of left atrial and LV pressures during diastole, which, in turn, leads to a shorter PHT and, therefore, over-estimation of MVA[4,19] (**Fig. 8**).

In terms of color Doppler, the proximal isovelocity surface area (PISA) method is another method for evaluating the effective mitral orifice area in both rheumatic and calcific MS. In contradistinction to the PISA method in MR, the color Doppler baseline is shifted in the opposite direction (ie, the baseline is shifted in the direction of inflow) for the assessment of MS. This calculation requires the measurement of the radius of the convergence hemisphere (centimeters), the aliasing velocity (centimeters per second), the peak mitral inflow velocity assessed by continuous wave Doppler (centimeters per second), and the opening leaflet angle relative to flow direction.[19] Although this method may be used in the setting of significant MR, it is technically difficult, requires multiple measurements, and is easily susceptible to manual measurement errors.[19]

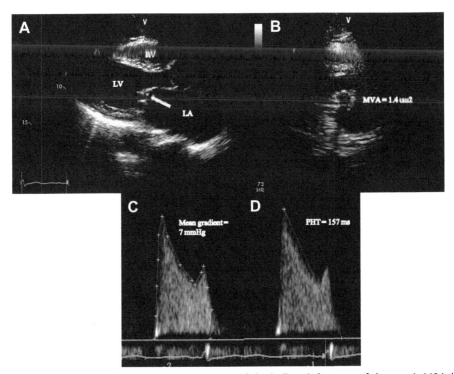

Fig. 7. Quantitative assessment of rheumatic MS. (*A*) One of the hallmark features of rheumatic MS is leaflet tip fusion with a hockey stick deformity of the anterior mitral valve leaflet in diastole (*arrow*). In this transthoracic parasternal long-axis view, note the lack of annular calcification and the limiting orifice confined to the leaflet tips. (*B–D*) Taken from the same patient, these 3 images demonstrate consistency among the 3 key methods for assessing rheumatic MS severity. Planimetry results in a MVA of 1.4 cm², consistent with moderate MS. A mean gradient of 7 mm Hg and a PHT-derived valve area of 1.4 cm² are also consistent with moderate MS. LA, left atrium; LV, left ventricle; RV, right ventricle.

To address the challenges of MVA assessment in calcific MS, Chu and colleagues[18] investigated the role of transthoracic RT3DE. The study goal was to identify a method that lacks the abovementioned limitations of planimetry and PHT in the context of calcific MS. Using the continuity equation as the reference standard to calculate MVA, the investigators compared PHT-derived MVA and RT3DE-derived MVA among 34 patients with calcific MS and a minimum mean transmitral gradient of 4 mm Hg. The 3D assessment first involved a full-volume 3D color acquisition. Offline analysis was then performed to view the mitral valve en face; from this view, MVA was determined by tracing the narrowest annular orifice. Compared with the reference standard, PHT-derived MVA overestimated MVA ($P = .037$), as anticipated, but RT3DE-derived MVA showed no significant difference ($P = .61$). RT3DE-derived MVA measurements also correlated better with the reference standard than PHT-derived MVA values ($r = 0.86$ vs 0.58, respectively). Taken together, these results indicate that transthoracic RT3DE is

a reliable method for MVA evaluation in calcific MS. This practical technique may serve a complimentary role to mean mitral valve gradient assessment and the PISA method, and consideration should be given to incorporating this approach into routine clinical practice. The same 3D protocol for MVA assessment may be performed using TEE, as illustrated in **Fig. 9**.

Radiation-Associated Calcific MS

Radiation therapy is an important treatment modality for several different malignancies. The dose, field size, and frequency of radiation are affected by the specific type and stage of the malignancy. Thoracic malignancies that are frequently treated with radiation include Hodgkin's disease and breast cancer. Current strategies for radiation therapy are designed to maximize therapeutic effect while minimizing short-term and long-term complications. Longitudinal studies indicate that cardiovascular effects from radiation confer a 2- to 3-fold increase in the

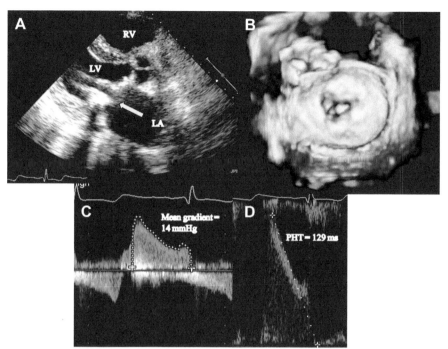

Fig. 8. Quantitative assessment of calcific MS. (A) Severe MAC extending onto both the anterior and posterior mitral valve leaflets is shown in this transthoracic parasternal long-axis view. This diastolic frame highlights the basal origin (*arrow*) of calcific MS and the lack of leaflet tip fusion. Calcific changes of the aortic valve are also appreciated in this view. (B) Planimetry of the MVA is unreliable on 2-dimensional imaging because the limiting orifice, unlike rheumatic MS, is not located at the leaflet tips. Planimetry may be performed, however, using 3-dimensional echo because this modality allows more accurate visualization of the limiting basal orifice. This 3-dimensional TEE image of the mitral valve, as viewed from the left atrial perspective, was acquired from a patient with ESRD requiring dialysis. Note the extensive annular calcification limiting the orifice size. (C) Mean mitral valve diastolic gradient may be used to assess the severity of calcific MS. The mean gradient of 14 mm Hg in this patient is consistent with severe MS. (D) PHT assessment of MVA is unreliable in calcific MS. Images (C) and (D) were acquired from the same patient. The PHT measurement corresponds to aN MVA of 1.7 cm², which is consistent with only mild MS. This discrepancy is typically caused by coexisting LV compliance abnormalities, which lead to more rapid equalization of LV and LA pressures during diastole and, therefore, overestimation of MVA. LA, left atrium; LV, left ventricle; RV, right ventricle.

risk of cardiac death among cancer survivors.[20] These effects are particularly prominent among adult long-term survivors of Hodgkin's disease, many of whom were treated during an era when high success rates were achieved with radiation strategies that were later found to confer deleterious cardiovascular consequences.[21] Such effects include accelerated CAD, restrictive myocardial disease, constrictive pericardial disease, conduction abnormalities, and valvular dysfunction.[20,21]

Autopsy studies report a 70% to 80% prevalence of valve fibrosis in patients treated with chest radiation doses exceeding 35 Gy.[22] Clinically significant radiation-induced valve disease, however, is present in only 6% to 15% of treated patients.[21,23] The risk is presumably dose related and tends to manifest more than 20 years following radiation exposure.[21,24] The left-sided cardiac valves are most commonly affected.[22] The mechanism of radiation-induced valve degeneration is poorly understood; however, the hypothesis is that radiation results in a decreased population of endothelial progenitor cells and directly induces valve thickening, fibrosis, calcification, and leaflet restriction.[23–25]

Valve regurgitation is the most frequently detected lesion, although aortic and MS do occur. Hallmark features of radiation-induced MS include severe MAC and thickening and calcification of the aorto-mitral curtain that extends along the anterior leaflet. In some cases, the posterior leaflet remains mobile, which distinguishes this entity from the degenerative calcific form of MS previously discussed.[20,23] Unlike rheumatic MS, there is no commissural fusion and the subvalvular apparatus is typically unaffected[20,23] (**Figs. 10** and **11**).

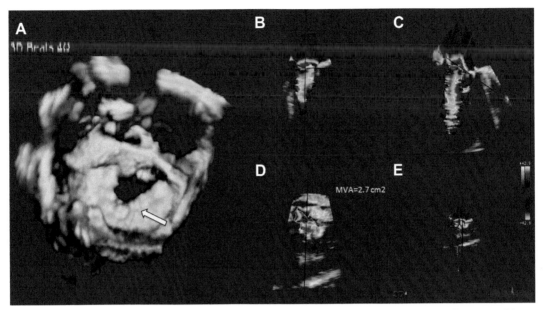

Fig. 9. Three-dimensional transesophageal echo assessment of calcific MS. (*A*) Full-volume 3-dimensional image of the mitral valve, as viewed from the left atrial perspective. There is severe MAC with extension along the length of the posterior leaflet (*arrow*) and subsequent narrowing of the mitral orifice area at the level of the annulus. (*B–E*) Offline 3-dimensional assessment and planimetry of the mitral orifice. Imaging planes are aligned in a perpendicular fashion at the level of the smallest orifice of the mitral valve using color Doppler as a guide (*B, C*). Planimetry is then performed on the en face view of the orifice (*D*). The MVA is 2.7 cm², consistent with mild stenosis.

Quantification of stenosis severity in MS caused by radiation is similar to any form of calcific MS. Three-dimensional TEE has been shown to be particularly useful because of the ability to demonstrate complete commissural opening and direct visualization of valve morphology from both the left atrial and LV perspectives.[23] Findings such as these are critical to the management of non-rheumatic MS because they preclude candidacy for balloon valvuloplasty and warrant referral for surgical mitral valve replacement, if clinically appropriate.

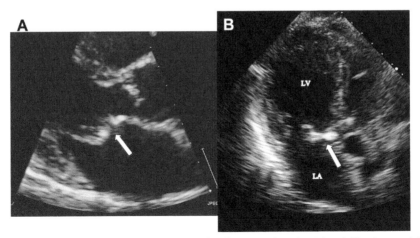

Fig. 10. Radiation-induced calcific MS. A key feature of radiation-induced MS is calcification and thickening of the aorto-mitral curtain that extends along the anterior mitral valve leaflet (*arrow*), which is seen in parasternal long-axis (*A*) and 4-chamber (*B*) views acquired from the same patient with a history of mediastinal radiation. The morphology and mobility of the posterior leaflet appears normal. LA, left atrium; LV, left ventricle.

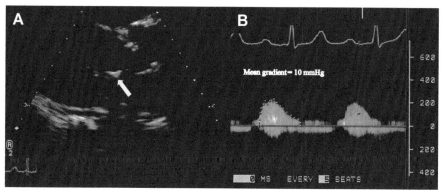

Fig. 11. This echo demonstrates typical echo findings in a patient with severe radiation-induced calcific MS. (*A*) There is calcification and thickening of the aorto-mitral curtain with secondary calcification and restriction of the anterior mitral valve leaflet (*arrow*). (*B*) The mean mitral valve gradient of 10 mm Hg suggests severe MS.

SUMMARY

MAC is a common finding in many patients, particularly those with traditional risk factors for cardiovascular disease. The presence of MAC is associated with a higher rate of adverse cardiovascular events. MAC can also lead to mitral valve dysfunction. The most common lesion is MR, although MS can also develop in heavily calcified valves. Risk factors for developing calcific MS include age, ESRD, and prior chest radiation therapy. The anatomy of the mitral valve with calcific MS is distinct from that of rheumatic disease. As a result, optimal methods of quantification of the severity of MS by echo also differ. In particular, PHT methods and planimetry are less reliable in calcific MS compared with rheumatic MS. RT3DE is well suited for the evaluation of calcific MS because of its ability to demonstrate en face views of the valve and allow for quantification of the orifice size at the level of the annulus.

REFERENCES

1. Silbiger JJ. Anatomy, mechanics, and pathophysiology of the mitral annulus. Am Heart J 2012; 164(2):163–76.
2. Harpaz D, Auerbach I, Vered Z, et al. Caseous calcification of the mitral annulus: a neglected, unrecognized diagnosis. J Am Soc Echocardiogr 2001; 14(8):825–31.
3. Deluca G, Correale M, Ieva R, et al. The incidence and clinical course of caseous calcification of the mitral annulus: a prospective echocardiographic study. J Am Soc Echocardiogr 2008;21(7):828–33.
4. Bonou M, Vouliotis AI, Lampropoulos K, et al. Continuity equation is the echocardiographic method of choice to assess degenerative mitral stenosis. Cardiol J 2011;18(5):577–80.
5. Willens HJ, Ferreira AC, Gallagher AJ, et al. Mobile components associated with rapidly developing mitral annulus calcification in patients with chronic renal failure: review of mobile elements associated with mitral annulus calcification. Echocardiography 2003;20(4):363–7.
6. Ribeiro S, Ramos A, Brandão A, et al. Cardiac valve calcification in haemodialysis patients: role of calcium-phosphate metabolism. Nephrol Dial Transplant 1998;13(8):2037–40.
7. Fox CS, Larson MG, Vasan RS, et al. Cross-sectional association of kidney function with valvular and annular calcification: the Framingham Heart Study. J Am Soc Nephrol 2006;17(2):521–7.
8. Atar S, Jeon DS, Luo H, et al. Mitral annular calcification: a marker of severe coronary artery disease in patients under 65 years old. Heart 2003;89:161–4.
9. Adler Y, Herz I, Vaturi M, et al. Mitral annular calcium detected by transthoracic echocardiography is a marker for high prevalence and severity of coronary artery disease in patients undergoing coronary angiography. Am J Cardiol 1998;82:1183–6.
10. Fox CS, Vasan RS, Parise H, et al, Framingham Heart Study. Mitral annular calcification predicts cardiovascular morbidity and mortality: the Framingham Heart Study. Circulation 2003;107:1492–6.
11. Willens HJ, Chirinos JA, Schob A, et al. The relation between mitral annular calcification and mortality in patients undergoing diagnostic coronary angiography. Echocardiography 2006;23:717–22.
12. Pujadas R, Arboix A, Anguera N, et al. Mitral annular calcification as a marker of complex aortic atheroma in patients with stroke of uncertain etiology. Echocardiography 2008;25:124–32.
13. Benjamin EJ, Plehn JF, D'Agostino RB, et al. Mitral annular calcification and the risk of stroke in an elderly cohort. N Engl J Med 1992;327:374–9.
14. Aronow WS, Koenigsberg M, Kronzon I, et al. Association of mitral anular calcium with thromboembolic

stroke and cardiac events at 39-month follow-up in elderly patients. Am J Cardiol 1990;65:1511–2.

15. Kizor R, Wiebers D, Whisnant J, et al. Mitral annular calcification, aortic valve sclerosis, and incident stroke in adults free of clinical cardiovascular disease. The Strong Heart Study. Stroke 2005;36: 2533–7.

16. Adler Y, Vaturi M, Fink N, et al. Association between mitral annulus calcification and aortic atheroma: a prospective transesophageal echocardiographic study. Atherosclerosis 2000;152:451–6.

17. Roberts WC, Perloff JK. A clinicopathologic survey of the conditions causing the mitral valve to function abnormally. Ann Intern Med 1972;77:939–75.

18. Chu JW, Levine RA, Chua S, et al. Assessing mitral valve area and orifice geometry in calcific mitral stenosis: a new solution by real-time three-dimensional echocardiography. J Am Soc Echocardiogr 2008; 21(9):1006–9.

19. Baumgartner H, Hung J, Bermejo J, et al, American Society of Echocardiography, European Association of Echocardiography. Echocardiographic assessment of valve stenosis: EAE/ASE recommendations for clinical practice. J Am Soc Echocardiogr 2009; 22(1):1–23.

20. Adabag AS, Dykoski R, Ward H, et al. Critical stenosis of aortic and mitral valves after mediastinal irradiation. Catheter Cardiovasc Interv 2004;63(2):247–50.

21. Hull MC, Morris CG, Pepine CJ, et al. Valvular dysfunction and carotid, subclavian, and coronary artery disease in survivors of Hodgkin lymphoma treated with radiation therapy. JAMA 2003;290(21): 2831–7.

22. Adams MJ, Hardenbergh PH, Constine LS, et al. Radiation-associated cardiovascular disease. Crit Rev Oncol Hematol 2003;45(1):55–75.

23. Malanca M, Cimadevilla C, Brochet E, et al. Radiotherapy-induced mitral stenosis: a three-dimensional perspective. J Am Soc Echocardiogr 2010;23(1):108.

24. Wethal T, Lund MB, Edvardsen T, et al. Valvular dysfunction and left ventricular changes in Hodgkin's lymphoma survivors. A longitudinal study. Br J Cancer 2009;101(4):575–81.

25. Carlson RG, Mayfield WR, Normann S, et al. Radiation-associated valvular disease. Chest 1991;99(3): 538–45.

The Role of 3-Dimensional Echocardiography in the Diagnosis and Management of Mitral Valve Disease
Myxomatous Valve Disease

Wendy Tsang, MD[a], Benjamin H. Freed, MD[b], Roberto M. Lang, MD[c],*

KEYWORDS

- Myxomatous mitral valve disease • Barlow's disease • Fibroelastic deficiency
- Three-dimensional echocardiography

KEY POINTS

- Myxomatous/degenerative mitral valve (MV) disease comprises a spectrum, with its most severe form recognized as Barlow's disease and the mildest form known as fibroelastic deficiency.
- Three-dimensional echocardiography has improved diagnosis and localization of mitral leaflet pathology, as well as quantification of regurgitation.
- Accurate localization of leaflet pathology is important in determining surgical repair strategy or in using a percutaneous approach.

INTRODUCTION

Myxomatous/degenerative MV disease is the most common cause of mitral regurgitation (MR) in developed countries.[1] This disease process comprises a spectrum, with its most severe form recognized as Barlow's disease and the mildest form known as fibroelastic deficiency (**Table 1**). This article discusses the etiology, presentation, diagnosis, and management of myxomatous MV disease.

ETIOLOGY

Barlow's disease results from an excess of myxomatous tissue, which is an abnormal accumulation of mucopolysaccharides in one or both the leaflets and many or only few of the chordae.[2] This myxoid infiltration results in thick, bulky, redundant billowing leaflets and elongated chordae, which often lead to bileaflet, multisegmental prolapse (**Fig. 1**). Barlow's disease is usually diagnosed in young women who are typically followed for many years with well-preserved left ventricular size, until indications for surgery are met in the fourth or fifth decade of life.

In contrast, fibroelastic deficiency results from acute loss of mechanical integrity due to abnormalities of connective tissue structure and/or function.[2] It usually results in a localized or unisegmental prolapse due to elongated chordae or flail leaflet due to ruptured chordae (see **Fig. 1**). Patients most commonly present in the sixth decade of life with a short, almost acute history of MR. Typically, the cause of this presentation is the rupture of a

[a] Division of Cardiology, Toronto General Hospital, University Health Network, University of Toronto, 200 Elizabeth Street, Toronto, Ontario M5G 2C4, Canada; [b] Northwestern Memorial Hospital, 201 East Huron Street, Chicago, IL 60611, USA; [c] University of Chicago Medical Center, 5841 South Maryland Avenue, MC 5084, Chicago, IL 60637, USA
* Corresponding author.
E-mail address: rlang@medicine.bsd.uchicago.edu

Cardiol Clin 31 (2013) 203–215
http://dx.doi.org/10.1016/j.ccl.2013.03.002
0733-8651/13/$ – see front matter © 2013 Elsevier Inc. All rights reserved.

Table 1
Differences between Barlow's disease and fibroelastic deficiency

Differentiating Characteristics	Barlow's Disease	Fibroelastic Deficiency
Pathology	Excess leaflet tissue due to accumulation of mucopolysaccharides	Loss of mechanical integrity due to impaired production of connective tissue
Typical age of diagnosis	Young (<40 y old)	Old (>60 y old)
Duration of disease	Years to decades	Days to months
Physical examination	Midsystolic click and late systolic murmur	Holosystolic murmur
Leaflet involvement	Multisegmental	Unisegmental
Leaflet lesions	Leaflet billowing and thickening	Thin leaflets with thickened involved segment
Chordae lesions	Chordal thickening and elongation	Chordal elongation and chordal rupture
Carpentier classification	Type II	Type II
Type of dysfunction	Bileaflet prolapse	Prolapse and/or flail
Complexity of valve repair	More complex	Less complex

single mitral chordae tendinae. This entity is the most common form of organic MV disease for which MV repair surgery is required.

There is considerable overlap between these 2 entities, and it is difficult to reliably distinguish between them based on either the gross or the histologic appearance of the MV. Some valves may represent a forme fruste of Barlow's disease and demonstrate myxoid infiltration on subsequent histologic examination.[3] Despite the challenges in definitively diagnosing these 2 entities, the preoperative differentiation between Barlow's disease and fibroelastic deficiency is a crucial aspect for referral, determination of the optimal surgical strategy, and postoperative outcome. The lesions resulting from Barlow's disease are complex and

frequently require expert surgical skills to achieve a successful repair, whereas lesions resulting from fibroelastic deficiency are more localized and can typically be undertaken by simple resection of the unsupported leaflet tissue by a less experienced surgeon. Difficulties with presurgical planning may lead to either unsuccessful repair or conversion to replacement with less favorable outcomes.[4,5]

DIAGNOSIS

Diseases that affect the MV are best described by defining the cause of the disease (ie, primary/direct vs secondary/indirect), the specific lesions caused by the disease, and the dysfunction it creates on

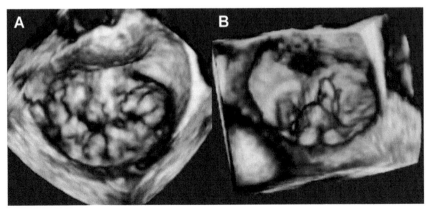

Fig. 1. Three-dimensional transesophageal echocardiographic images of the mitral valve demonstrating Barlow's disease (A) with bileaflet, multisegmental prolapse and fibroelastic deficiency (B) with P2 prolapse and chordal rupture.

the MV apparatus. This "pathophysiologic triad," first described by Carpentier in the early 1980s, is still extremely useful today in characterizing the different types of MV disorders.[6]

No matter what the cause of the MV disease, each disease process frequently results in one or more lesions. For example, degenerative diseases such as Barlow's disease and fibroelastic deficiency result in multiple types of lesions including excess myomatous leaflet tissue, chordal elongation, thinning, and rupture. These lesions in turn lead to MV dysfunction. Instead of classifying this dysfunction as simply MV stenosis or regurgitation, the Carpentier classification scheme has been developed to aid in the surgical strategy based on the type of leaflet motion (**Table 2**).[7] Patients with mitral annular dilatation or leaflet perforation usually have normal leaflet motion and are categorized as type I dysfunction. Type II dysfunction includes patients with prolapse (free edge of one or both leaflets overriding the plane of the annulus during valve closure) and flail (excessive motion of the leaflet margin above the plane of the annulus) due to excessive and redundant leaflet tissue or chordal rupture, respectively (**Fig. 2**). Leaflet restriction during valve closure due to fusion of various components of the MV apparatus is defined as type IIIa dysfunction, whereas leaflet restriction during valve opening resulting from leaflet tethering is defined as type IIIb dysfunction. In addition to these classifications, a modification to this system has added systolic anterior motion of the leaflets (type IVa) and hybrid conditions (type V).[8]

Although the Carpentier classification for MR lesions provided a systematic method to categorize the mechanisms of MR to determine the surgical strategy, it must be emphasized that even with recent modifications, this classification system neglects to include papillary muscle motion abnormalities.[8] For example, "mitral papillary muscle traction," a phenomenon described in Barlow's disease, occurs when excess systolic loading on the chordae causes the tips of the papillary muscles to move toward the mitral annulus during systole rather than toward the left ventricular apex, causing regurgitation.[9,10] In addition, the development of three-dimensional (3D) transesophageal echocardiography (TEE) has highlighted weaknesses in this classification. 3D TEE provides in greater detail information regarding the pathomorphologic changes to the MV, allowing a tailored approach rather than a standard approach in which a preestablished operation is performed according to the Carpentier classification system. This method is an especially important change in the surgical approach to myxomatous MV disease because patients often have more than a single

mechanism of MR, which reduces the utility of the Carpentier classification system.

UTILITY OF THREE-DIMENSIONAL ECHOCARDIOGRAPHY

Three-dimensional echocardiography (3DE) has considerably improved the ability of physicians to both diagnose and treat patients with myxomatous MV disease.[11] Multiple studies have shown that 3DE is superior to two-dimensional echocardiography (2DE) in accurately diagnosing myxomatous MV disease.[3,12,13] 3DE is less operator dependent and more reproducible than 2DE at any expertise level. The diagnostic accuracy of 3D TEE was compared with that of 2D TEE in a large number of patients undergoing repair for MV prolapse in which echocardiographic findings were compared with the surgical ones. 3D TEE correctly identified prolapse in 92% of patients versus 78% of patients using 2D TEE.[14]

In addition to its superior accuracy in diagnosing myxomatous MV disease, 3DE also has the ability to differentiate between Barlow's disease and fibroelastic deficiency. When 3D quantitative parameters were used to differentiate between patients with and without degenerative MV disease, billowing height and volume were the strongest predictors for the presence of degenerative MV disease, and results were highly reproducible.[12] A 3D billowing height cutoff value of 1.0 mm differentiated between normal and degenerative disease without overlap and a 3D billowing volume cutoff value of 1.15 mL differentiated between Barlow's disease and fibroelastic deficiency without overlap.

Application of 3DE quantification to patients with myxomatous valve disease undergoing MV repair has found that (1) mitral annular dimensions with 3DE were accurate and reproducible compared with direct intraoperative measurements; (2) patients with myxomatous valve disease have significantly larger annular dimensions than controls during diastole; (3) control patients have early-systolic anteroposterior and area contraction, increased annular height, deeper saddle-shaped depth, and unchanged intercommissural diameter, whereas patients with myxomatous valve disease have mostly unchanged annular dimensions but significant intercommissural dilation, and (4) post-repair, the annulus is smaller in patients with myxomatous valve disease but continues to lack systolic saddle-shaped accentuation.[15]

Parametric maps transform the 3D images of the MV into color-encoded topographic displays of MV anatomy, in which the color gradations indicate the distance of the leaflet from the mitral

Table 2
Carpentier's functional classification for mitral valve dysfunction with modification

	Type I	Type II	Type IIIa	Type IIIb	Type IVa	Type V
Motion of leaflet margin	Normal	Prolapse or flail	Restricted leaflet opening	Restricted leaflet closure	Systolic anterior leaflet motion	Hybrid conditions
Associated disease processes	Chronic atrial fibrillation Bacterial endocarditis	Degenerative disease (Barlow's disease or fibroelastic deficiency)	Rheumatic disease	Myocardial infarction Dilated cardiomyopathy	Hypertrophic cardiomyopathy Post–mitral valve repair Hemodynamic-induced (eg, hypovolemia, tachycardia)	Combined rheumatic valve disease and infective endocarditis
Associated lesions	Annular dilatation Leaflet perforation	Leaflet thickening Leaflet billowing Leaflet elongation Chordal thickening Chordal rupture	Commissure fusion Leaflet thickening Chordae thickening	Papillary displacement Chordae tethering Annular dilatation	Asymmetric septal hypertrophy Anterior leaflet enlargement Undersized mitral annuloplasty ring	Tethered, restricted small posterior leaflet with flail anterior leaflet Anterior leaflet systolic anterior motion with flail or prolapsing posterior leaflet

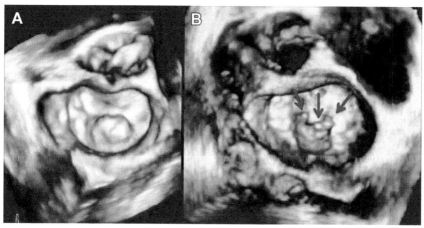

Fig. 2. Three-dimensional transesophageal echocardiographic images of the mitral valve demonstrating isolated P2 prolapse (A) and P2 prolapse with multiple ruptured chords (arrows, B).

annular plane toward the left atrium. It has been shown that, with the use of 3D parametric maps, the diagnostic accuracy and reproducibility In novice readers is significantly improved compared with the use of 2DE (**Fig. 3**).[13] In addition, parametric maps improve the differentiation of MV billowing, where the leaflet body but not the tips prolapses beyond the mitral annular plane, versus prolapse, where the leaflet body and the tips prolapse beyond the mitral annular plane. With the aid of 3D parametric maps, it has been shown that in degenerative MV disease, prolapsing height and anterior leaflet surface were the strongest predictors of surgical repair complexity, irrespective of the cause of MR.[16]

3DE has also highlighted the different conformational changes that occur between Barlow's disease and fibroelastic deficiency after MV repair. The annular diameters and MV area were

significantly reduced for both disease entities postrepair. However, the MV annulus was found to be larger in patients with Barlow's disease, consistent with the different mean sizes of the implanted prosthetic rings.[17] In addition, the greater reduction in posterior leaflet area in patients with Barlow's disease compared with those with fibroelastic deficiency is in agreement with the higher rate of posterior leaflet resection and sliding performed for this type of degenerative disease.

The propensity for developing post-MV repair systolic anterior motion, in part, depends on the degree of mitroaortic and septoaortic angles, presence of excess tissue, and displacement of the mitral coaptation line toward the posterior leaflet, all of which are well characterized by 3DE (**Fig. 4**).[18–21] By quantifying the extent of the excess anterior and posterior leaflet length,

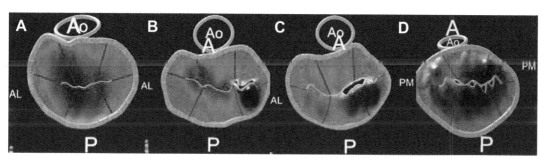

Fig. 3. Three-dimensional parametric maps of the mitral valve demonstrating (A) normal anatomy, (B) P3 flail scallop, (C) P2 and P3 prolapse, and (D) Barlow's disease. (Reprinted from Tsang W, Weinert L, Sugeng L, et al. The value of three-dimensional echocardiography derived mitral valve parametric maps and the role of experience in the diagnosis of pathology. J Am Soc Echocardiogr Copyright 2011;24:860–7; with permission from Elsevier.)

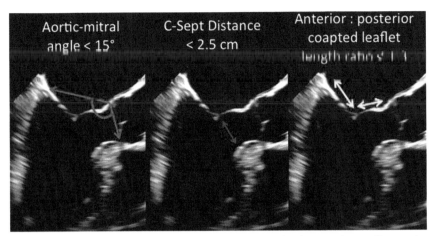

Fig. 4. Echocardiographic indicators of increased risk for post–mitral valve repair systolic anterior motion. (1) Aortic–mitral annular angle <15°; (2) leaflet coaptation point to septum (C-Sept) distance <2.5 cm; and (3) anterior to posterior leaflet length ratio <1.3.

surface area, and billowing volume before and after surgery, 3DE analysis helps identify patients who are most at risk for developing systolic anterior motion.

3DE ACQUISITION AND DISPLAY OF THE MYXOMATOUS MITRAL VALVE
Transthoracic 3D Echocardiographic Acquisition

3D transthoracic echocardiographic (TTE) images of a myxomatous MV should be acquired from either the parasternal long-axis view or the apical 4-chamber view (**Table 3**). The MV should be located in the center of the pyramidal 3D volume and should include a section of the left atrium, the left ventricle base from the papillary muscles, and a portion of the aortic valve for image orientation postacquisition. The 3D TTE image of the myxomatous MV should be presented en face from either the left atrial or left ventricular perspective, with the aortic valve located at the 12 o'clock position so that sites of prolapsed leaflets and flail

chords can be identified. In addition, 3DE multi-plane imaging is used to confirm normal and abnormal leaflet segment findings, as structures visualized in one plane can be examined in real time by checking a second orthogonal plane.

Transesophageal 3D Echocardiography Acquisition

3D TEE images of a myxomatous MV are best obtained from either the 60° mitral bicommissural or the 120° long-axis midesophageal views (**Fig. 5**).[22] When examining the MV chords, the transgastric short-axis view of the MV is best used with the multi-planar mode. As described earlier, the MV should be presented en face visualization from either the left ventricular or the left atrial perspectives to localized regions of prolapse or flail. These views facilitate communication between the imager and the surgeon because the MV can be displayed in a manner similar to the way the surgeon visualizes the valve in the operating room when approaching the valve from the left atrium.

Table 3
Three-dimensional echocardiography acquisition of the myxomatous mitral valve

	Transthoracic Echocardiography	Transesophageal Echocardiography
Acquisition view	Parasternal long axis Apical 4 chamber	Midesophageal 60° (4 chamber) Midesophageal 120° (long axis)
Mode	Zoom ±Color	Narrow-angle or zoom ±Color
Display	Orient the aortic valve at the 12 o'clock position regardless of whether viewed from the left atrium or the left ventricle	Orient the aortic valve at the 12 o'clock position regardless of whether viewed from the left atrium or the left ventricle

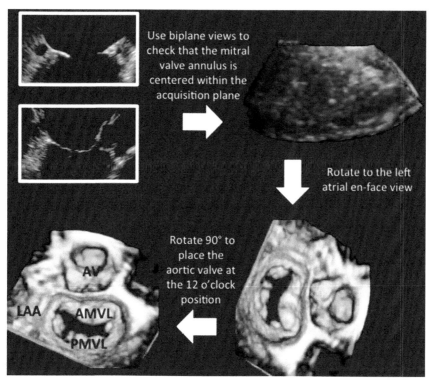

Fig. 5. Acquisition and presentation of the mitral valve. See text for details. AMVL, anterior mitral valve leaflet; AV, aortic valve; LAA, left atrial appendage; PMVL, posterior mitral valve leaflet.

Three-Dimensional Color Doppler Echocardiography

Color Doppler 3D imaging should also be performed to detect the presence and severity of MR in patients with myxomatous MV disease. The uses and limitations of 3D color Doppler assessments are discussed in the following section.

THREE-DIMENSIONAL QUANTIFICATION OF MITRAL REGURGITATION

Determining MR severity by quantitative analysis is an important step in the management of myxomatous MV disease. 3DE is uniquely suited for this purpose as leaflet and chordal changes in myxomatous MV disease culminate in effective regurgitant orifice areas, vena contracta area, proximal isovelocity surface area, and anatomic regurgitant surface areas with a complex 3D geometry (**Table 4**).[23]

3D Vena Contracta Area

Myxomatous MV disease often results in eccentric MR jets with asymmetric vena contracta areas, which are better assessed by 3DE as cross-sectional; this is because single-plane vena

contracta width measurements may miss the true vena contracta width and so underestimate MR severity.[24] Multiple studies have compared vena contracta area measurements by 3DE to various 2D quantitative parameters and have consistently found that the accuracy and reproducibility for MR severity is far superior when 3D vena contracta is used.[25–27] Typically, measurement of the 3DE vena contracta area is performed from an en face cut plane (**Fig. 6**), which is reliable and has been proved to classify MR severity comparable to the American Society of Echocardiography–recommended 2D integrative method.[28]

3D Proximal Isovelocity Surface Area

The asymmetric regurgitant orifice areas present in myxomatous MV patients also result in a nonhemispherical proximal flow convergence region.[29] Thus, studies have demonstrated that hemiellipsoidal models rather than hemispheric models of proximal flow convergence result in a much more accurate estimation of the effective regurgitant orifice area.[30,31] Alternatively, 3DE multiplanar reconstruction techniques can be used to obtain the largest radius for proximal isovelocity surface area measurements for calculation of

Table 4
3DE quantitative assessment of mitral regurgitation

	Problems with 2DE	Strengths	Weaknesses
Vena contracta	Myxomatous leaflets form an asymmetric jet, which violates symmetric vena contracta assumption	True cross-sectional vena contracta measurement Multiplanar, cross-sectional width assessment Direct measure of effective regurgitant orifice area avoiding geometric assumptions More accurate and reproducible	Requires proper selection of the systolic frame Displayed area is affected by user settings Poor correlation with mild regurgitant flows 3DE color Doppler limitations (limited spatial and temporal resolution, risk of stitch artifact)
Proximal isovelocity surface area	Asymmetric orifice formed by the myxomatous leaflets results in nonhemispheric proximal isovelocity surface area	Convergence is nonhemispherical More accurate assessment of radius without geometric assumptions	Greater Doppler angle dependence defines the lateral margins of the isovelocity surface area Not validated for multiple jets Requires significant off-line processing 3DE color Doppler limitations (see earlier)
Regurgitant orifice area	Myxomatous leaflets result in asymmetric, nonplanar anatomic orifice	Direct en face visualization of the mitral valve Can be calculated in real time	Requires proper selection of the systolic frame
Stroke volume		Integration of flow velocities throughout the cardiac cycle More accurate and reproducible	Not valid with concomitant valvular disease or intracardiac shunting

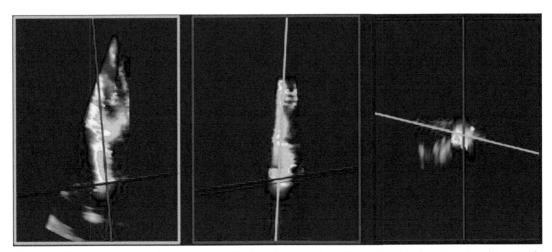

Fig. 6. Multiplanar analysis of mitral regurgitation from a three-dimensional color Doppler dataset. The true cross-sectional vena contracta area can be measured from the en face plane (*blue plane*) identified using orthogonal cut planes (*green, red, and blue planes*).

effective regurgitant orifice area. Although this allows a more accurate assessment of the effective regurgitant orifice area, it still relies on geometric assumptions regarding the proximal flow convergence region. However, currently available software allows the direct tracing of the convergence zone in multiple radial imaging planes with reconstructions of the total surface area, obviating geometric assumptions.[30,32]

3D Anatomic Regurgitant Orifice Area

Because 2D planimetry of the effective regurgitant orifice area in patients with myxomatous MR is inaccurate due to the complex, nonplanar 3D geometry of the orifice, 3D anatomic regurgitant orifice area measurement may provide a reasonable alternative to determine the severity of MR.[33] Although there are several methods for determining the anatomic regurgitant orifice area, one method that manually traces the leaflet edges within a 3D data set to obtain a 3D orifice area (**Fig. 7**) has demonstrated good correlation with 2D proximal isovelocity surface area–derived effective regurgitant orifice area. This method has better reproducibility than the other methods, including the ones in which the planar anatomic regurgitant orifice area is measured from 3D data acquired using real-time zoom mode.[33,34]

3D Mitral Inflow and Left Ventricular Outflow Tract Stroke Volume

A different approach to quantification of myxomatous MR is to directly measure stroke volume. This measurement obviates the assessment of the complex geometry of the myxomatous MV orifice

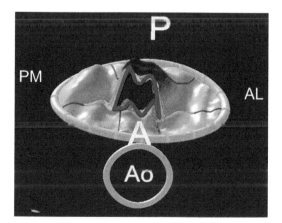

Fig. 7. Three-dimensional parametric map of the mitral valve demonstrating the nonplanar, asymmetric anatomic regurgitant orifice (*red outline*) in a patient with P2 and P3 leaflet prolapse. A, anterior; AL, anterolateral; Ao, aorta; P, posterior; PM, posteromedial.

area and the resultant jet. Compared with 2DE, 3DE allows stroke volume quantification without geometric assumptions, flow profile assumptions, or reliance on single-plane measurements. Stroke volume is calculated by measuring 3D color Doppler data within a region of interest, and studies have demonstrated that 3D-derived left ventricular outflow and mitral inflow stroke volume measurements are accurate.[35,36]

A new method for quantifying MV regurgitant volume was developed using a single 3D TTE volume data set to obtain both 3D-derived left ventricular outflow and MV inflow stroke volumes.[37] This study demonstrated that left ventricular outflow and MV inflow stroke volume measurements, using real-time 3DE, were significantly more accurate and reproducible than those obtained with 2DE. In addition, this technique was highly feasible and rapid.

Limitations of 3D-Derived Quantitative Measurements for MR

Despite the improved accuracy and reproducibility in the assessment of myxomatous MR with 3DE, there are still multiple limitations with each technique. 3D-derived vena contracta area is subject to color Doppler limitations and also depends on the proper selection of the systolic frame as it can significantly affect accurate and reproducible measurements.[38] Proximal isovelocity surface area still requires significant off-line processing and is not practical in a busy clinical setting. Although 3D proximal velocity flow convergence is angle independent, the lower temporal resolution of 3D color Doppler might affect proper selection of the largest flow convergence region. Anatomic regurgitant orifice area requires proper selection of the systolic frame and is limited by the poor temporal resolution of 3DE. 3D mitral inflow and left ventricular outflow tract stroke volume holds great promise, but this method still requires further validation in patients with MR.

MANAGEMENT
Surgical Intervention

Current American College of Cardiology/American Heart Association guidelines recommend performing MV repair over replacement at experienced centers when the likelihood of repair success is greater than or equal to 90%.[39,40] The 2 main surgical techniques performed for MV repair are (1) the Carpentier technique, which involves leaflet resection to restore normal leaflet geometry and implantation of a rigid or semirigid annuloplasty ring, and (2) the American Correction technique where the MV leaflets are never resected, but artificial polytetrafluoroethylene chordae are used instead to correct localized leaflet prolapse and a completely flexible annuloplasty ring implanted. The American Correction technique has been shown to have a freedom from reoperation at 10 years of 90% and freedom from recurrent MR at 10 years of 94%.[41] This result is because the technique is aimed at reducing postoperative leaflet and chordal stress and ultimately restoring dynamic valve function. 3D TEE studies have demonstrated that early postoperatively more dynamic changes in the structure of the mitral annulus are maintained during the cardiac cycle with the American Correction.[42–44] In particular, the use of a flexible annuloplasty ring has been shown to preserve physiologic mitral annular folding dynamics, which may be important in long-term valve function and prevention of left ventricular outflow tract obstruction.[45]

In degenerative MR, mitral annular, leaflet, and subvalvular measurements from 3D TEE may modify the type of operation performed. Choice of technique used ultimately requires great input from 3D TEE, as it has been shown that a near 100% repair rate can be achieved when a single technique is not used to repair all valves and that the surgeon adapts resectional and nonresectional techniques to the lesions seen in each valve.[46]

To improve surgical outcomes, an individualized surgical plan for each patient, directed toward the predominant MR mechanism, should be developed. The 3 fundamental principles guiding MV reconstruction are (1) to preserve or restore normal leaflet motion, (2) to create a large surface of leaflet coaptation, and (3) to remodel and stabilize the annulus.[47] 3D TEE measurements can be used by the surgeon to tailor surgical choices with respect to annuloplasty ring characteristics, ring size, the need for leaflet resection, and papillary neochord or chord-cutting implantation.[48,49] For instance, quantitative 3D TEE measurements obtained before and after surgery of the mitral annular shape, height, and intercommissural diameter helps predict the likelihood of success given how close the postrepair mitral annulus is restored to its natural saddle shape and function. In turn, this knowledge might provide prognostic information on the durability of various approaches to MV repair and may further improve surgical repair techniques. However, there are still immeasurable variables affecting leaflet position postannuloplasty. Some areas of prolapse may be resolved with placement of the annuloplasty ring, but others may appear, which increases the intraoperative complexity and the level of skill needed. Thus, MV repairs require not only accurate intraoperative imaging but also an experienced surgeon.

Mitral Valve Percutaneous Procedures

The past decade has witnessed significant advances in percutaneous MV treatment of patients with MR. Edge-to-edge repair of MR using a "clip" device guided by 3DE is gaining popularity.[50] This intervention results in a double-orifice MV with significant reduction in the total regurgitant orifice and improvement in the patient's symptoms and functional capacity. Before the procedure, 3DE is useful in determining eligibility for this procedure (**Table 5**). During the procedure, 3DE aids in transseptal puncture guidance, optimal clip positioning, and accurate assessment of MR severity before and after clip deployment. Occasionally, based on echocardiographic guidance, placement of a second clip may be required. 3DE is best at visualizing the precise site of the residual lesion for proper clip placement.[51]

Several other percutaneous procedures such as MV annuloplasty and replacement are currently being developed for the treatment of myxomatous MV disease, which clearly benefit from 3D imaging. In addition, transcatheter occlusion of paravalvular leaks is commonly being performed with 3DE guidance (**Fig. 8**).

Table 5 Echocardiographic criteria for mitral valve clip	
Calcification	No significant calcifications on A2 and P2 scallops, especially at grasping sites
Clefts	No significant clefts present at A2 and P2 scallops
Coaptation length	Vertical length >2 mm
Mitral valve orifice area	>4.0 cm^2
Flail segment	Width ≤15 mm Gap ≤10 mm
Regurgitant jet	Primary jet originates from A2 and P2 scallop malcoaptation Any secondary jet should be mild in severity

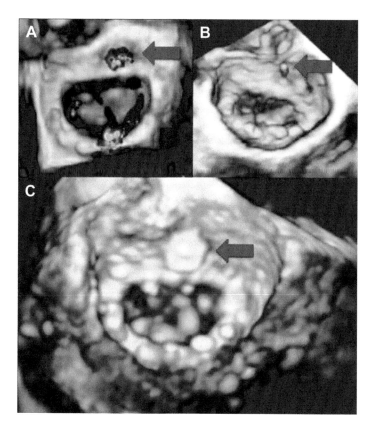

Fig. 8. Three-dimensional transesophageal echocardiographic images of a bioprosthetic mitral valve demonstrating identification of paravalvular regurgitation (*A*), guidance of the catheter wire during percutaneous intervention (*B*), and closure with an Amplatzer device (St. Jude Medical, St. Paul, MN, USA) (*C*).

SUMMARY

In summary, myxomatous MV disease is a spectrum that ranges from fibroelastic deficiency to Barlow's disease. Diagnosis has been greatly aided by the use of 3DE, improving accuracy of not only lesion localization but also quantification of the associated MR. These improvements in turn have altered MV surgical repair techniques and percutaneous interventions.

REFERENCES

1. Salgo IS, Tsang W, Ackerman W, et al. Geometric assessment of regional left ventricular remodeling by three-dimensional echocardiographic shape analysis correlates with left ventricular function. J Am Soc Echocardiogr 2012;25(1):80–8.
2. Anyanwu AC, Adams DH. Etiologic classification of degenerative mitral valve disease: Barlow's disease and fibroelastic deficiency. Semin Thorac Cardiovasc Surg 2007;19(2):90–6.
3. Adams DH, Anyanwu AC, Sugeng L, et al. Degenerative mitral valve regurgitation: surgical echocardiography. Curr Cardiol Rep 2008;10(3):226–32.
4. Gillinov AM, Cosgrove DM, Blackstone EH, et al. Durability of mitral valve repair for degenerative disease. J Thorac Cardiovasc Surg 1998;116(5):734–43.
5. Lee EM, Shapiro LM, Wells FC. Superiority of mitral valve repair in surgery for degenerative mitral regurgitation. Eur Heart J 1997;18(4):655–63.
6. Carpentier A. Pathophysiology, preoperative valve analysis, and surgical indications. Maryland Heights (MO): Saunders-Elsevier; 2012.
7. Carpentier A. Cardiac valve surgery–the "French correction". J Thorac Cardiovasc Surg 1983;86(3):323–37.
8. Shah PM, Raney AA. Echocardiography in mitral regurgitation with relevance to valve surgery. J Am Soc Echocardiogr 2011;24(10):1086–91.
9. Sanfilippo AJ, Harrigan P, Popovic AD, et al. Papillary muscle traction in mitral valve prolapse: quantitation by two-dimensional echocardiography. J Am Coll Cardiol 1992;19(3):564–71.
10. Lee TM, Su SF, Huang TY, et al. Excessive papillary muscle traction and dilated mitral annulus in mitral valve prolapse without mitral regurgitation. Am J Cardiol 1996;78(4):482–5.
11. Sugeng L, Shernan SK, Salgo IS, et al. Live 3-dimensional transesophageal echocardiography initial experience using the fully sampled matrix array probe. J Am Coll Cardiol 2008;52(6):446–9.

12. Chandra S, Salgo IS, Sugeng L, et al. Characterization of degenerative mitral valve disease using morphologic analysis of real-time three-dimensional echocardiographic images: objective insight into complexity and planning of mitral valve repair. Circ Cardiovasc Imaging 2011;4(1):24–32.

13. Tsang W, Weinert L, Sugeng L, et al. The value of three-dimensional echocardiography derived mitral valve parametric maps and the role of experience in the diagnosis of pathology. J Am Soc Echocardiogr 2011;24(8):860–7.

14. La Canna G, Arendar I, Maisano F, et al. Real-time three-dimensional transesophageal echocardiography for assessment of mitral valve functional anatomy in patients with prolapse-related regurgitation. Am J Cardiol 2011;107(9):1365–74.

15. Grewal J, Suri R, Mankad S, et al. Mitral annular dynamics in myxomatous valve disease: new insights with real-time 3-dimensional echocardiography. Circulation 2010;121(12):1423–31.

16. Chikwe J, Adams DH, Su KN, et al. Can three-dimensional echocardiography accurately predict complexity of mitral valve repair? Eur J Cardiothorac Surg 2012;41(3):518–24.

17. Maffessanti F, Marsan NA, Tamborini G, et al. Quantitative analysis of mitral valve apparatus in mitral valve prolapse before and after annuloplasty: a three-dimensional intraoperative transesophageal study. J Am Soc Echocardiogr 2011;24(4):405–13.

18. Lee KS, Stewart WJ, Lever HM, et al. Mechanism of outflow tract obstruction causing failed mitral valve repair. Anterior displacement of leaflet coaptation. Circulation 1993;88(5 Pt 2):II24–9.

19. Carpentier A, Chauvaud S, Fabiani JN, et al. Reconstructive surgery of mitral valve incompetence: ten-year appraisal. J Thorac Cardiovasc Surg 1980;79(3):338–48.

20. Flameng W, Meuris B, Herijgers P, et al. Durability of mitral valve repair in Barlow disease versus fibroelastic deficiency. J Thorac Cardiovasc Surg 2008;135(2):274–82.

21. Jebara VA, Mihaileanu S, Acar C, et al. Left ventricular outflow tract obstruction after mitral valve repair. Results of the sliding leaflet technique. Circulation 1993;88(5 Pt 2):II30–4.

22. Lang RM, Badano LP, Tsang W, et al. EAE/ASE recommendations for image acquisition and display using three-dimensional echocardiography. J Am Soc Echocardiogr 2012;25(1):3–46.

23. Bhave NM, Lang RM. Quantitative echocardiographic assessment of native mitral regurgitation: two- and three-dimensional techniques. J Heart Valve Dis 2011;20(5):483–92.

24. Kahlert P, Plicht B, Schenk IM, et al. Direct assessment of size and shape of noncircular vena contracta area in functional versus organic mitral regurgitation using real-time three-dimensional echocardiography. J Am Soc Echocardiogr 2008; 21(8):912–21.

25. Zeng X, Levine RA, Hua L, et al. Diagnostic value of vena contracta area In the quantification of mitral regurgitation severity by color Doppler 3D echocardiography. Circ Cardiovasc Imaging 2011;4(5): 506–13.

26. Marsan NA, Westenberg JJ, Ypenburg C, et al. Quantification of functional mitral regurgitation by real-time 3D echocardiography: comparison with 3D velocity-encoded cardiac magnetic resonance. JACC Cardiovasc Imaging 2009;2(11):1245–52.

27. Yosefy C, Hung J, Chua S, et al. Direct measurement of vena contracta area by real-time 3-dimensional echocardiography for assessing severity of mitral regurgitation. Am J Cardiol 2009;104(7):978–83.

28. Little SH, Pirat B, Kumar R, et al. Three-dimensional color Doppler echocardiography for direct measurement of vena contracta area in mitral regurgitation: in vitro validation and clinical experience. JACC Cardiovasc Imaging 2008;1(6):695–704.

29. Shiota T, Jones M, Delabays A, et al. Direct measurement of three-dimensionally reconstructed flow convergence surface area and regurgitant flow in aortic regurgitation: in vitro and chronic animal model studies. Circulation 1997;96(10):3687–95.

30. Matsumura Y, Saracino G, Sugioka K, et al. Determination of regurgitant orifice area with the use of a new three-dimensional flow convergence geometric assumption in functional mitral regurgitation. J Am Soc Echocardiogr 2008;21(11):1251–6.

31. Shiota T, Sinclair B, Ishii M, et al. Three-dimensional reconstruction of color Doppler flow convergence regions and regurgitant jets: an in vitro quantitative study. J Am Coll Cardiol 1996;27(6):1511–8.

32. Little SH, Igo SR, Pirat B, et al. In vitro validation of real-time three-dimensional color Doppler echocardiography for direct measurement of proximal isovelocity surface area in mitral regurgitation. Am J Cardiol 2007;99(10):1440–7.

33. Chandra S, Salgo IS, Sugeng L, et al. A three-dimensional insight into the complexity of flow convergence in mitral regurgitation: adjunctive benefit of anatomic regurgitant orifice area. Am J Physiol Heart Circ Physiol 2011;301(3):H1015–24.

34. Altiok E, Hamada S, van Hall S, et al. Comparison of direct planimetry of mitral valve regurgitation orifice area by three-dimensional transesophageal echocardiography to effective regurgitant orifice area obtained by proximal flow convergence method and vena contracta area determined by color Doppler echocardiography. Am J Correct 2011;107(3):452–8.

35. Lodato JA, Weinert L, Baumann R, et al. Use of 3-dimensional color Doppler echocardiography to measure stroke volume in human beings: comparison with thermodilution. J Am Soc Echocardiogr 2007;20(2):103–12.

36. Pemberton J, Jerosch-Herold M, Li X, et al. Accuracy of real-time, three-dimensional Doppler echocardiography for stroke volume estimation compared with phase-encoded MRI: an in vivo study. Heart 2008;94(9):1212–3.

37. Thavendiranathan P, Liu S, Datta S, et al. Automated quantification of mitral inflow and aortic outflow stroke volumes by three-dimensional real-time volume color-flow Doppler transthoracic echocardiography: comparison with pulsed-wave Doppler and cardiac magnetic resonance imaging. J Am Soc Echocardiogr 2012;25(1):56–65.

38. Buck T, Plicht B, Kahlert P, et al. Effect of dynamic flow rate and orifice area on mitral regurgitant stroke volume quantification using the proximal isovelocity surface area method. J Am Coll Cardiol 2008;52(9):767–78.

39. Bonow RO, Carabello BA, Chatterjee K, et al. 2008 focused update incorporated into the ACC/AHA 2006 guidelines for the management of patients with valvular heart disease: a report of the American College of Cardiology/American Heart Association Task Force on Practice Guidelines (Writing Committee to revise the 1998 guidelines for the management of patients with valvular heart disease). Endorsed by the Society of Cardiovascular Anesthesiologists, Society for Cardiovascular Angiography and Interventions, and Society of Thoracic Surgeons. J Am Coll Cardiol 2008;52(13):e1–142.

40. McCarthy PM. When is your surgeon good enough? When do you need a "referent surgeon"? Curr Cardiol Rep 2009;11(2):107–13.

41. Lawrie GM, Earle EA, Earle N. Intermediate-term results of a nonresectional dynamic repair technique in 662 patients with mitral valve prolapse and mitral regurgitation. J Thorac Cardiovasc Surg 2011;141(2):368–76.

42. Ben Zekry S, Nagueh SF, Little SH, et al. Comparative accuracy of two- and three-dimensional transthoracic and transesophageal echocardiography in identifying mitral valve pathology in patients undergoing mitral valve repair: initial observations. J Am Soc Echocardiogr 2011;24(10):1079–85.

43. Ben Zekry S, Lang RM, Sugeng L, et al. Mitral annulus dynamics early after valve repair: preliminary observations of the effect of resectional versus non-resectional approaches. J Am Soc Echocardiogr 2011;24(11):1233–42.

44. Lawrie GM, Earle EA, Earle NR. Nonresectional repair of the Barlow mitral valve: importance of dynamic annular evaluation. Ann Thorac Surg 2009; 88(4):1191–6.

45. Dagum P, Timek T, Green GR, et al. Three-dimensional geometric comparison of partial and complete flexible mitral annuloplasty rings. J Thorac Cardiovasc Surg 2001;122(4):665–73.

46. Castillo JG, Anyanwu AC, Fuster V, et al. A near 100% repair rate for mitral valve prolapse is achievable in a reference center: implications for future guidelines. J Thorac Cardiovasc Surg 2012; 144(2):308–12.

47. Carpentier A. Pathophysiology, preoperative valve analysis, and surgical indications. Maryland, Heights, Missouri: Saunders-Elsevier; 2012.

48. Lang RM, Adams DH. 3D echocardiographic quantification in functional mitral regurgitation. JACC Cardiovasc Imaging 2012;5(4):346–7.

49. Fedak PW, McCarthy PM, Bonow RO. Evolving concepts and technologies in mitral valve repair. Circulation 2008;117(7):963–74.

50. Feldman T, Foster E, Glower DD, et al. Percutaneous repair or surgery for mitral regurgitation. N Engl J Med 2011;364(15):1395–406.

51. Silvestry FE, Rodriguez LL, Herrmann HC, et al. Echocardiographic guidance and assessment of percutaneous repair for mitral regurgitation with the Evalve MitraClip: lessons learned from EVEREST I. J Am Soc Echocardiogr 2007;20(10):1131–40.

The Role of Echocardiography in the Management of Patients with Myxomatous Disease

David Messika-Zeitoun, MD, PhD[a,b], Yan Topilsky, MD[c],
Maurice Enriquez-Sarano, MD[d],*

KEYWORDS

- Mitral regurgitation • Echocardiography • Surgery • Mitral valve repair • Quantification

KEY POINTS

- Severe mitral regurgitation (MR) with left ventricular enlargement/dysfunction or pulmonary hypertension should be promptly referred for surgical management.
- Surgery should also be considered in cases of severe left atrial enlargement as assessed by volume measurement.
- An exercise stress test is strongly recommended in asymptomatic patients in combination with echocardiography (exercise stress echocardiography), as it seems to provide additional prognostic information.
- Anatomy, and more specifically the probability of successful repair, can be assessed by echocardiography, preferably transesophageal echocardiography, as this information can be useful when surgery is being considered, particularly in asymptomatic patients with no left ventricular or atrial consequences of MR.
- Three-dimensional echocardiography with the availability of real-time imaging seems promising not only for the assessment of valve anatomy but also for the quantification of MR severity.

INTRODUCTION

Degenerative mitral regurgitation (MR) is the leading cause of organic MR in western countries. Its mechanism is primarily characterized by mitral valve prolapse due to excessive movement (≥2 mm abnormal systolic movement beyond the saddle-shaped annular level) as classified by Carpentier (type II). The anatomic lesions of the degenerative MR etiology encompass a wide spectrum, including fibroelastic deficiency (localized and isolated prolapsed segment often associated with ruptured chordae with myxomatous degeneration limited to prolapsing segments) to extensive myxomatous disease (often called Barlow disease with

large valves comprising multiple degenerated segments presenting as thick and hooded with excess tissue and elongated chordae mostly). Myxomatous degeneration is defined by the accumulation of mucopolysaccharides responsible of the thickening and "proliferative" aspect of the valve tissue. Even if molecular disorders and pathophysiologic pathways may not be uniform, there is a continuum between the different anatomic aspects. In this article the role of echocardiography in the management of patients with degenerative MR as an entity is presented. Echocardiography is indeed the method of choice to evaluate patients with degenerative MR and plays a crucial role in clinical management.[1,2] It allows accurate assessment of

[a] Department of Cardiology, AP-HP, Bichat Hospital, 46 rue Henri Huchard, Paris 75018, France; [b] University Paris 7, Diderot, Paris, France; [c] Division of Cardiology, Tel-Aviv Medical Center, 6 Weizman Street, Tel-Aviv 64239, Israel; [d] Division of Cardiovascular Diseases and Internal Medicine, Mayo Clinic, 200 First Street Southwest, Rochester, MN 55905, USA
* Corresponding author.
E-mail address: sarano.maurice@mayo.edu

Cardiol Clin 31 (2013) 217–229
http://dx.doi.org/10.1016/j.ccl.2013.03.009
0733-8651/13/$ – see front matter © 2013 Elsevier Inc. All rights reserved

MR severity, left ventricular and atrial consequences, cause, mechanisms, and anatomic lesions and consequently defines the probability of successful for mitral valve repair.

ASSESSMENT OF THE DEGREE OF MR SEVERITY
General Principles

The assessment of MR severity is essential because MR degree is the main determinant of outcome irrespective of the underlying cause and mechanism. This assessment should therefore rely on an integrative approach based on a combination of semi-quantitative and quantitative methods in addition to the underlying mechanism of the regurgitation. There is now a general consensus as reflected in the recent guidelines by both the American Society of Echocardiography and the European Association of Echocardiography, that color flow jet assessment should only be used for diagnosing MR and not for MR quantification.[3,4] Although color Doppler assessment of MR severity can be obvious at both extremes of the spectrum, precise quantification is crucial in most cases for appropriate clinical decision-making. In particular, the recent European Association of Echocardiography guidelines highlight the importance of the quantification of MR severity using the vena contracta width and the flow convergence method.[4]

The Vena Contracta Width

The vena contracta (VC) is the narrowest neck of the regurgitant flow through or immediately below the regurgitant orifice.[5,6] The VC width is thus the diameter of the effective regurgitant orifice (ERO). For the determination of the VC, the ultrasound beam should be positioned perpendicular to the MR flow (usually in parasternal long axis view but in some patients with very eccentric jets in the apical views to benefit from the axial resolution). The 3 components of the regurgitant jet—the proximal flow convergence, the VC, and the downstream extension of the jet—should be clearly visualized within a zoomed image (**Fig. 1**). A VC ≥7 mm is associated with severe MR with high sensitivity and specificity. Less than 3 mm, severe MR can be excluded with high specificity but intermediate VC values—between 3 and 7 mm—fall within a gray zone and may need further confirmation using a quantitative method.

The Proximal Isovelocity Surface Area Method or PISA Method

MR severity can also be quantified using the ERO, a measure of the valve lesion and the regurgitant volume (RVol), a measure of the volume overload. The PISA method is simple, fast, and reproducible and has been proven to be reliable by multiple investigators.[7,8] It is based on the principle of conservation of mass. The principle of PISA has been described elsewhere[7] and is out of the scope of the present review but several technical rules should be emphasized (**Fig. 2**), as follows:

- *Incidence.* The measurement of the radius of the flow convergence along the beam of ultrasound, which should be aligned with the centerline of the regurgitant flow (opposite to VC measurement, perpendicular to regurgitant flow), usually the apical views but occasionally in the parasternal long axis view in case of very eccentric jets.[7]
- *Aliasing velocity.* The aliasing velocity should be shifted down (in the direction of the

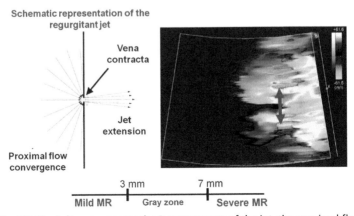

Fig. 1. Principle of the VC. The left part presents the 3 components of the jet, the proximal flow convergence, the VC, and the downstream extension of the jet. Measurement of the VC should be performed perpendicularly to the regurgitant jet. The threshold for mild and severe mitral regurgitation is presented in the bottom part.

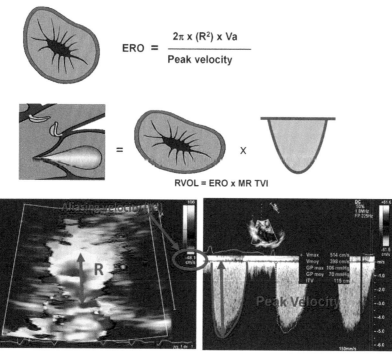

Fig. 2. Calculation of the effective regurgitant orifice (ERO) and regurgitant volume (RVol) using the PISA method. MR, mitral regurgitation; TVI, time-velocity integral.

regurgitant jet) and adjusted to obtain an appropriate hemispheric proximal flow convergence. Higher velocities should be used in severe MR than in mild or moderate MR and aliasing velocities >40 cm/s are commonly used.

- *Zoom*. Measurements of the radius of the flow convergence should be performed using a focused zoomed view to avoid small measurement errors that may translate into large ERO/RVol errors and lead to misclassification of MR severity.
- *Timing*. In patients with mitral valve prolapse, phasic changes of MR are observed and the ERO increases throughout systole. These changes can lead to an underestimation or overestimation of the overall degree of regurgitation. However, properly timed measurements—measurement of the radius of the flow convergence at the level of the T wave and use of the peak velocity of the regurgitant jet—allow accurate estimation of the ERO and of the RVol.[9]

PISA measurements are usually performed using transthoracic echocardiography (TTE) but can also be performed using transesophageal echocardiography (TEE) in patients with poor echocardiographic windows. The same rules apply for TTE

and TEE. A severe MR is defined by a regurgitant volume (RVol) $\geq$60 mL or a regurgitant orifice (ERO) $\geq$0.40 cm^2.[3,4] It is worth noting that the prognostic value of these thresholds have been validated prospectively and that the prognostic value of quantitative measurements supersede those of semi-quantitative measurements.[10]

Specific Situations in Degenerative MR

Mid late systolic MR

In patients with bileaflet prolapse or Barlow disease, MR may occur predominantly or purely in the later phase of systole (mid-late systolic MR as opposed to classical holosystolic MR). Comparison of the clinical characteristics and outcomes for 111 patients with mid-late MR and 90 patients with holosystolic MR matched for age, gender, ejection fraction (EF), rhythm, and ERO (calculated as the RVol using the PISA method) was recently reported.[11] Despite similar effective regurgitant orifice by design (and similar jet area), the regurgitant volume of patients with mid-late systolic MR was smaller as the consequence of shorter regurgitant duration and smaller time-velocity was integral. Mid-late systolic MR was also associated with lower MR sequelae (less left ventricle and left atrial enlargement) and better mid-term outcomes. Interestingly, ERO in contrast to RVol was not linked to outcome. These results clearly demonstrate that in patients with mid-late systolic MR, the ERO calculated using the PISA method may be misleading and that the RVol provides information more reflective of MR severity

Multiple jets

In patients with mitral valve prolapse, especially very redundant valve with diffuse myxomatous changes, multiple jets are common (**Fig. 3**) and assessment of MR severity can be challenging. The PISA method can still be used but the ERO and the RVol should be calculated for each jet and the sum of the effective regurgitant orifices and regurgitant volumes retained. Other quantitative methods such as the quantitative Doppler and the quantitative 2-dimensional echocardiography can also be used in the absence of concomitant aortic regurgitant and very irregular rhythm.[12] The quantitative Doppler method is based on the calculation of the mitral and aortic stroke volumes (**Fig. 4**). This method is accurate and reproducible in experienced hands. The quantitative 2-dimensional echocardiography method is based on the calculation of the end-systolic and end-diastolic left ventricular volumes using the Simpson rules. The volume difference between the 2 phases is equal to the forward stroke volume plus the RVol. Thus the RVol can be obtained by subtracting the aortic stroke volume from this difference. Accuracy and reproducibility of left ventricular volume measurements can be improved by the use of contrast.[13]

Usefulness of 3D Echocardiography

Vena contracta

Three-dimensional echocardiography can provide true otherwise unobtainable cross-sectional views, allowing measuring the vena contracta area (VCA). Two-dimensional images should be first optimized and 3D acquisition performed using live 3D or zoom 3D mode (single beat mode). The VCA is the narrowest cross-sectional area of the color Doppler jet at the valve level or immediately below and thus corresponds to the ERO[14–16] but measurement of the VCA is free of any geometric or flow assumption. In degenerative MR, the regurgitant orifice is roughly circular in contrast to rheumatic or functional MR, where it appears rather elongated along the mitral coaptation line and noncircular.

3D PISA

The ERO and the RVol can also be assessed using the PISA method and 3D echocardiography. Acquisition should be performed in single beat mode with baseline aliasing velocity shifted in the direction of the MR jet. The shape of the proximal flow convergence may be hemi-elliptic rather than hemispheric, which theoretically favors 3D PISA but shape alterations due to angle-dependency of color Doppler represent important limitations. Other limitations are the current poor spatial and temporal resolutions of 3D color Doppler.

Anatomic regurgitant orifice area

The anatomic effective orifice area can also be derived from echocardiography (**Fig. 5**).[17,18] Although current measurement of anatomic regurgitant orifice area relies on manual tracing in multiple planes and is time-consuming, future automation is expected. Such automation may also yield direct anatomic regurgitant area measurements throughout systole.

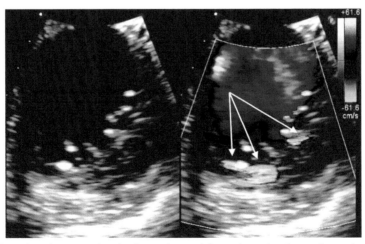

Fig. 3. Patient with Barlow disease and multiple jets (*arrows*) (transthoracic echocardiography, parasternal short-axis view).

Rvol = Mitral stroke volume - Aortic stroke volume

Mitral stroke volume = mitral annulus diameter x mitral TVI
Aortic stroke volume = LVOT diameter x LVOT TVI

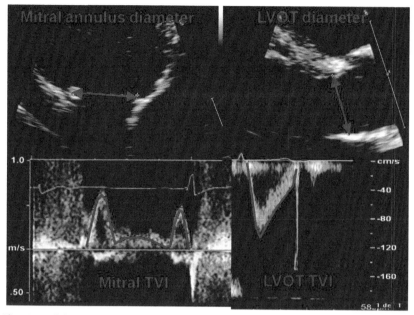

Fig. 4. Quantification of the severity of mitral regurgitation using the uantitative Doppler method. LVOT, left ventricular outflow tract; Rvol, regurgitant volume; TVI, time-velocity integral.

Overall, additional value and clinical implications of 3D assessment of MR degree deserve further validation but with technological improvements, there is little doubt that these promising methodologies will eventually be implemented in routine echocardiographic practice with time.

ECHOCARDIOGRAPHIC ASSESSMENT OF THE CONSEQUENCES OF MR

In addition to symptoms and the presence of atrial fibrillation, the clinical decision-making process in patients with severe degenerative MR relies on the assessment of the consequences of MR on the left ventricular size (LV) and function, left atrial (LA) size, and systolic pulmonary artery pressure (SPAP). Echocardiography can also be coupled to an exercise test to obtain additional and complementary prognostic information.

Left Ventricular Size and Function

Traditional parameters
LV enlargement (eccentric hypertrophy) is the compensatory response to the volume overload

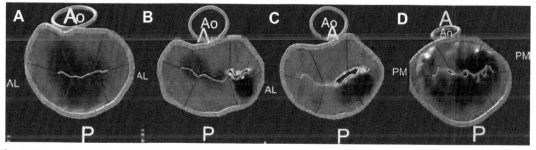

Fig. 5. Examples of anatomic effective orifice derived from 3-dimensional echocardiography. A, anterior; AL, anterolateral; Ao, aortic valve; P, posterior; PM, posteromedial. (*Data from* Tsang W, Weinert L, Sugeng L, et al. The value of three-dimensional echocardiography derived mitral valve parametric maps and the role of experience in the diagnosis of pathology. J Am Soc Echocardiogr 2011;24(8):860–7.)

related to MR. During the chronic and compensated phase, LV ejection remains normal or is increased. In the decompensated phase, LV end-systolic dimensions (diameter or volume) increase and LV EF and forward stroke volume decrease. Based on outcome studies,[19,20] surgery is recommended when LV EF is ≤60%.[1,2] While a LV end-systolic diameter threshold of 45 mm was the common threshold in past guidelines iterations, LV end-systolic diameter ≥40 mm is the new standard for surgery in US guidelines and may be considered in patients with flail leaflet, high likelihood of repair, low surgical risk (class IIa recommendation for European guidelines).[1] Indeed recent data from the Mitral Regurgitation International DAtabase (MIDA) registry (large multicenter registry of patients with organic MR due to flail leaflets, diagnosed in routine clinical practice in 5 US and European centers) have shown that an LV end-systolic diameter ≥40 mm was independently associated with increased mortality under medical management.[21] Postoperatively, patients with LV end-systolic diameter ≥40 mm continue to incur excess (albeit reduced) risk; hence, LV end-systolic diameter 36 to 39 mm may be a safer threshold for surgery. It is worth noting that women often present with smaller LV size despite similar MR degree[22] but no specific size-adjusted thresholds have been validated in MR.

Role of new echocardiographic methods— speckle tracking

LV EF is generally considered a crude estimate of myocardial contractility. Recently, 2-dimensional speckle tracking strain imaging was developed with the aim of providing a more sensitive method to evaluate LV myocardial contractility.[23] Results from several studies suggest that low global longitudinal strain is associated with postoperative LV dysfunction[24] and event-free survival in addition to LA size and brain natriuretic peptide level.[26] More data are clearly needed to confirm the potential clinical usefulness of longitudinal strain in the clinical decision-making process in asymptomatic patients with severe MR and preserved LVEF.

Left Atrial Size

LA enlargement is also a pathophysiologic response to volume overload in organic MR, which allows LA pressure homeostasis. Several studies have shown that LA diameter is a marker for developing future heart failure[26] or atrial fibrillation[27] with or without mitral valve surgery.[28] Recently, in the MIDA registry, patients in sinus rhythm with LA diameter ≥55 mm and MR caused by flails leaflets incurred increased mortality under medical treatment, independently of symptoms or ventricular dysfunction.[29]

LA enlargement in patients with MR is frequently asymmetric. LA size assessed by M-mode echocardiography using a single-diameter measurement has limited accuracy with frequent underestimation of LA volume and wide range of error.[30] In contrast, accurate echocardiographic LA volume measurements can be obtained using 2D echocardiography. In a previous study the authors validated echocardiographic LA volume measurements using computed tomography as the reference method.

Biplane area–length method and a vertical longitudinal-length

$$\text{LA volume} = 0.85 \times A1 \times A2 / (L1 + L2) / 2$$

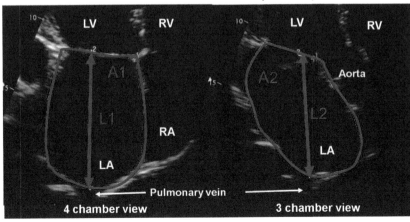

Fig. 6. Measurement of the left atrial volume using the biplane area–length method (4-chamber and 3-chamber views) and a vertical longitudinal-length, which provided the highest accuracy compared with computed tomography. RV, right ventricle.

Biplane area–length method and a vertical longitudinal length provided the highest correlation and accuracy (**Fig. 6**). LA index ≥ 40 mL/m^2 was beyond the normal range and more importantly predicted superiorly and independently to LA diameter the occurrence of atrial fibrillation and of the combined endpoint of death or need for mitral surgery. More recently, it has been shown that LA index at diagnosis predicted long-term outcome, incrementally to known predictors of outcome. This marker of risk was particularly important because mitral surgery performed in patients with severely enlarged LA (LA index ≥ 60 mL/m^2) markedly improved outcome and restored life expectancy.[31] In the recently updated European Society of Cardiology Guidelines, a severely enlarged LA (LA index ≥ 60 mL/m^2) is now considered a criterion to consider surgery in asymptomatic patients with severe MR, preserved LV function, low surgical risk, and high likelihood of durable repair (class IIb recommendation).

Systolic Pulmonary Artery Pressure

The presence of tricuspid regurgitation even of a mild degree allows the estimation of SPAP. Elevated SPAP (≥ 50 mm Hg) is a marker of poor prognosis and should lead to consideration for surgery. Even after mitral valve surgery, an increased risks persist (albeit reduced); therefore, those with borderline pulmonary hypertension (45–49 mm Hg) should be monitored closely.

Role of Exercise Echocardiography

Reduced functional capacity is an independent predictor of subsequent high risk of clinical events and an important indicator of the need for surgical intervention.[32] A functional assessment obtained from a patient is usually subjective and may not accurately reflect the true exercise tolerance particularly in patients who are often sedentary. In particular, exercise stress testing is highly recommended in asymptomatic patients with severe MR, to unmask symptomatic impairment and functional limitation unrecognized from the physical examination.

Exercise echocardiography may also provide prognostic information. In addition to resting SPAP, exercise-induced pulmonary hypertension seems associated with a markedly reduced 2-year symptom-free survival,[33] with an SPAP >60 mm Hg during exercise suggested as a threshold value above which asymptomatic patients with severe asymptomatic MR might be referred for surgery (class IIb recommendation). Moreover, in patients with unclear symptoms and disproportionate MR severity, exercise MR has been suggested to be a valuable test. Indeed, not only functional regurgitation but also degenerative MR are dynamic and increase in a substantial proportion of patients. Marked changes in MR severity have also been linked with exercise-induced changes in systolic PAP and reduced symptom-free survival.[34] Generally, pilot studies have been of limited size and quality control remains challenging, so that hemodynamic exercise echocardiography has gained limited clinical use.

MITRAL VALVE LESIONS AND ANATOMY

Mitral valve repair is the procedure of choice for patients with degenerative MR who undergo mitral valve surgery. Mitral valve repair as opposed to mitral valve replacement is associated with better quality of life, lower morbidity (at least partially due to preservation of LV function and the freedom from anticoagulation therapy), and better long-term survival. It may restore a normal life-expectancy when timely performed.[10,35–38] In asymptomatic patients with severe MR, but no LV and LA enlargement and normal SPAP and therefore at a low surgical risk, indication for mitral valve surgery is still debated with different levels of recommendations proposed by the European (IIb) and North American Cardiology Societies (IIa).[1,2] The crux of the controversy regarding the timing of surgery centers around the balance between the inherent risks of major surgery, especially in the case of valve replacement versus the risks of irreversible myocardial remodeling due to MR, such as sudden death and heart failure. Thus, assessment of the likelihood of successful durable repair plays an important role in the clinical decision-making process, especially in asymptomatic patients with severe degenerative MR. However, it is also worth noting that the probability of successful repair depends not only on the anatomic lesion but also on surgical expertise.[39–41]

Morphologic Assessment

The success of mitral valve repair rests on accurate mitral valve anatomic assessment and characterization of the leaflets' lesions. Thus, a precise morphologic assessment is mandatory if one wants to predict the probability of successful mitral valve repair accurately. This evaluation relies on the assessment of the cause and disease localization and identification of the diseased segment(s) or scallops of the leaflets involved. A systematic approach is recommended because a combination of lesions may coexist and only the correction of all valve dysfunction will allow for a successful repair.

The anterior leaflet is attached to one-third of the annulus circumference and the posterior leaflet is attached to the remaining two-thirds of the annulus circumference. Each mitral leaflet is usually divided into 3 segments (1 = lateral, 2 = middle, and 3 = medial). The posterior leaflet is divided into 3 scallops (P1, P2, and P3 from the lateral to the medial aspect) separated by incisures of widely variable depth between the individual scallops, so that this segmentation is based on anatomic features. In contrast, the anterior leaflet is usually a single structure and the corresponding parts facing P1, P2, and P3 are labeled A1, A2, and A3, respectively (**Fig. 7**). This anterior segmentation also correlates to the insertions of major secondary chords on the ventricular side of the leaflet. The region between the anterior and posterior valve is referred to as anterolateral and posteromedial commissures. Thus according to the modified Carpentier classification, 8 segments can be individualized. However, size and number of scallops may vary, especially in Barlow disease with additional scallops exceeding the conventional nomenclature, and it is not always possible using echocardiography to visualize a clear separation between scallops.

Transthoracic Echocardiography

The localization of diseased segments can be achieved using TTE. In parasternal long axis, A2 and P2 are visualized but A1P1 can also be visualized by inclining the probe laterally and A3P3 medially in this view. The parasternal short axis is particularly helpful to identify the segments that are prolapsing. Use of color Doppler also helps to identify the diseased segments. In the apical 4-chamber view, A2 and P2 are usually seen, whereas the 2-chamber view reproduces the intercommissural TEE view.

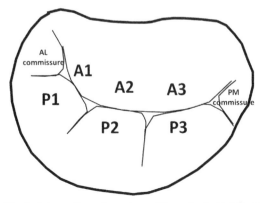

Fig. 7. Schematic en face view of the mitral valve from the left atrium as the surgical view after atriotomy. A, anterior valve; AL, anterolateral; P, posterior valve; PM, posteromedial.

Is Transesophageal Echocardiography Mandatory?

Transesophageal echocardiography provides a more precise anatomic assessment and detection of finer details. Several studies have shown that in patients with satisfactory images, TTE could correctly identify most of the leaflets lesions,[42] avoiding the need for preoperative TEE. Nevertheless, TEE is useful intra-operatively to provide the surgeon with a view of the anatomic lesions and to monitor the surgical results. Segments visualized in the different incidences (transesophageal or transgastric) and angles using TEE are presented in **Fig. 8**.

Role of Three-dimensional Echocardiography

Despite its excellent accuracy compared with surgery as the gold standard, 2D-TEE requires manually manipulation of the transducer to examine all leaflets and segments and to reconstruct the mitral valve mentally from multiple 2D views. Real-time 3-dimensional transesophageal echocardiography (RT-3DTEE) is a relatively new echocardiographic modality providing an immediate and intuitive assessment of the anatomy of the mitral valve. En face views of the mitral valve can be viewed from the position of the left ventricular surface or left atrial surface (as seen by the surgeon after left atriotomy) and may provide useful information to the surgeon preoperatively. Several studies have compared the agreement between 2-dimensional and 3-dimensional echocardiography to actual surgical findings.[43,44] RT-3DTEE provided a better prolapse localization than other imaging modalities (2DTEE, 2DTTE, and 3DTTE) even in patients with complex lesions and multiple prolapse segments. The incremental value of RT-3DTEE seems especially important in the subset of patients with complex multisegment mitral valve disease. Whether RT-3DTEE improves the actual repair rate has yet to be demonstrated. In the authors' opinion, RT-3DTEE should be considered an adjunct to 2D-TEE in providing a precise description of anatomic lesions and regarded as complementary. Similar to the case of 2DTEE, RT-3DTEE is also operator-dependent and requires specific training, but in experienced hands, excellent intra-observer and interobserver agreement can be achieved. Different examples of disease segments are presented in **Fig. 9**.

Predictors of Successful Repair

In expert centers, a mitral valve repair success rate of more than 95% can be achieved in patients undergoing the procedure with rates of mortality as

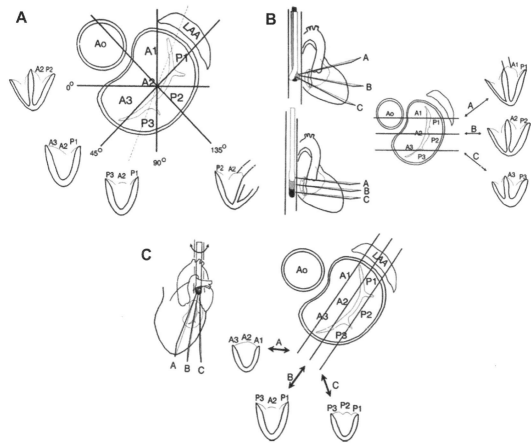

Fig. 8. Examination of the mitral valve using transesophageal echocardiography. Probe in the mid esophageal position, segments visualized in the different angles' planes. (*B*) Segments visualized moving the probe (*A–C*) from a high-esophageal to a low-esophageal position (*C*) intercommissural view. LAA, Left atrial appendage; (*From* Foster GP, Isselbacher EM, Rose GA, et al. Accurate localization of mitral regurgitant defects using multiplane transesophageal echocardiography. Ann Thorac Surg 1998;65:1025–31; with permission.)

low as 1% in asymptomatic patients younger than 75 years with normal EF. Although the rate of adverse events are higher in elderly patients (≥75 years), the operative rate of mortality has significantly declined over time from 25% to 30% in the 1980s to less than 5% nowadays. Furthermore, the feasibility of valve repair has also increased across all age groups, with successful outcomes reaching >90% regardless of age.[45] Such low operative rates of mortality have also been reported by several groups with the survival benefit of valve repair significantly improved over valve replacement in this subset of elderly patients.[46] However this low operative rate of mortality may be biased due to the low surgical referral rate of elderly patients in community practices. Such patients are often denied a curative treatment despite having a very acceptable rate of mortality, not because of severe comorbidities but often only because of age.[47] Thus, early surgery

should be carefully considered in elderly patients with severe MR before the onset of severe symptoms.

Anterior or bileaflet prolapse is significantly more difficult to repair than isolated posterior leaflet prolapse. Severe annular dilatation (≥50 mm) and involvement of multiple scallops, especially if the anterior leaflet is involved, are also predictors of unsuccessful repair. Calcifications of the leaflets or annulus and restrictive leaflet motion may also pose as a significant challenge to mitral valve repair. However, in centers that have refined mitral repair strategies, very high repair rates have been reported even with these difficult cases. Recent studies have reported high repair rates and durable results in patients with bileaflet prolapse.[48,49] Even in patients with Barlow disease (**Fig. 10**) characterized by severe annular dilatation, excess of leaflet tissue, and multiple sites of leaflet prolapse, mitral valve reconstruction is often possible with

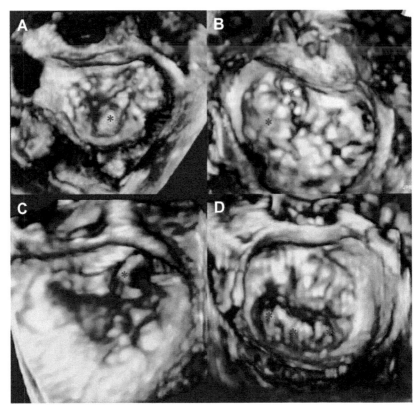

Fig. 9. Examples of prolapsed segments visualized using three-dimensional transesophageal echocardiography. (*A*) P2 prolapse. Note the rupture of chordar. (*B*) P1/A1 flail (*right*), (*C*) A3 prolapse, and (*D*) large complete (P1P2P3) prolapse. The *asterisk* show the prolapsing segment (s).

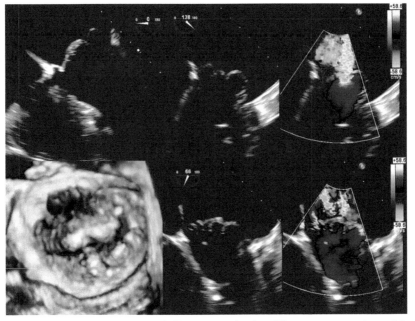

Fig. 10. Barlow disease. Note the billowing of all segments in the different transesophageal incidences with multiple jets. The diffuse disease is well appreciated using 3-dimensional echocardiography.

excellent long-term results.[50] However, these results cannot be extrapolated to many cardiac surgery departments. It is sobering to note that if overall the rate of mitral valve replacement tends to decrease it remains too frequently performed even in developed countries.[51]

In degenerative MR, lack of valve tissue is usually not an issue but very redundant leaflets with excessive anterior leaflet tissue can lead to the occurrence of systolic anterior motion after mitral valve surgery, especially if the left ventricle is not dilated and the left ventricle is hyperdynamic, or if there is a short distance between the mitral valve coaptation point and the ventricular septum. Careful measurement of the height of the anterior leaflet and subsequent appropriate ring selection helps reduce the risk of systolic anterior motion.[52]

SUMMARY

Echocardiography allows an accurate and quantitative assessment of MR severity and of MR consequences. Severe MR with left ventricular enlargement/dysfunction or pulmonary hypertension should be promptly referred for surgical management. Surgery should also be considered in cases of severe LA enlargement as assessed by volume measurement. An exercise stress test is strongly recommended in asymptomatic patients in combination with echocardiography (exercise stress echocardiography) as it seems to provide additional prognostic information. The anatomy, and more specifically, the probability of successful repair can also be assessed by echocardiography, preferably TEE, as this information can be useful when surgery is being considered, particularly in asymptomatic patients with no left ventricular or atrial consequences of MR. Three-dimensional echocardiography with the availability of real-time imaging seems very promising not only for the assessment of valve anatomy but also for the quantification of MR severity. In the near future, with technological improvements, there is little doubt that 3-dimensional echocardiography will become part of routine clinical practice for the evaluation of patients with degenerative MR. In conclusion, echocardiography plays a crucial role in the assessment and management of patients with degenerative MR as information that can be obtained using echocardiography is unique and unparalleled when considered alongside other imaging modalities.

REFERENCES

1. Vahanian A, Alfieri O, Andreotti F, et al. Guidelines on the management of valvular heart disease (version 2012): the Joint Task Force on the Management of Valvular Heart Disease of the European Society of Cardiology (ESC) and the European Association for Cardio-Thoracic Surgery (EACTS). Eur Heart J 2012;33(19):2451–96.

2. Nishimura RA, Carabello BA, Faxon DP, et al. ACC/AHA 2008 guideline update on valvular heart disease: focused update on infective endocarditis: a report of the American College of Cardiology/American Heart Association Task Force on Practice Guidelines: endorsed by the Society of Cardiovascular Anesthesiologists, Society for Cardiovascular Angiography and Interventions, and Society of Thoracic Surgeons. Circulation 2008; 118(8):887–96.

3. Zoghbi WA, Enriquez-Sarano M, Foster E, et al. Recommendations for evaluation of the severity of native valvular regurgitation with two-dimensional and Doppler echocardiography. J Am Soc Echocardiogr 2003;16(7):777–802.

4. Lancellotti P, Moura L, Pierard LA, et al. European Association of Echocardiography recommendations for the assessment of valvular regurgitation. Part 2: mitral and tricuspid regurgitation (native valve disease). Eur J Echocardiogr 2010;11(4): 307–32.

5. Tribouilloy C, Shen WF, Quere JP, et al. Assessment of severity of mitral regurgitation by measuring regurgitant jet width at its origin with transesophageal Doppler color flow imaging. Circulation 1992;85(4):1248–53.

6. Hall SA, Brickner ME, Willett DL, et al. Assessment of mitral regurgitation severity by Doppler color flow mapping of the vena contracta. Circulation 1997;95(3):636–42.

7. Enriquez-Sarano M, Miller FJ, Hayes S, et al. Effective mitral regurgitant orifice area: clinical use and pitfalls of the proximal isovelocity surface area method. J Am Coll Cardiol 1995;25:703–9.

8. Vandervoort P, Rivera J, Mele D, et al. Application of color Doppler flow mapping to calculate effective regurgitant orifice area. An in vitro study and initial clinical observations. Circulation 1993;88:1150–6.

9. Enriquez-Sarano M, Sinak L, Tajik A, et al. Changes in effective regurgitant orifice throughout systole in patients with mitral valve prolapse. A clinical study using the proximal isovelocity surface area method. Circulation 1995;92:2951–8.

10. Enriquez-Sarano M, Avierinos JF, Messika-Zeitoun D, et al. Quantitative determinants of the outcome of asymptomatic mitral regurgitation. N Engl J Med 2005;352(9):875–83.

11. Topilsky Y, Michelena H, Bichara V, et al. Mitral valve prolapse with mid-late systolic mitral regurgitation: pitfalls of evaluation and clinical outcome compared with holosystolic regurgitation. Circulation 2012;125(13):1643–51.

12. Enriquez-Sarano M, Bailey K, Seward J, et al. Quantitative Doppler assessment of valvular regurgitation. Circulation 1993;87:841–8.

13. Thomson HL, Basmadjian AJ, Rainbird AJ, et al. Contrast echocardiography improves the accuracy and reproducibility of left ventricular remodeling measurements: a prospective, randomly assigned, blinded study. J Am Coll Cardiol 2001; 38(3):867–75.

14. Yosefy C, Hung J, Chua S, et al. Direct measurement of vena contracta area by real-time 3-dimensional echocardiography for assessing severity of mitral regurgitation. Am J Cardiol 2009;104(7): 978–83.

15. Zeng X, Levine RA, Hua L, et al. Diagnostic value of vena contracta area in the quantification of mitral regurgitation severity by color Doppler 3D echocardiography. Circ Cardiovasc Imaging 2011;4(5): 506–13.

16. Little SH, Pirat B, Kumar R, et al. Three-dimensional color Doppler echocardiography for direct measurement of vena contracta area in mitral regurgitation: in vitro validation and clinical experience. JACC Cardiovasc Imaging 2008;1(6):695–704.

17. Chandra S, Salgo IS, Sugeng L, et al. A three-dimensional insight into the complexity of flow convergence in mitral regurgitation: adjunctive benefit of anatomic regurgitant orifice area. Am J Physiol Heart Circ Physiol 2011;301(3):H1015–24.

18. Tsang W, Weinert L, Sugeng L, et al. The value of three-dimensional echocardiography derived mitral valve parametric maps and the role of experience in the diagnosis of pathology. J Am Soc Echocardiogr 2011;24(8):860–7.

19. Enriquez-Sarano M, Tajik A, Schaff H, et al. Echocardiographic prediction of survival after surgical correction of organic mitral regurgitation. Circulation 1994;90:830–7.

20. Enriquez-Sarano M, Tajik A, Schaff H, et al. Echocardiographic prediction of left ventricular function after correction of mitral regurgitation: results and clinical implications. J Am Coll Cardiol 1994;24: 1536–43.

21. Tribouilloy C, Grigioni F, Avierinos JF, et al. Survival implication of left ventricular end-systolic diameter in mitral regurgitation due to flail leaflets a long-term follow-up multicenter study. J Am Coll Cardiol 2009;54(21):1961–8.

22. Avierinos JF, Inamo J, Grigioni F, et al. Sex differences in morphology and outcomes of mitral valve prolapse. Ann Intern Med 2008;149(11):787–95.

23. Mor-Avi V, Lang RM, Badano LP, et al. Current and evolving echocardiographic techniques for the quantitative evaluation of cardiac mechanics: ASE/EAE consensus statement on methodology and indications endorsed by the Japanese Society of Echocardiography. J Am Soc Echocardiogr 2011;24(3):277–313.

24. Lancellotti P, Cosyns B, Zacharakis D, et al. Importance of left ventricular longitudinal function and functional reserve in patients with degenerative mitral regurgitation: assessment by two-dimensional speckle tracking. J Am Soc Echocardiogr 2008;21(12):1331–6.

25. Magne J, Mahjoub H, Pierard LA, et al. Prognostic importance of brain natriuretic peptide and left ventricular longitudinal function in asymptomatic degenerative mitral regurgitation. Heart 2012; 98(7):584–91.

26. Ling H, Enriquez-Sarano M, Seward J, et al. Clinical outcome of mitral regurgitation due to flail leaflets. N Engl J Med 1996;335:1417–23.

27. Grigioni F, Avierinos JF, Ling LH, et al. Atrial fibrillation complicating the course of degenerative mitral regurgitation: determinants and long-term outcome. J Am Coll Cardiol 2002;40(1):84–92.

28. Kernis SJ, Nkomo VT, Messika-Zeitoun D, et al. Atrial fibrillation after surgical correction of mitral regurgitation in sinus rhythm: incidence, outcome, and determinants. Circulation 2004;110(16):2320–5.

29. Rusinaru D, Tribouilloy C, Grigioni F, et al. Left atrial size is a potent predictor of mortality in mitral regurgitation due to flail leaflets: results from a large international multicenter study. Circ Cardiovasc Imaging 2011;4(5):473–81.

30. Messika-Zeitoun D, Bellamy M, Avierinos JF, et al. Left atrial remodelling in mitral regurgitation–methodologic approach, physiological determinants, and outcome implications: a prospective quantitative Doppler-echocardiographic and electron beam-computed tomographic study. Eur Heart J 2007;28(14):1773–81.

31. Le Tourneau T, Messika-Zeitoun D, Russo A, et al. Impact of left atrial volume on clinical outcome in organic mitral regurgitation. J Am Coll Cardiol 2010;56(7):570–8.

32. Messika-Zeitoun D, Johnson BD, Nkomo V, et al. Cardiopulmonary exercise testing determination of functional capacity in mitral regurgitation: physiologic and outcome implications. J Am Coll Cardiol 2006;47(12):2521–7.

33. Magne J, Lancellotti P, Pierard LA. Exercise pulmonary hypertension in asymptomatic degenerative mitral regurgitation. Circulation 2010;122(1): 33–41.

34. Magne J, Lancellotti P, Pierard LA. Exercise-induced changes in degenerative mitral regurgitation. J Am Coll Cardiol 2010;56(4):300–9.

35. Mohty D, Orszulak TA, Schaff HV, et al. Very long-term survival and durability of mitral valve repair for mitral valve prolapse. Circulation 2001; 104(12 Suppl 1):I1–7.

36. Braunberger E, Deloche A, Berrebi A, et al. Very long-term results (more than 20 years) of valve repair with carpentier's techniques in non-rheumatic mitral valve insufficiency. Circulation 2001;104(12 Suppl 1):I8–11.

37. Kang DH, Kim JH, Rim JH, et al. Comparison of early surgery versus conventional treatment in asymptomatic severe mitral regurgitation. Circulation 2009;119(6):797–804.

38. Enriquez-Sarano M, Schaff H, Orszulak T, et al. Valve repair improves the outcome of surgery for mitral regurgitation. Circulation 1995,91.1264–5.

39. Gillinov AM, Blackstone EH, Nowicki ER, et al. Valve repair versus valve replacement for degenerative mitral valve disease. J Thorac Cardiovasc Surg 2008;135(4):885–93, 893.e1–2.

40. Gammie JS, O'Brien SM, Griffith BP, et al. Influence of hospital procedural volume on care process and mortality for patients undergoing elective surgery for mitral regurgitation. Circulation 2007;115(7):881–7.

41. Bolling SF, Li S, O'Brien SM, et al. Predictors of mitral valve repair: clinical and surgeon factors. Ann Thorac Surg 2010;90(6):1904–11 [discussion: 1912].

42. Monin JL, Dehant P, Roiron C, et al. Functional assessment of mitral regurgitation by transthoracic echocardiography using standardized imaging planes diagnostic accuracy and outcome implications. J Am Coll Cardiol 2005;46(2):302–9.

43. Grewal J, Mankad S, Freeman WK, et al. Real-time three-dimensional transesophageal echocardiography in the intraoperative assessment of mitral valve disease. J Am Soc Echocardiogr 2009; 22(1):34–41.

44. La Canna G, Arendar I, Maisano F, et al. Real-time three-dimensional transesophageal echocardiography for assessment of mitral valve functional anatomy in patients with prolapse-related regurgitation. Am J Cardiol 2011;107(9):1365–74.

45. Detaint D, Sundt TM, Nkomo VT, et al. Surgical correction of mitral regurgitation in the elderly: outcomes and recent improvements. Circulation 2006; 114(4):265–72.

46. Chikwe J, Goldstone AB, Passage J, et al. A propensity score-adjusted retrospective comparison of early and mid-term results of mitral valve repair versus replacement in octogenarians. Eur Heart J 2011;32(5):618–26.

47. Mirabel M, Iung B, Baron G, et al. What are the characteristics of patients with severe, symptomatic, mitral regurgitation who are denied surgery? Eur Heart J 2007;28(11):1358–65.

48. Chan V, Ruel M, Chaudry S, et al. Clinical and echocardiographic outcomes after repair of mitral valve bileaflet prolapse due to myxomatous disease. J Thorac Cardiovasc Surg 2012;143(Suppl 4):S8–11.

49. Okada Y, Nasu M, Koyama T, et al. Outcomes of mitral valve repair for bileaflet prolapse. J Thorac Cardiovasc Surg 2012;143(Suppl 4):S21–3.

50. Jouan J, Berrebi A, Chauvaud S, et al. Mitral valve reconstruction in Barlow disease: long-term echographic results and implications for surgical management. J Thorac Cardiovasc Surg 2012; 143(Suppl 4):S17–20.

51. Gammie JS, Sheng S, Griffith BP, et al. Trends in mitral valve surgery in the United States: results from the Society of Thoracic Surgeons Adult Cardiac Surgery Database. Ann Thorac Surg 2009; 87(5):1431–7 [discussion: 1437–9].

52. Adams DH, Anyanwu AC, Rahmanian PB, et al. Large annuloplasty rings facilitate mitral valve repair in Barlow's disease. Ann Thorac Surg 2006; 82(6):2096–100 [discussion: 2101].

Ischemic (Functional) Mitral Regurgitation

Judy W. Hung, MD

KEYWORDS

- Mitral regurgitation • Myocardial infarction • Papillary muscle • Echocardiography

KEY POINTS

- The main mechanism of ischemic mitral regurgitation (MR) relates to distortion of the spatial relationships between the mitral valve and papillary muscles secondary to ventricular remodeling, frequently as a result of myocardial infarction of the segments underlying the papillary muscles. Annulus dilatation is also usually present.
- This process can then become self-perpetuating as MR leads to ventricular dilatation, which in turn leads to further papillary muscle displacement, annular dilatation, and then more MR.
- Echocardiography provides mechanistic insights into the complex pathophysiology that involves the myocardium, the mitral subvalvular apparatus, and mitral annulus.
- Echocardiography may provide a more directed approach where the surgeon and cardiologist can tailor the operative strategy in individual patients.
- The evidence that treatment of ischemic MR improves long-term survival remains unclear, and further studies are needed to determine whether correcting ischemic MR will improve survival and/or symptoms.

INTRODUCTION AND DEFINITION

Mitral regurgitation (MR) is a frequent complication of myocardial infarction and coronary artery disease that is associated with adverse prognosis.[1–3] "Ischemic mitral regurgitation" (IMR) is a commonly used but poorly defined term in the medical literature and refers to MR that has developed in setting of coronary disease. The mitral valve leaflets in IMR are intrinsically normal, and concomitant valvular pathology such as flail leaflet, endocarditis, and/or severe calcific mitral valve disease should be distinguished.

In most patients, the initiating insult in IMR relates to ventricular remodeling following myocardial infarction or ischemia, rather than being due to active or reversible acute ischemia. In addition, there is considerable clinical heterogeneity of IMR. IMR is associated with several clinical situations. The most dramatic presentation is that of new, acute MR secondary to a ruptured papillary muscle following myocardial infarction. Associated with high mortality, it is fortunately a rare presentation of ischemic MR with an incidence of less than 1% of acute myocardial infarctions. Another uncommon clinical presentation of IMR is secondary to transient acute myocardial and/or papillary muscle ischemia. This situation relates temporarily due to acute ischemia, and the MR resolves once the acute ischemia improves. By far, the most common clinical situation encountered for IMR is chronic MR due to geometric changes of the left ventricle (LV) secondary to remodeling from ischemic heart disease.

Chronic IMR is characterized mechanistically by valve leaflets that coapt apically within the LV, restricting leaflet closure In a pattern known as incomplete mitral leaflet closure.[4,5] It is important to emphasize that mitral valve function should be understood in terms of its relationship to its ventricular support structures and not as freestanding

Echocardiography, Blake 256, Division of Cardiology, Massachusetts General Hospital, Harvard Medical School, 55 Fruit Street, Boston, MA 02114-2696, USA
E-mail address: jhung@partners.org

Cardiol Clin 31 (2013) 231–236
http://dx.doi.org/10.1016/j.ccl.2013.04.003
0733-8651/13/$ – see front matter © 2013 Published by Elsevier Inc.

leaflets attached at the annulus. The mitral valve apparatus includes anterior and posterior mitral leaflets, the mitral annulus, papillary muscles, and associated chordae tendineae. The mitral leaflets are attached to the mitral annulus and tethered to the ventricle by the papillary muscles via the chordae tendineae. The posteromedial and anterolateral papillary muscles, located along the inferior and posterolateral surfaces of the LV, respectively, give off chordae to each mitral leaflet. The papillary muscles and chordae tendineae serve to anchor the leaflets at the annular level during coaptation. The mechanism underlying functional MR relates to an altered mitral valve geometry resulting from the underlying left ventricular (LV) remodeling process. Although a spectrum of morphologic abnormalities of the LV and papillary muscles exists, considerable evidence points to the central and predominant role of tethering as the final common pathway in inducing functional MR.[4,6,7]

With infarction, the papillary muscles and surrounding LV remodel, becoming thinned and dilated, and resulting in posterolateral displacement of the papillary muscles. Posterolateral displacement of the papillary muscles leads to stretching of the chordae tendineae and increased tethering forces on the mitral valve leaflets. In turn, an increase in mitral leaflet tethering leads to more apical leaflet coaptation and restricted leaflet closure, with resultant regurgitation (**Fig. 1**). Because of the posterolateral location of the papillary muscles, infarctions in this coronary territory have a greater incidence of associated MR compared with anterior infarctions.[5] In patients who develop diffuse LV dysfunction, and global LV dilation,

either from a nonischemic myopathic process or from multiple infarctions, similar papillary muscle displacement occurs. Dilation of the mitral annulus also plays a role in the development of functional MR.[8,9] Annular dilation results in stretching of the mitral leaflets causing incomplete closure of the mitral leaflets.

The term "functional" MR is often used interchangeably with ischemic MR, and broadly defined it as MR without any abnormality of the mitral valve leaflets. Functional MR generally includes patients with both idiopathic nonischemic cardiomyopathy and ischemic cardiomyopathy and is therefore a broader and less-specific term than IMR. Mechanistically, however, both functional and chronic ischemic MR mentioned earlier are similar.

As previously mentioned, mitral leaflet morphology is essentially normal in IMR. During the past decade, experimental investigations have contributed to a better understanding of the pathophysiology of IMR. Recent studies suggest that the primary cause of IMR is ventricular distortion of the normal spatial relationship of the mitral valve apparatus and LV.[4,6,7,9–14] With adverse LV remodeling (dilatation and change of shape), one or both of the mitral leaflets are pulled apically into the LV as a consequence of the outward displacement of the papillary muscles resulting from the remodeling. This results in incomplete mitral leaflet closure where the leaflet coaptation point is apically displaced. The IMLC pattern is more difficult to assess in the long axis views in which the continuity between the anterior mitral leaflet and aortic valve is demonstrated as the mitral annular plane is not defined in this view.

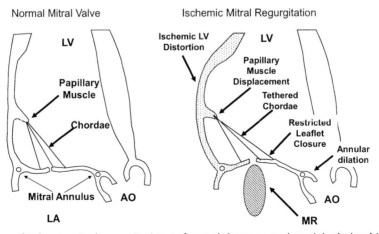

Fig. 1. Mechanism of ischemic mitral regurgitation. Left panel shows normal spatial relationship between mitral valve apparatus and left ventricle. Right panel shows mechanism of ischemic mitral regurgitation, which develops from ischemic LV distortion leading to papillary muscle displacement, tethered mitral leaflets, and restricted leaflet closure. Annular dilation also contributes to this process. Ao, aorta; LA, left atrium.

This pattern is best seen in the apical 4-chamber view (**Fig. 2**). The leaflets are apically displaced, tethered, and may have restricted mobility, especially the posterior leaflet. There are several methods to quantify the degree of tethering. The most common is a simple area measurement from the leaflets to the annular plane (tenting area), typically performed at midsystole where the area is at a minimum. Another measure is coaptation height or depth, which simply measures the maximal distance from the leaflet tips to the annular plane and appears to correlate with the presence and severity of ischemic MR.[15] More recently, 3-dimensional echocardiography has been applied to quantify leaflet tethering by measuring the tethering distance from papillary muscle tip to the mitral annulus,[4,16] and measurement of tenting volume (volume from leaflets to annular plane) add reference and may provide additional data to assess tethering.

Tethering of the basal or strut chordae can lead to a bend in the body of the anterior leaflet, contributing to tethering and impaired coaptation (**Fig. 3**). Mitral annulus dilatation may also be a contributing factor of IMR.[8,12,13] However, the degree of dilatation can vary and does not necessarily correlate with the degree of MR. In addition, the nonplanar saddle-shape of the annulus is important to minimize stress on the valve leaflets and contributes to valve competence. In IMR, the annulus becomes flatter, which may alter the closing mechanics of the mitral valve.

Annular dilatation occurs primarily due to dilatation of the posterior mitral annulus. Although most of the dilatation is in the posterior annulus, the anterior (fibrous) annulus also dilates although to a lesser extent.[17] In addition, annular dilatation is asymmetric, especially in the region of the posterior commissure (P2–P3 segment).[8] Echocardiographic assessment of IMR should also include an assessment of LV function and quantitation of the degree of MR. LV function should include ejection fraction, LV dimensions, assessment of wall-motion abnormalities, and structural abnormalities of the mitral valve chordae and papillary muscles. An integrative approach to the quantitation of MR should be performed including Doppler techniques for direct quantitation as well as supportive echo data (left atrial size, LV chamber size, pattern of pulmonary vein flow) in the overall assessment.

PROGNOSIS

The presence of IMR is associated with a poor prognosis. Increased mortality with development of MR has been shown in patients post-infarction, post–transluminal coronary angioplasty, and post–coronary artery bypass surgery.[17–21] In fact, the impact of IMR on mortality occurs in a dose-dependent manner, with even mild MR having an effect.[3,20]

MANAGEMENT OF IMR

The treatment of ischemic MR remains unclear. Surgical treatment options for IMR include coronary artery bypass grafting alone[22,23] or with concomitant mitral valve annuloplasty[24,25] or replacement.[26] Currently, the most common technique to repair IMR is the placement of an undersized annuloplasty ring (reduction annuloplasty) to reduce annular size. Although effective in reducing IMR acutely, there is a significant incidence of up to 30% of recurrent IMR following ring annuloplasty.[27–29] Importantly, ring annuloplasty has not been associated with improvement in survival in IMR. This may be because of several factors including significant recurrence rate of IMR and or continued ventricular remodeling.

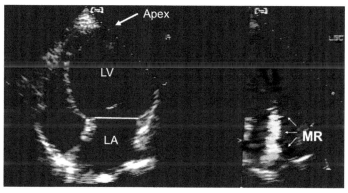

Fig. 2. Echocardiographic assessment of incomplete mitral leaflet closure pattern is best seen in the apical 4-chamber view. Mitral leaflets coapt apically, above the annular plane (*solid line-left panel*), resulting in mitral regurgitation (*small arrows*).

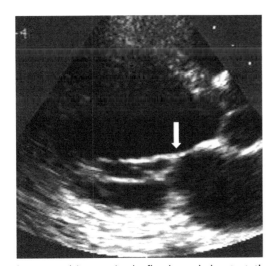

Fig. 3. Bend in anterior leaflet (*arrow*) due to tethering of the body of the leaflet from basal chord.

Ischemic MR is a complex lesion with multiple mechanistic variables that may vary in individual patients. Echocardiography provides important mechanistic insights for optimal management. However, multiple mechanisms may be present and their relative contribution may not be clear. Uncertainty and dissatisfaction with surgical ring annuloplasty has led to alternative approaches to treatment of IMR including transection of basal chordae secondary,[30–32] posterior leaflet patch extension,[33] annular cinching,[12] infarct plication,[34] papillary muscle sling,[35] and external restraints.[36] These alternate approaches have been mostly applied in small series or in conjunction with ring annuloplasty. In the absence of evidence-based randomized trials and until the controversy over the optimal treatment of ischemic MR is clarified, the choice of procedure will continue to be based on patients' clinical status, the severity of MR, and institutional and individual surgeons' expertise. The intended or planned approach may also be affected by the course of surgery. Coronary artery bypass surgery typically precedes MV surgery, and if adverse events occur during the earlier part of the operation, additional surgery may be abandoned.

The degree of MR is central to decision making, and characterization of the severity of valve regurgitation is among the most difficult problems in valvular heart disease. Preoperative transthoracic echocardiography by experienced laboratories is preferred to intraoperative transesophageal echocardiography to reflect the true degree of MR, because MR is often artificially underestimated by the altered hemodynamics in anesthetized patients. Moreover, as recommended by the American Society of Echocardiography,[37] a comprehensive, multifaceted, integrated approach to quantitating MR should be performed.

SUMMARY

The main mechanism of ischemic MR relates to distortion of the spatial relationships between the mitral valve and papillary muscles secondary to ventricular remodeling. This frequently results from myocardial infarction of the segments underlying the papillary muscles. Annulus dilatation is also usually present. This process can then become self-perpetuating as MR leads to ventricular dilatation, which in turn leads to further papillary muscle displacement, annular dilatation, and then more MR. Echocardiography provides mechanistic insights into the complex pathophysiology that involves the myocardium, the mitral subvalvular apparatus, and mitral annulus. Therefore, echocardiography may provide a more directed approach where the surgeon and cardiologist can tailor the operative strategy in individual patients. Finally, the evidence that treatment of ischemic MR improves long-term survival remains unclear, and further studies are needed to determine whether correcting ischemic MR will improve survival and/or symptoms.

REFERENCES

1. Tcheng JE, Jackman JD Jr, Nelson CL, et al. Outcome of patients sustaining acute ischemic mitral regurgitation during myocardial infarction. Ann Intern Med 1992;117:18–24.
2. Lehmann KG, Francis CK, Dodge HT. Mitral regurgitation in early myocardial infarction. Ann Intern Med 1992;117:10–7.
3. Lamas GA, Mitchell GF, Flaker GC, et al. Clinical significance of mitral regurgitation after acute myocardial infarction. Circulation 1997;96:827–33.
4. Otsuji Y, Handschumacher MD, Liel-Cohen N, et al. Mechanism of ischemic mitral regurgitation with segmental left ventricular dysfunction: three-dimensional echocardiographic studies in models of acute and chronic progressive regurgitation. J Am Coll Cardiol 2001;37:641–8.
5. Kumanohoso T, Otsuji Y, Yoshifuku S, et al. Mechanism of higher incidence of ischemic mitral regurgitation in patients with inferior myocardial infarction: quantitative analysis of left ventricular and mitral valve geometry in 103 patients with prior myocardial infarction. J Thorac Cardiovasc Surg 2003; 125:135–43.
6. Godley RW, Wann LS, Rogers EW, et al. Incomplete mitral leaflet closure in patients with papillary muscle dysfunction. Circulation 1981;63:565–71.

7. Levine RA, Schwammenthal E. Ischemic mitral regurgitation on the threshold of a solution. From paradoxes to unifying concept. Circulation 2005; 112:745–58.

8. Kaji S, Nasu M, Yamamuro A, et al. Annular geometry in patients with chronic ischemic mitral regurgitation. Three-dimensional magnetic resonance imaging study. Circulation 2005;112(Suppl I):I409–44.

9. Tibayan FA, Rodriquez F, Langer F, et al. Does septal-lateral annular cinching work for chronic ischemic mitral regurgitation? J Thorac Cardiovasc Surg 2004;127:654–63.

10. Gorman JH, Jackson BM, Gorman RC, et al. Papillary muscle discoordination rather than increased annular area facilitates mitral regurgitation after acute posterior myocardial infarction. Circulation 1997;96(Suppl II):124–7.

11. Gorman JH III, Gorman RC, Plappert T, et al. Infarct size and location determine development of mitral regurgitation in the sheep model. J Thorac Cardiovasc Surg 1998;115:15–22.

12. Tibayan FA, Rodriquez F, Zasio MK, et al. Geometric distortions of the mitral valvular-ventricular complex in chronic ischemic mitral regurgitation. Circulation 2003;108(Suppl II):116–21.

13. Kwan J, Shiota T, Agler DA, et al. Geometric differences of the mitral apparatus between ischemic and dilated cardiomyopathy with significant mitral regurgitation: real-time three dimensional echocardiographic study. Circulation 2003; 107:1135–40.

14. Carabello BA. Ischemic mitral regurgitation and ventricular remodeling. J Am Coll Cardiol 2004;43: 384–5.

15. Calafiore AM, Gallina S, Di Mauro M, et al. Mitral valve procedure in dilated cardiomyopathy: repair or replacement? Ann Thorac Surg 2001;71:1146–52.

16. Watanabe N, Ogasawara Y, Yamaura Y, et al. Quantitation of mitral valve tenting in ischemic mitral regurgitation by transthoracic real-time three-dimensional echocardiography. J Am Coll Cardiol 2005;45:763–9.

17. Ahmad RM, Gillinov AM, McCarthy PM, et al. Annular geometry and motion in human ischemic mitral regurgitation: novel assessment with there-dimensional echocardiography and computer reconstruction. Ann Thorac Surg 2004;78:2063–8.

18. Ellis SG, Whitlow PL, Raymond RE, et al. Impact of mitral regurgitation on long-term survival after percutaneous coronary intervention. Am J Cardiol 2002; 89:315–8.

19. Bursi F, Enriquez-Sarano M, Nkomo VT, et al. Heart failure and death after myocardial infarction in the community. The emerging role of mitral regurgitation. Circulation 2005;111:295–301.

20. Grigioni F, Detaint D, Avierinos JF, et al. Contribution of ischemic mitral regurgitation to congestive heart failure after myocardial infarction. J Am Coll Cardiol 2005;45:260–7.

21. Lam BK, Gillinov AM, Blackstone EH, et al. Importance of moderate ischemic mitral regurgitation. Ann Thorac Surg 2005;79:462–70.

22. Trichon BH, Glower DD, Shaw LK, et al. Survival after coronary revascularization, with and without mitral valve surgery, in patients with ischemic mitral regurgitation. Circulation 2003;108(Suppl I): 11103–10.

23. Tolis GA Jr, Korkolis DP, Kopf GS, et al. Revascularization alone (without mitral valve repair) suffices in patients with advanced ischemic cardiomyopathy and mid-to-moderate mitral regurgitation. Ann Thorac Surg 2002;74:1476–80.

24. Filsoufi F, Aklog L, Byrne JG, et al. Current results of combined coronary artery bypass grafting and mitral annuloplasty in patients with moderate ischemic mitral regurgitation. J Heart Valve Dis 2004;13:747–53.

25. Mihaljevic T, Lam BK, Rajeswaran J, et al. Impact of mitral valve annuloplasty combined with revascularization in patients with functional ischemic mitral regurgitation. J Am Coll Cardiol 2007;49: 2191–201.

26. Gillinov AM, Wierup PN, Blackstone EH, et al. Is repair preferable to replacement for ischemic mitral regurgitation? J Thorac Cardiovasc Surg 2001;122: 1125–41.

27. Tahta SA, Oury JH, Maxwell JM, et al. Outcome after mitral valve repair for functional ischemic mitral regurgitation. J Heart Valve Dis 2002;11:11–8.

28. McGee EC, Gillinov AM, Blackstone EH, et al. Recurrent mitral regurgitation after annuloplasty for functional ischemic mitral regurgitation. J Thorac Cardiovasc Surg 2004;128:916–24.

29. Diodato MD, Moon MM, Pasque MK, et al. Repair of ischemic mitral regurgitation does not increase mortality or improve long-term survival in patients undergoing coronary artery revascularization. a propensity analysis. Ann Thorac Surg 2004;78: 794–9.

30. Messas E, Guerrero JL, Handschumacher MD, et al. Chordal cutting: a new therapeutic approach for ischemic mitral regurgitation. Circulation 2001;104: 1958–63.

31. Messas E, Pouzot B, Touchot B, et al. Efficacy of chordal cutting to relieve chronic persistent ischemic mitral regurgitation. Circulation 2003; 108(Suppl II):111–5.

32. Borger MA, Murphy PM, Alim A, et al. Initial results of the chordal-cutting operation for ischemic mitral regurgitation. J Thorac Cardiovasc Surg 2007;133: 1483–92.

33. Varennes B, Chaturvedi R, Sidhu S, et al. Initial results of posterior leaflet extension for severe type IIIb ischemic mitral regurgitation. Circulation 2009; 119:2837–43.

34. Timek TA, Lai DT, Liang D, et al. Effects of paracommissural septal-lateral annular cinching on acute ischemic mitral regurgitation. Circulation 2004; 110(Suppl II):79–84.

35. Hvass U, Tapia M, Baron F, et al. Papillary muscle sling: a new functional approach to mitral repair in patients with ischemic left ventricular dysfunction and functional mitral regurgitation. Ann Thorac Surg 2003;75:809–11.

36. Hung J, Guerrero JL, Handschumacher MD, et al. Reverse ventricular remodeling reduces ischemic mitral regurgitation: echo-guided device application in the beating heart. Circulation 2002;106:2594–600.

37. Zoghbi WA, Enriquez-Sarano M, Foster E, et al. Recommendations for evaluation of native valvular regurgitation with two dimensional and Doppler echocardiography. J Am Soc Echocardiogr 2003; 16:777–803.

The Role of Echocardiography During Mitral Valve Percutaneous Interventions

Nina C. Wunderlich, MD[a,b], Roy Beigel, MD[c,d,e], Robert J. Siegel, MD[c],*

KEYWORDS

- Echocardiography • Mitral stenosis • Mitral regurgitation • Paravalvular leak
- Percutaneous intervention

KEY POINTS

- As the mitral leaflets cannot be assessed by fluoroscopy, preprocedural assessment, procedural guidance, and postprocedural assessment of percutaneous mitral interventions for mitral valve stenosis (MS), mitral regurgitation (MR), and mitral valve (MV) paravalvular leaks (PVLs) rely heavily on echocardiography.
- Although two-dimensional (2D) transesophageal echocardiography (TEE) has played a major role in guidance of the procedures, three-dimensional (3D) TEE provides more detailed information on MV anatomy and catheter and device positions.
- Combining 2D and 3D TEE improves results and reduces procedure time.

INTRODUCTION

TEE is routinely used to guide percutaneous interventions involving the MV. The most common percutaneous procedures are (1) percutaneous mitral balloon valvuloplasty (PMBV) for rheumatic MS, (2) edge-to-edge repair with the MitraClip (Abbott Laboratories, Abbott Park, IL, USA) for MR, and (3) closure of prosthetic paravalvular mitral leakages (PVML). 3D TEE has become an important adjunct in patient selection and is, in some cases, critical for intraprocedural guidance for percutaneous mitral interventions.

PERCUTANEOUS MITRAL BALLOON VALVULOPLASTY

PMBV, a safe and effective treatment of MS,[1 0] is the preferred treatment option for selected symptomatic patients with MS.[10–12] Rheumatic fever, the leading cause of MS,[13,14] causes commissural fusion of the valve, narrowing of the valve orifice, and valve obstruction. Commissural fusion (Fig. 1A, B) is the requisite lesion for PMBV to be effective. PMBV is not effective for degenerative calcific MS, where heavy mitral annular calcification is the main lesion.

Preprocedural Assessment of MS Severity

Evaluation of MS includes assessment of the valve area, the mean Doppler gradients, and pulmonary artery pressure (Table 1).[10,11,15] 2D planimetry of the mitral valve area (MVA) is performed from the parasternal short axis view when the maximal diastolic orifice is present (see Fig. 1B). The entire MV orifice should be seen. High gain settings should be avoided, as they may lead to underestimation

Conflict of Interest: None.
[a] Cardiovascular Center, Darmstadt, Germany; [b] University Hospital, Mainz, Germany; [c] The Heart Institute, Cedars Sinai Medical Center, 8700 Beverly Blvd, Los Angeles, CA 90048, USA; [d] The Leviev Heart Center, Sheba Medical Center, Tel-Hashomer 52621, Israel; [e] Sackler School of Medicine, Tel Aviv University, Tel Aviv, Israel
* Corresponding author.
E-mail address: siegel@cshs.org

Cardiol Clin 31 (2013) 237–270
http://dx.doi.org/10.1016/j.ccl.2013.03.003
0733-8651/13/$ – see front matter © 2013 Elsevier Inc. All rights reserved.

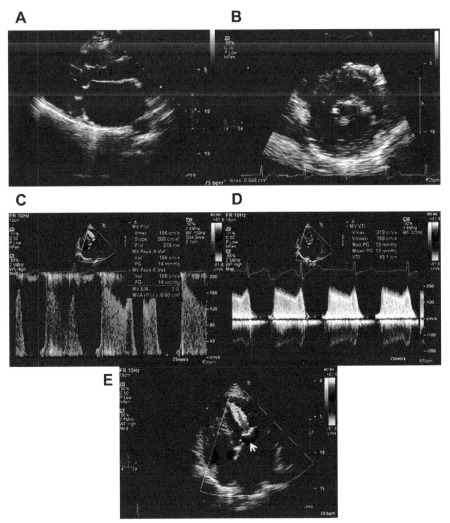

Fig. 1. Transthoracic 2D parasternal long axis view (*A*) demonstrating commissural fusion with a restricted mitral valve. In the short axis view (*B*), 2D planimetry of the mitral valve area is performed in the parasternal short axis view at the tip of the leaflets when maximal excursion of the leaflets is seen. The inner edge of the MV orifice is traced in middiastole. Doppler echocardiography using the pressure half-time ($T_{1/2}$) method (*C*). $T_{1/2}$ is obtained by tracing the deceleration slope of the E-wave on Doppler spectral display of transmitral inflow, and in the case shown it is 279 ms, resulting in an estimated valve area of 220/279 = 0.8 cm². The MV area can be calculated from the following formula: $220/(T_{1/2})$. (*D*) Doppler measurements using the continuous wave Doppler signal across the mitral valve showing a mean pressure gradient of 12 mm Hg consistent with severe mitral stenosis. (*E*) The continuity equation and proximal isovelocity surface area (PISA; *white arrow*) methods can also be used for quantification of MS severity.

of MVA. Planimetry correlates with the anatomic valve area as assessed on explanted valves.[16] Some reports indicate planimetry by 3D echo is more accurate and reproducible than 2D echocardiography.[17–19]

Mitral maximal and mean Doppler gradients are also calculated. The maximal gradient, derived from peak mitral velocity, is influenced by left atrial (LA) compliance and left ventricular (LV) diastolic function.[20] However, the mean MV gradient more accurately reflects MS severity. Continuous wave (CW) Doppler measurements across the MV have good correlation with invasive measurements using transseptal (TS) catheterization (see **Fig. 1**D).[21] Mitral transvalvular gradients are highly rate and flow dependent, as the transmitral gradient is a function of the square of the transvalvular flow. Thus, heart rate and cardiac output significantly affect the transmitral diastolic gradient (see **Table 1**, Appendix A—MS assessment).[22]

Table 1
Methods and quantification of mitral valve stenosis severity

	Quantification of Severity	Method	Limitations
Valve area (cm^2)			
Pressure half-time ($T_{1/2}$) (see **Fig. 1C**, Appendix A)	Mild >1.5 Moderate 1–1.5 Severe <1	$220/(T_{1/2})$	Aortic regurgitation Atrial septal defects Previous surgical/ percutaneous mitral valvuloplasty
Planimetry (see **Fig. 1B**)		Tracing the inner edge of the MV orifice in middiastole	Underestimation due to high gain
Continuity equation (Appendix A)		$\pi\left(\dfrac{D2}{4}\right)\left(\dfrac{VTI\ aorta\ (cm)}{VTI\ mitral\ (cm)}\right)$	Limited accuracy and reproducibility Atrial fibrillation Aortic and/or mitral regurgitation
Proximal isovelocity (PISA) (Appendix A)		$\pi\,(r^2)(V_{alias})/Peak\ V_{mitral} \times \alpha/180°$	Technically demanding
Mean gradient (mm Hg) (see **Fig. 1D**)	Mild <5 Moderate 5–10 Severe >10	Tracing of the Doppler diastolic mitral flow profile	Heart rate and flow dependent
Pulmonary artery systolic pressure (mm Hg)	Mild <30 Moderate 30–50 Severe >50	Tricuspid regurgitation gradient + right atrial pressure	Underestimation due to malalignment Inaccurate estimation of right atrial pressure

Assessment of Valve Anatomy and Suitability for PMBV

Echocardiographic evaluation of the mitral valve anatomy and pathology dictates the feasibility and likelihood of successful PMBV (**Figs. 2 and 3, Table 2**).

- The Wilkins score (see **Table 2**)[23] is most commonly used for transthoracic echocardiographic (TTE) assessment; 2D echo is used to evaluate valve morphologic leaflet mobility, flexibility, thickness, calcification, subvalvular fusion, commissural fusion, and calcification. The features that determine suitability for PMBV have been used to develop different scoring systems.[1,23–27] Each feature is graded on a 1 to 4 scale yielding a maximum score of 16. A score greater than 8 suggests the valve may not be suitable for PMBV.
- Assessment of commissural calcium[27] (see **Figs. 2 and 3**): The extent of commissural calcification is quantified by giving each half commissure (anterolateral and posteromedial) with detection of high-intensity bright echos a score of 1. Commissural calcification can, therefore, range from grade 0 to grade 4 (see **Fig. 3**). The grade of intercommissural calcium is a significant predictor of achieving

an MVA post-PMVB[28] greater than 1.5 cm^2 without creating significant MR.[29] The usefulness is greatest in patients with a Wilkins score of 8 or less (= patients with relatively "good" valves), whereas in patients with a score greater than 8, calcium scoring does not add additional predictive value. Patients with commissural calcification grade 0/1 had larger valve areas and better improvement of symptoms than patients with grade 2/3.
- Echocardiographic grouping (**Table 3**)[1]

The echocardiographic grouping is based on the echocardiographic and fluoroscopic (calcification) assessment of the following characteristics: valve mobility, fusion of the subvalvular apparatus, and the amount of leaflet calcification (see **Table 3**).

In a subset of 40 patients, a Wilkins score of 7 to 9 correlated with the echocardiographic group 1, range 8 to 12 correlated with group 2, and range 10 to 15 with group 3.[30]

- Real-time 3D transthoracic echocardiographic (RT-TT3DE) score (**Table 4**)[31]: this score evaluates both mitral leaflets and the subvalvular apparatus. The RT-TT3DE score seems to be highly reproducible with good interobserver and intraobserver agreement

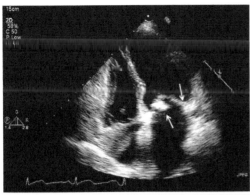

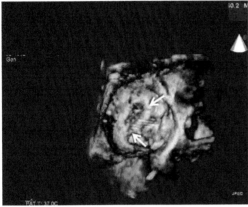

Fig. 2. Transthoracic 2D apical 4-chamber view (*top*) and 3D TEE reconstruction (*bottom*) showing severe commissural calcification (*arrows*), which makes the patient high risk for percutaneous balloon valvuloplasty.

in the assessment of MV morphology in patients with MS. RT-TT3DE is reported to be superior for detection of calcification and commissural splitting. Predictors of optimal PMBV were leaflet mobility and the involvement of the subvalvular apparatus. The incidence and severity of postprocedural MR was associated with a high calcification RT-TT3DE score.

No scoring system has been proved to be superior; thus, they should be used in conjunction with one another as part of a comprehensive echocardiographic assessment of the valve pathology.

Intraprocedural Guidance

Different types of balloons are available (single balloon, double balloon, and Inoue balloon [Toray Medical Co, Ltd, Chiba, Japan]) for PMBV. The Inoue balloon, the most commonly used, had low intraprocedural and periprocedural mortality and a success rate of 95% or more. On average, MVA increases to 1.9 to 2.0 cm^2, and New York Heart Association (NYHA) functional improves to class I–II in 90% of the cases.[8]

When anticoagulation therapy is withheld before PMBV, thrombi can develop rapidly in patients with MS. Thus, before TS puncture, TEE should be done to exclude an LA thrombus and to reassess contraindications for PMBV (**Box 1**). Most interventionalists exclude patients with an LA thrombus (**Fig. 4**) for PMBV. If a thrombus is detected, the authors postpone the procedure until it has resolved on repeat TEE. Cases with excessive and/or nonresolving LA thrombus should be considered for surgery rather than for PMBV.[10,11]

For most PMBV cases, the preferred TS puncture site is in the posterior, a more inferior region of the fossa ovalis. TEE or alternatively intracardiac echo guidance is helpful, especially in patients with dilated atria or unusual morphology of the interatrial septum (IAS) such as a large atrial septal aneurysm, prior IAS surgery, or distortion of the IAS from scoliosis or prior pneumectomy. The tip of the needle for TS puncture can be identified by a tentlike indentation of the IAS on TEE (**Fig. 5**). The height above the valve is best appreciated in the 4-chamber view (~0°), the anterior-posterior orientation is obtained using a short axis view at the base (30°–45°), and the superior-inferior orientation is seen on a long axis view (90°–100°). X-plane imaging facilitates the TS

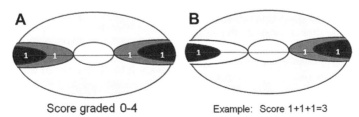

Score graded 0-4   Example: Score 1+1+1=3

Fig. 3. Schematic of the evaluation of commissural calcification score. Commissural calcification is quantified by giving half commissure each (anterolateral and posteromedial) with detection of high-intensity bright echos a score of 1. Commissural calcification can therefore range from grade 0 (no calcification) to grade 4 (*A*) (both commissures are completely calcified). (*B*) gives an example where half a commissure is calcified on the left side and the entire commissure is calcified on the right side. The added score is therefore 3.

Table 2
Echocardiographic scoring of the mitral valve (adapted from the Wilkins score)

Imaging Modality	Views	Mitral Valve Scoring
2D	Parasternal long axis 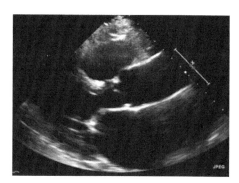	The following characteristics are scored: Leaflet mobility 1 = Mobile valve, only leaflet tips restriction 2 = Leaflet mid and base portions with normal mobility 3 = Valve continues to move forward in diastole, mainly from the base 4 = Immobile or minimal mobile valve in diastole
	Parasternal short axis 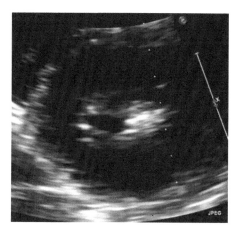	Leaflet thickening 1 = Leaflet thickness 4–5 mm 2 = Mid leaflets normal, thickening of margins 5–8 mm 3 = Entire leaflet thickening 5–8 mm 4 = Thickening of all leaflet tissue >8–10 mm
	Apical 4-chamber 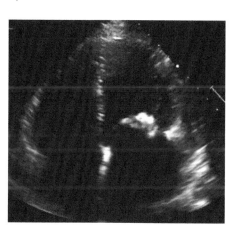	Leaflet calcification 1 = Single area of increased echo brightness 2 = Scattered areas of brightness confined to leaflet margins 3 = Brightness extending into midportions of the leaflets 4 = Extensive brightness throughout much of the tissue

(continued on next page)

Table 2
(continued)

Imaging Modality Views	Mitral Valve Scoring
Apical 2-chamber 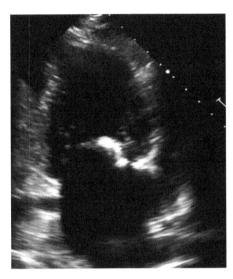	Subvalvular involvement 1 = Minimal thickening just below the MV leaflets 2 = Thickening up to 1/3 of chordal length 3 = Thickening extending to distal 1/3 of the chords 4 = Extensive thickening of all chordal structures Maximal score: 16. A score >8 suggests the valve may not be suitable to percutaneous mitral balloon valvuloplasty

puncture by showing simultaneous anterior-posterior and superior-inferior orientations.

After TS puncture, the PMBV catheter and the balloon are placed across the mitral valve leaflets

Table 3
Description of the 3 group grading of mitral valve anatomy as assessed by 2D echocardiography and fluoroscopy

Echocardiographic Group	Mitral Valve Anatomy
Group 1	Pliable, noncalcified anterior mitral leaflet and mild subvalvular disease, ie, thin chordate ≥10 mm long
Group 2	Pliable noncalcified anterior mitral leaflet and severe subvalvular disease, ie, thickened chordate <10 mm long
Group 3	Calcification of MV of any extent, as assessed by fluoroscopy, whatever the state of the subvalvular apparatus

(**Fig. 6**). 2D and 3D TEE are useful in guiding delivery of catheters and wires across the MV, positioning the balloon within the mitral valve orifice, and confirming that the balloon is optimally positioned between the mitral leaflets. Inflation of the balloon in the subvalvular region should be avoided, as this may lead to valvular, chordal, or papillary muscle rupture (**Fig. 7**). As shown in **Fig. 8**, during balloon inflation, the mitral valve orifice is completely occluded, stasis is evident by echo, and hemodynamic deterioration may occur. Close monitoring of hemodynamic parameters is mandatory during this phase of the procedure. Dilation of the MV orifice due to splitting of the commissures is evident by echo and fluoroscopy—the constriction of the balloon, visible at its waist at the level of the mitral leaflets, suddenly disappears.

Subsequently, echocardiographic reassessment is done for the following:

- Severity and location of MR (newly developed MR emerging from the commissures indicate a rupture of the valve leaflets) (1.4%–9.4% develop significant MR[32,33])
- Mitral valve leaflet mobility
- Post-PMBV MVA using mean Doppler gradients, 2D and 3D MV planimetry (**Fig. 9**)
- Commissural opening (see **Fig. 9**D, E)

Table 4
Real-time transthoracic 3D echocardiographic score for the evaluation of mitral valve stenosis before percutaneous mitral balloon valvuloplasty

	Anterior Mitral Leaflet			Posterior Mitral Leaflet		
	A1	A2	A3	P1	P2	P3
Thickness (0–6) (0 = normal, 1 = thickened)[a]	0–1	0–1	0–1	0–1	0–1	0–1
Mobility (0–6) (0 = normal, 1 = thickened)[a]	0–1	0–1	0–1	0–1	0–1	0–1
Calcification (0–10) (0 = no, 1–2 = calcified)[b]	0–2	0–1	0–2	0–2	0–1	0–2

Subvalvular Apparatus[b]			
	Proximal Third	Middle Third	Distal Third
Thickness (0–3) (0 = normal, 1 = thickened)	0–1	0–1	0–1
Separation (0–6) (0 = normal, 1 = partial, 2 = no)	0,1,2	0,1,2	0,1,2

Each leaflet is divided into 3 segments (anterior leaflet: A1 [lateral], A2 [middle], A3 [medial]; posterior leaflet: P1 [lateral], P2 [middle], P3 [lateral]). Each segment is scored separately for thickness, mobility, and calcification. Normal thickness and mobility are scored as 0, whereas abnormal thickness or mobility is scored as 1. Absence of calcification is scored as 0, calcification in A2 or P2 (middle segments) is scored as 1, and calcification of commissural segments of both leaflets (A1, A3, and P1 and P3) is scored as 2. In addition, the anterior and posterior chordae are scored at a proximal (mitral valve level), a middle, and a distal (papillary muscle level) level. At each level, the anterior and the posterior leaflets are scored for thickness and separation in between. Normal thickness gets a score of 0, abnormal thickness a score of 1. Normal chordal separation (defined as distance in between >5 mm) is scored as 0, partial separation (defined as distance in between <5 mm) as 1, and absence of separation as 2. The individual score points are added up, the calculated total score ranges from 0 to 31 points. Mild mitral valve involvement was defined as <8 points, moderate MV involvement 8 to 13, and severe MV involvement ≥14.
  [a] Normal = 0, mild = 1–2, moderate 3–4, severe ≥5.
  [b] Normal = 0, mild = 1–2, moderate 3–5, severe ≥6.
  Adapted from Anwar AM, Attia WM, Nosir YF, et al. Validation of a new score for the assessment of mitral stenosis using real-time three-dimensional echocardiography. J Am Soc Echocardiogr 2010;23(1):13–22.

- Assessment of complications such as pericardial effusion and left-to-right shunt through the artificial atrial septal defect (ASD) secondary to the TS puncture.

The pressure half-time method (see **Fig. 1C**) post-PMBV is unreliable for calculation of MVA because of multiple factors: atrial compliance, a newly created ASD, and changes in hemodynamics influence this measurement.[5,34–37]

Box 1
Contraindications to percutaneous mitral balloon valvuloplasty

- Mitral valve area greater than 1.5 cm²
- Left atrial thrombus
- More than mild mitral regurgitation
- Severe or bicommissural calcification
- Absence of commissural fusion
- Severe concomitant aortic valve disease or severe combined tricuspid stenosis and regurgitation
- Concomitant coronary artery disease requiring bypass surgery

RT 3D echocardiography is reported as having better accuracy and agreement with invasively determined MVA compared with conventional 2D planimetry[38] and superior in assessing commissural opening than 2D echo.

Successful PMBV has been defined as an MVA 1.5 cm² or more or 1.0 cm² or more, MR 2+ or less, and absence of complications.[10,11] **Table 5** lists predictors of outcome after PMBV, which include a variety of clinical, morphologic, and hemodynamic parameters. **Box 2** summarizes the periinterventional role of echocardiography.

EDGE-TO-EDGE REPAIR WITH THE MITRACLIP FOR MITRAL REGURGITATION

Alfieri[45] developed a surgical technique of suturing the free edges of the mid portions of the anterior (A2) and posterior (P2) mitral valve scallops to create a double mitral valve orifice to treat MR. St. Goar developed the MitraClip as a catheter-based approach to create a double MV orifice and thereby reduce MR (St. Goar, personal communication, 2005).

The MitraClip system (**Fig. 10**) is the only percutaneous method available to alter the mitral valve morphology and annulus diameter and reduce

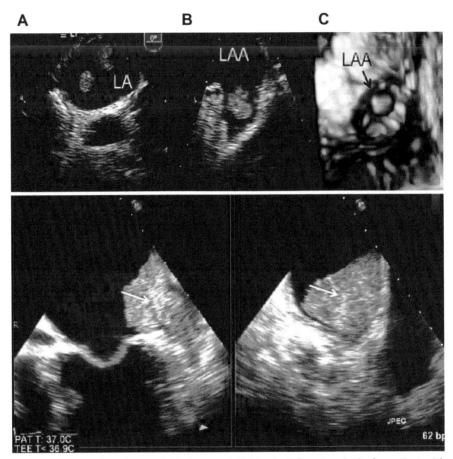

Fig. 4. (*Top*) In (*A*), 2 mobile thrombi are visible in 2D TEE (0°) in the left atrium (LA) of a patient with mitral stenosis before surgery. In (*B*), a large thrombus (2D TEE 70°) in the left atrial appendage (LAA) is shown, and in (*C*), a 3D TEE en face view of the LAA orifice reveals a thrombus close to the LAA ostium (*arrow*). (*Bottom*) 2D TEE x-plane images showing a large thrombus in the LAA (*arrows*).

MR.[46,47] A TS approach (**Fig. 11**) is used to enter the left atrium and gain access to the MV. This catheter system has 2 arms that form a Clip when closed (see **Fig. 10**). During the procedure, the Clip arms are opened in the LV and during a pullback into the LA, the central portions of the MV anterior and posterior leaflets are entrapped in the Clip arms, creating a double mitral orifice (**Fig. 12**) and a reduction in MR. **Box 3** lists echocardiographic parameters essential for evaluation before and during MitraClip placement.

Patient Selection

Patients with MitraClip often have comorbidities such as impaired LV function and reduced left ventricular ejection fraction (LVEF) (<40%) that make them poor surgical candidates. Franzen and colleagues[48] showed that MitraClip implantation can be safely performed with good results even in patients with LVEF less than 20%.

For the MitraClip procedure, patients need to have moderate to severe or severe MR (≥3+ to 4+) (**Table 6**) and the appropriate MV morphology. As seen in **Fig. 13**A, there is P2 prolapse and flail with a flail gap that is not excessive. **Fig. 13**B shows severe functional MR with appropriate coaptation depth and normal leaflet morphology. **Fig. 13**C shows severe MR due to anterior leaflet prolapse with a trivial flail gap. **Table 7** shows MV morphologic characteristics that identify optimal patients for MV Clip therapy.[46,49]

Imaging of the MV

Echocardiography is the best method to assess MR severity, mechanism, repairability, and hemodynamic consequences.[50,51] 2D TTE is used to assess MR severity, whereas TEE is used to assess valve morphology. Important 2D TEE views (**Fig. 14**) are used to characterize valve abnormalities. In the 0° views (from the upper esophagus),

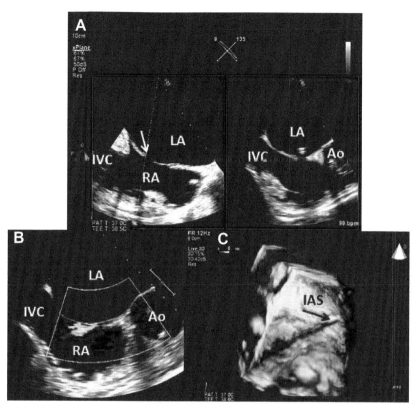

Fig. 5. (*A*) TEE x-plane image shows intraatrial septum (IAS; *white arrow*) from 2 aspects; the left panel shows the IAS in the long axis view with the inferior vena cava (IVC) to the left. The right panel identifies the aorta (Ao), an anterior structure, helping to avoid puncturing it by the transseptal (TS) needle. (*B*) Color flow in this view allows identification of a stretched patent foramen ovale (PFO) with left-to-right shunting. Puncture of the IAS at this site should be avoided (see text for more details). (*C*) 3D en face view of the IAS after the TS puncture and passage of the catheter and wire (*black arrow*). IVC, inferior vena cava; LA, left atrium; RA, right atrium.

A1 and P1 segments are seen in the superior position, A2 and P2 segments in the midesophagus, and A3 and P3 segments in the distal esophagus. In intercommissural views (~60°), the P1, A2, and P3 segments are seen when the plane cuts both commissures. With a clockwise rotation of the probe, the anterior leaflet segments A1 to 3 are seen, and with a counterclockwise rotation, the posterior leaflet segments P1 to 3 are seen. The left ventricular outflow tract (LVOT) view (additional 90° to the intercommissural view) demonstrates the A2 and the P2 segment. Transgastric short axis imaging shows all segments of both leaflets when optimal images are obtained.

3D TEE is superior to 2D for assessing mitral valve anatomy.[50–53] X-plane imaging of the intercommissural view allows additional scanning of the valve segments from medial to lateral as well as assessment of the posteromedial and the anterolateral commissures as shown in **Fig. 13**C. 3D TEE provides detailed en face views

from the LA perspective ("surgical view") of the mitral valve scallops. 3D images of the submitral apparatus from a ventricular view are especially helpful in assessing the anterior mitral leaflet as well as restricted posterior leaflet motion. In addition, 3D TEE is used to evaluate adjacent structures.[50]

Posterior leaflet prolapses are best visualized from the LA view, and the anterior leaflet is also well seen from the LV (see **Fig. 13**D). Assessment of anterior prolapse (see **Fig. 13**E, F) can be more difficult than that of posterior prolapse (see **Fig. 13**A, B), as scallops are less pronounced on the anterior leaflet.[54] 3D TEE is more accurate in identifying which segments of the mitral valve are abnormal, prolapsed, or flail than 2D TEE.[52–54] In addition, identifying perforations, clefts, and gaps is more accurate with 3D TEE.[52,55]

In gated 3D echocardiography, multiple volumes are acquired (usually over 2–7 heart beats) and combined to form a single volumetric data

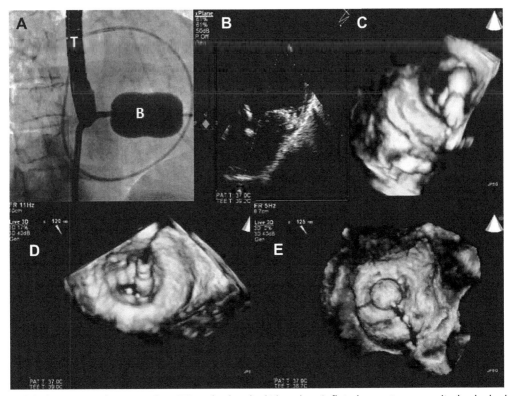

Fig. 6. (*A*) Fluoroscopy demonstrating TEE probe (marked T) and an inflated percutaneous mitral valvuloplasty balloon (marked B). (*B*) 2D TEE showing the balloon catheter across the mitral valve (MV). (*C*) An uninflated balloon is seen at the edge of the mitral orifice. (*D*) The balloon is seen entering the MV orifice. (*E*) The balloon is seen being inflated within the stenotic MV orifice.

set that has a higher temporal and spatial resolution. However, patient movement, respirations, or arrhythmias can cause artifacts with gated 3D imaging.[56]

Guiding of the MitraClip Procedure

The MitraClip procedure is highly technical and is best performed when there is active collaboration and good communication between the echocardiologist and the interventionalist. 2D TEE can be used to guide MitraClip implantation; however, 3D TEE adds substantial information[57] regarding the position of catheters, wires, devices, and target structures in a single 3D view. 3D echo and x-plane imaging can optimize TS puncture, steering of the delivery catheter in a 3D space (LA) toward the mitral valve, and proper MitraClip positioning perpendicular to the line of coaptation in the middle segments of the mitral valve (see **Fig. 11**; **Figs. 15–20**). In one study, the addition of 3D TEE resulted in nearly a 30% reduction in procedure time[58] compared with 2D TEE and fluoroscopy.

As the initial intraprocedural evaluation of the MitraClip is done under general anesthesia, the type of anesthesia and the medications that influence preload and afterload should be kept constant to ensure that preprocedural, intraprocedural, and postprocedural assessments of MR are performed under similar hemodynamic conditions. For preprocedural and postprocedural MR assessment, ultrasound settings including color scale and gain should be identical.

The MitraClip procedure is divided into 7 steps, which are outlined in **Box 4**.[59]

Transseptal puncture

The optimal puncture site, located superiorly and posteriorly in the IAS, is determined by 2D TEE imaging planes: short axis view at the base for anterior-posterior orientation (30°–45°), a bicaval view for superior (cranial)-caudal orientation (90°–120°), and a 4-chamber view (0°–20°) to identify the height above the mitral valve for TS puncture. 3D x-plane allows imaging in a short axis view at the base and in a bicaval view simultaneously

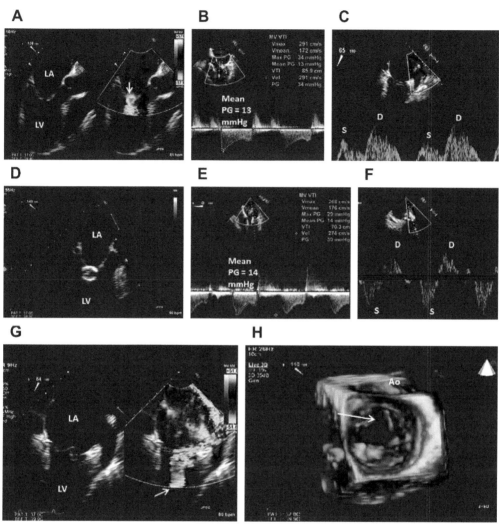

Fig. 7. (A) 2D TEE long axis view of a stenotic mitral valve; a diastolic PISA is present (*arrow*). (B) The mean diastolic pressure gradient (PG) is 13 mm Hg. (C) Doppler imaging of the pulmonary vein (PV) flow showing blunted systolic flow (marked S) and elevated diastolic flow (marked D), consistent with elevated left atrial filling pressures. (D) Percutaneous mitral valvuloplasty balloon is not at the valve level; rather it is too apical and inflated in the chordal apparatus. (E) The mean PG has gone up, the continuous wave Doppler now shows mitral regurgitation (MR) with a V-wave cutoff sign indicating acute MR. (F) There is associated systolic flow reversal in the PV. (G) A large PISA (*arrow*) in the left ventricle (LV) and severe eccentric, laterally directed, MR is shown. (H) 3D TEE in the surgical view of the left atrium (LA) shows that the anterior mitral leaflet, in addition to the commissures, has been split (*large arrow*). Ao, aorta.

(see **Fig. 11**). In cases with MV prolapse or flail MV (degenerative disease), the puncture site should be 4 to 5 cm above the mitral annulus to allow room for catheter and MitraClip system manipulation. With functional MR, the plane of MV coaptation is generally below the mitral annulus due to valve tethering. In these cases, the site of TS puncture is more apical, closer to the plane of the MV annulus, namely, ∼3.5 cm above the annular plane. TS access should not be across a persistent

foramen ovale, as this site is too anterior. With suboptimal TS puncture site, the procedure is more difficult, complex, and generally takes longer due to the need for more catheter manipulations with the large MitraClip delivery system (CDS).

Introduction of the steerable guide catheter into the LA

The steerable guide catheter (SGC) is advanced with the dilator into the LA over a stiff guidewire,

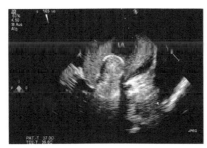
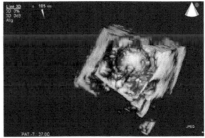

Fig. 8. (*Left*) 2D TEE showing the balloon being inflated within the stenotic MV orifice and the development of severe stasis in the left atrium (LA). (*Right*) 3D surgical view of the LA shows a fully inflated percutaneous mitral valvuloplasty balloon.

which is placed in the left upper pulmonary vein with fluoroscopic and TEE guidance (see **Fig. 15**). The dilator is identified by a cone-shaped tip with echogenic ridges. A radiopaque, echo bright, double ring characterizes the tip of the guide catheter. To prevent damaging the LA wall, advancement of the SGC is done with continuous 2D and 3D TEE guidance and fluoroscopy (see **Fig. 15**).

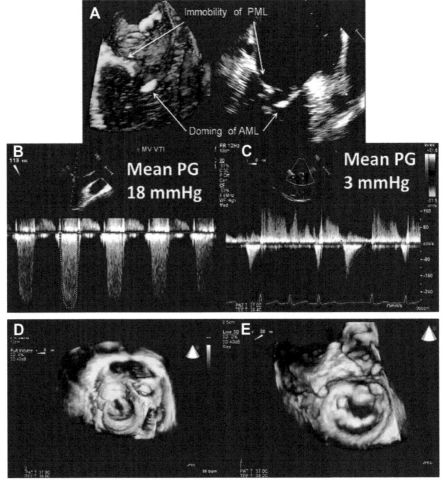

Fig. 9. (*A*) 2D and 3D TEE images post–balloon valvuloplasty. (*B, C*) Continuous wave Doppler showing the mean gradient (*B*) before and (*C*) after valvuloplasty, which has dropped from 18 to 3 mm Hg, indicating a successful procedure. (*D, E*) 3D images from the left atrium of the mitral valve orifice (*D*) before and (*E*) after successful valvuloplasty. AML, anterior mitral leaflet; PML, posterior mitral leaflet.

Table 5
Predictors of results after percutaneous mitral balloon valvuloplasty

Predictors of Good Immediate Results	Predictors of Good Long-term Results
Commissural calcium grade 0/1[27,28]	Complete commissural opening[39]
Wilkins score <8[3,23]	Larger MV area post-PMBV[39]
Presence of sinus rhythm[6]	Presence of sinus rhythm[40]
Good leaflet mobility[31]	Absence of calcium at fluoroscopy[40]
No involvement of the subvalvular apparatus[31]	Low MR grade after PMBV[6]
	Wilkins score ≤ 8[32]

Predictors of Poor Immediate Results	Predictors of Poor Long-term Results
Older age[1,30]	Higher cardiothoracic index[30]
Smaller initial MV area[1,30]	Lower MV area post-PMBV[30]
Use of the double-balloon technique[30]	Previous open heart (surgical) commissurotomy[30,41]
Higher echocardiographic group[30]	Immediate post-PMBV mean PAP (cutoff >25 mm Hg) predicts mitral reintervention[42]
Commissural calcium grade 2/3[27,28]	Increasing preprocedural and postprocedural MR[43]
Wilkins score >8[3,23]	Wilkins score >8[32,41]
Valvular calcification and severe subvalvular lesions[3]	Post-PMBV mitral regurgitation ≥ 3+[41]
Previous commissurotomy[1]	Older age[44]
Baseline mitral regurgitation[1]	NYHA functional class IV[41]
	Pre-PMBV mitral regurgitation ≥ 2+[41]
	Higher post-PMBV pulmonary artery pressure[41]

Abbreviation: PAP, pulmonary artery pressure.

After the SGC is in the LA, the dilator and guidewire are removed.

Advancement of the clip delivery system into the LA

The CDS is placed in the LA under fluoroscopic guidance (see **Fig. 16**). 2D and 3D TEE monitoring are also used to maintain the end of the SGC across the IAS. The location of the CDS and the Clip are imaged continuously to ensure that the tip does not cause injury to the free LA wall. 3D TEE and x-plane imaging are useful to assess the distance of the CDS from the LA wall.

Box 2
Role of echocardiography during percutaneous mitral balloon valvuloplasty

- Reassessment of mitral valve pathology before the procedure (MS and MR) and identification of contraindications (see **Box 1**)
- Guidance of transseptal puncture
- Optimization of balloon placement across the MV orifice
- Assessment of residual MS after PMBV
- Assessment of MR severity after PMBV
- Assessment of complications

Steering and positioning of the MitraClip above the mitral valve

The positioning of the CDS above the mitral valve is best guided by 3D TEE. On 2D TEE medial-lateral Clip adjustments are monitored in the midesophageal intercommissural view and anterior-posterior adjustments in the orthogonal midesophageal long axis view (see **Fig. 17**). The MitraClip needs to be positioned in the LA at the mid portion of the MV leaflets and perpendicular to the line of MV coaptation. This is difficult to confirm with 2D TEE but straightforward with 3D TEE. The MitraClip should also split the regurgitation jet in both orthogonal views, and the tip of the Clip should be directed toward the largest proximal isovelocity surface area (PISA). A short axis transgastric view is used to assess Clip orientation when only 2D TEE imaging is available, as 3D TEE en face view generally allows precise orientation of the MitraClip arms in the LA. As shown in **Fig. 17**, the 3D en face view identifies when the Clip is positioned above the middle segments of the MV and oriented perpendicular to the line of MV coaptation.

Advancing the MitraClip into the LV

Advancing the MitraClip with the Clip arms open into the LV is well seen by fluoroscopy and with x-plane imaging in which the intercommissural view (60°–90°) and the LVOT view (110°–130°)

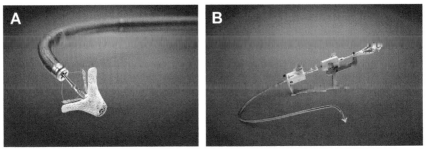

Fig. 10. (*A*) A close-up view showing the Teflon-covered MitraClip arms; the gripper arms are seen below. (*B*) The entire catheter delivery system is shown, and it includes the platform on which the catheter sits during the procedure, the anterior-posterior (A/P) knob, and the mediolateral (M/L) knob. The MitraClip is a 22F system, which fits inside a 24F catheter system. (*Courtesy of* Abbott Vascular, Santa Clara, CA; with permission. CAUTION: Investigational device. Limited by Federal (U.S.) law to investigational use only.)

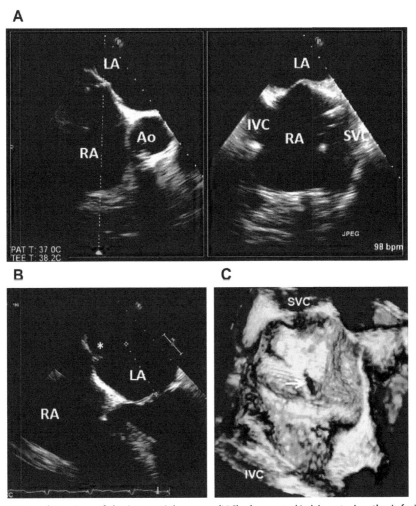

Fig. 11. (*A*) 2D TEE x-plane view of the intraatrial septum (IAS); the aorta (Ao) is anterior, the inferior vena cava (IVC) is caudal, and the superior vena cava (SVC) is cephalad. (*B*) The distance from the transseptal (TS) needle to the mitral annular plane is measured for optimal TS puncture site for the MitraClip (*asterisk*). It is more superior (≥4 cm) in degenerative mitral regurgitation (MR) and more apical (3.5–4 cm) with functional MR. Indentation from the TS needle (*asterisk*) is shown as well as in a (*C*) 3D en face view of the left atrium (LA) showing a left atrial aspect of the IAS immediately after a MitraClip procedure (*white arrow* marks the slitlike residual IAS defect after the TS puncture). RA, right atrium.

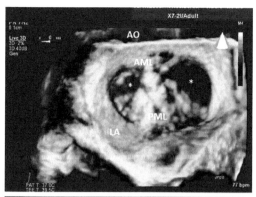

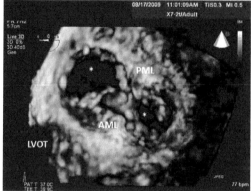

Fig. 12. 3D TEE images of the mitral valve after the MitraClip procedure from the atrial (*top*) and ventricular (*bottom*) views. Note the double orifices (*asterisk*). AML, anterior mitral leaflet; Ao, aorta; LA, left atrium; LVOT, left ventricular outflow tract; PML, posterior mitral leaflet.

Box 3
Echocardiographic parameters essential for evaluation before, during, and after MitraClip implantation

- Quantification of mitral valve morphology and MR severity
- Guidance of the MitraClip system during the procedure
- Assessing intraprocedural results
- Identification of complications during the procedure
- Assessment of final results post–Clip implantation in regard to MR severity and diastolic gradient
- Follow-up regarding MR severity, residual shunting through the atrial septum at the site of transseptal puncture, and pulmonary artery systolic pressure

---

are simultaneously visualized (see **Fig. 18**). The LVOT view is used to demonstrate and locate the open Clip arms. With the intercommissural view, no parts of the Clip arms should be seen. As demonstrated in **Fig. 18**, fluoroscopy and TEE guide the device across the MV into the LV, where orientation of the Clip arms and CDS are reassessed. As the guiding catheter and Clip may rotate during advancement from the LA to the LV, as shown in **Fig. 18**, 2D transgastric short axis view or 3D imaging from either the LA or the LV is used to reassess the Clip orientation in relation to the mitral valve and the line of coaptation. Using an en face LA view, the gain should be lowered to visualize the Clip in the LV and its orientation relative to the MV.

Grasping of the leaflets and assessment of proper leaflet insertion

As demonstrated in **Fig. 19**A, leaflets are usually grasped using the 2D LVOT view (see **Fig. 19**). The MitraClip is initially closed up to 60°–90°. Full closure is done after demonstrating that there is adequate insertion of both the anterior and posterior leaflets and a reduction in MR severity. Multiple imaging planes are used to assess leaflet insertion. As found in **Fig. 19**A, the posterior leaflet insertion is well seen in the LVOT view, and the anterior and posterior leaflet insertions are well seen in the 4-chamber view (see **Fig. 19**B). Slight rotations of the TEE probe are used to view the leaflet insertion from different angulations. The intercommissural view may help detect chordae tendinae that are entrapped within the Clip. After echo documentation that the leaflets are well inserted and positioned within the Clip and gripper arms along with a reduction in MR, the MitraClip is fully closed.

Assessment of result and MitraClip release

With each MitraClip procedure, the maximal possible reduction of MR should be strived for without creating residual MS (see **Fig. 20**; **Fig. 21**). Confirmation that both leaflets are adequately grasped and inserted in the MitraClip is essential. Placement of a MitraClip creates a tissue bridge between the two leaflets, which separates a medial and a lateral orifice. Identified in **Fig. 20**, the final orifice size and geometry can be evaluated in 3D en face aspects of the mitral valve from the left atrium and the left ventricle. An isosceles tissue triangle indicates uniform and symmetric placement of the MitraClip on both leaflets.

Qualitative and quantitative assessment of MR severity can be difficult due to the double mitral valve orifice (or triple orifice in some cases in which 2 Clips are implanted). There are no validated

Table 6
Assessment of MR severity

	Mild	Moderate	Severe
Qualitative			
MR color flow Doppler	Small central jet <4 cm² or <20% of LA volume	Signs of MR > mild but no criteria for severe MR	Large central jet >40% of LA volume/eccentric wall hugging jet
Proximal isovelocity (PISA)	No or minimal PISA	Signs of MR > mild but no criteria for severe MR	Large PISA
CW Doppler signal of MR jet	Non–echo dense/parabolic	Echo dense/parabolic	Dense/late systolic cutoff
Semiquantitative			
Vena contracta width (cm)	<0.3 cm	Signs of MR > mild but no criteria for severe MR	≥0.7 cm
Pulmonary vein flow	Systolic dominant flow	Intermediate signs	Blunted S-wave or systolic flow reversal
Mitral inflow	Dominant A-wave	Intermediate signs	Dominant E-wave (>1.2 m/s)
LA/LV size	Normal LV size	Intermediate signs	Enlarged LA and/or LV
Quantitative			
Regurgitant volume (R Vol) (mL/beat)	<30	Mild-moderate: 30–44 Moderate-severe: 45–59	≥60
Regurgitant fraction (%)	<30	Mild-moderate: 30–39 Moderate-severe: 40–49	>50
Effective regurgitant orifice area (cm²)	<0.2	Mild-moderate: 0.2–0.29 Moderate-severe: 0.3–0.39	≥0.4

studies or guidelines to grade severity of residual MR after Clip implantation. The authors use color flow, pulsed wave, and CW Doppler in concert to assess residual MR.[10,11,50]

At least trivial residual MR is always present post-MitraClip implantation. Color jet area is larger with multiple jets, commonly seen after a MitraClip procedure. There is potential to overestimate residual MR with multiple jets.[60] As the MitraClip is echo dense, it can cause artifacts and affect assessment of residual MR. The presence of small color jets, even if multiple, is generally consistent with mild MR.

Hemodynamically significant MR reduction reduces LA pressure. As seen in **Fig. 21**, pulmonary vein systolic flow reversal (if present pre-Clip) disappears and the S-wave should become more pronounced or even dominant with a successful Clip procedure.

Vena contracta and PISA methods have not been validated to assess MR severity post-MitraClip due to multiple jets and affected MV

orifice. Regurgitant volume in the absence of aortic regurgitation and ventricular septal defects can be calculated by subtracting the forward flow (velocity-time integral derived in the LVOT × LVOT area) from the total stroke volume (end-diastolic volume − end-systolic volume) for quantification of MR.[61] For LV volumes, 3D acquisition is reported to be superior to 2D.[57] Recent studies indicate that 3D echo has potential to quantify MR in the presence of irregularly shaped vena contracta areas; however, this needs further validation.[62,63] Evaluation of the severity of residual MR is supplemented by the catheterization laboratory data. With a reduction in MR, there is a decline in the LA or pulmonary capillary wedge pressure (PCWP) V wave, improved stroke volume, and reduced MR by contrast left ventriculography.

The mitral valve gradient is evaluated after each MV Clip to prevent the creation of significant MS. A transvalvular mean gradient of 5 mm Hg or less by CW Doppler is acceptable. Planimetry of the new orifices is done with 2D or standard transgastric

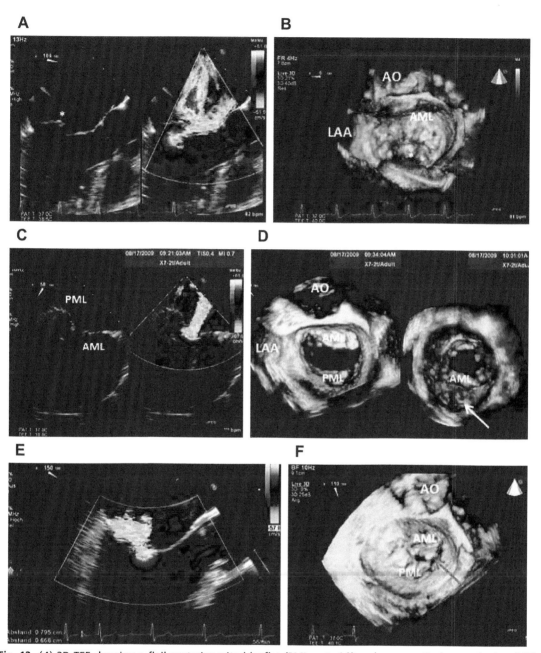

Fig. 13. (*A*) 2D TEE showing a flail posterior mitral leaflet (PML, *asterisk*) and severe mitral regurgitation (MR) confirmed by (*B*) 3D TEE demonstrating a flail midportion of the posterior leaflet (P2) (*asterisk*). (*C*) 2D TEE showing a dilated globular left ventricle and severe central MR. (*D*) 3D TEE confirms normal mitral valve leaflet morphology, but the LV 3D view suggests some restriction of the PML (*arrow* pointing at the left ventricular outflow tract). (*E*) 2D TEE long axis view showing severe MR with a large PISA and vena contracta and a posteriorly directed jet. (*F*) 3D TEE confirms prolapse of the anterior mitral leaflet (AML, *blue arrow*). Ao, aorta; LAA, left atrial appendage.

short axis view 3D TEE. If the sum of the planimetered orifices gives an area of less than 1.5 cm^2, this is criteria for significant MS.[46,49] After MitraClip deployment, there does not seem to be progression of MS based on a 2-year follow-up study.[64,65]

In cases with greater than 2+ MR, an additional Clip may be placed if the gradient is less than 3 to 4 mm Hg or the Clip can be moved to a more optimal site. After Clip deployment, MR needs to be reassessed as changes in MR can occur after

Table 7
Morphologic characterization for MitraClip eligibility

Ideal Valve Morphology for a MitraClip Procedure	Unsuitable Valve Morphology for a MitraClip Procedure
MR originating from the midportion of the valve (degenerative or functional etiology)	Perforated mitral leaflets or clefts Lack of primary and secondary chordal support
Lack of calcification in the grasping area	Severe calcification in the grasping area
Mitral valve area >4 cm²	Hemodynamically relevant mitral stenosis
Length of posterior leaflet ≥10 mm	Length of posterior leaflet <7 mm
Nonrheumatic or endocarditic valve disease	Rheumatic valve disease—with restriction in systole and diastole (Carpentier IIIa) or endocarditic valve disease
Flail width <15 mm Flail gap <10 mm	
Sufficient leaflet tissue for mechanical coaptation: Coaptation depth <11 mm Coaptation length >2 mm	Gap between the leaflets >2 mm

Adapted from the EVEREST criteria and the Abbott training center experience.

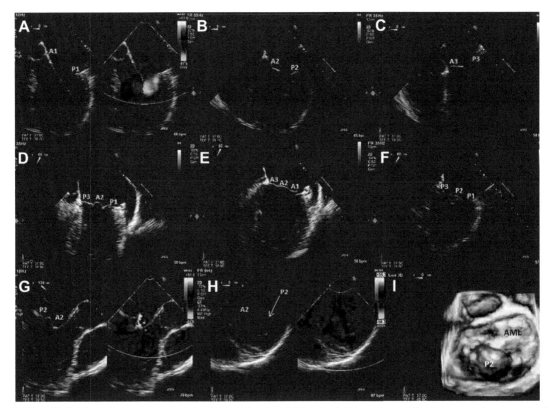

Fig. 14. 2D TEE imaging to evaluate mitral regurgitation (MR) morphology. Panels (*A–C*) show each segment of the anterior and posterior leaflet as described in the text. In the 5- and 4-chamber views, (*D–F*) show the bicommissural view for evaluating the anterior leaflet when the transducer is rotated clockwise and counterclockwise to bring out the leaflets. (*G*) Long axis 3-chamber view demonstrates clearly the midportion of the anterior and posterior leaflet (A2, P2). (*H*) The transgastric view demonstrates all segments of the anterior and posterior leaflets as well as the line of coaptation (*arrow* pointing to P2). (*I*) A single 3D TEE view demonstrates that it can be used to supplant the multiple imaging planes of 2D to identify the prolapsed middle scallop of the posterior leaflet.

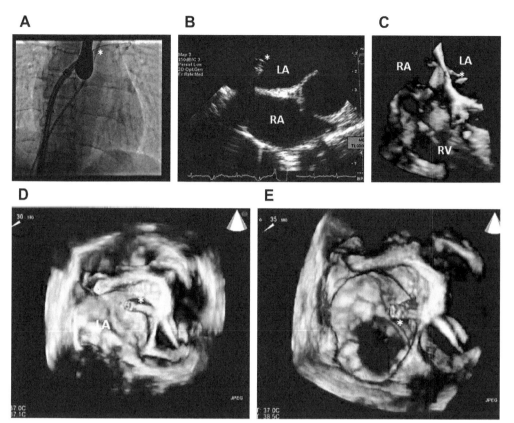

Fig. 15. (*A*) Fluoroscopic, (*B*) 2D TEE, and (*C–E*) 3D TEE images show advancement of the guide catheter (*asterisk*) into the left atrium (LA). RA, right atrium; RV, right ventricle.

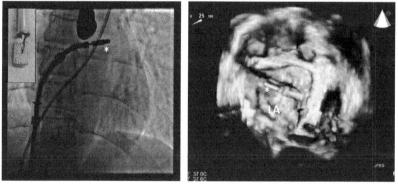

Fig. 16. (*Left*) Fluoroscopy and (*right*) 3D TEE show the advancement of the MitraClip (*upper left box*) into the left atrium (LA).

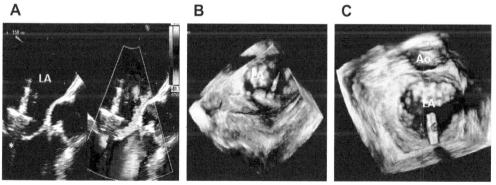

Fig. 17. (*A*) 2D TEE and (*B, C*) 3D TEE showing the MitraClip (*asterisk*) in the left atrium (LA). (*B*) The MitraClip is not in the midportion of the mitral valve (MV) or perpendicular to the MV line of coaptation. (*C*) After catheter manipulation, the Clip is now perfectly aligned. Ao, aorta.

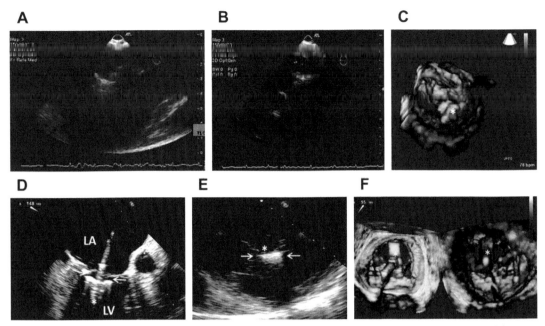

Fig. 18. The Clip (*asterisk*) is shown advanced into the left ventricle (LV) by (*A, B*) 2D TEE and (*C*) 3D TEE. (*B*) 2D TEE short axis view and (*C*) 3D view from the LV, which show the Clip to be perpendicular to the MV line of coaptation. (*D*) Long axis TEE view showing the valve at the time of grasping of the leaflets. (*E*) Short axis view and (*F*) 3D TEE also showing grasping of the anterior and posterior mitral valve leaflets (*arrows* show clip and leaflets in contact). LA, left atrium.

the Clip is released as the tension on the MV and the Clip changes when the CDS is released.

Additional MitraClip Implantation

During placement of a second MitraClip, its orientation in the LA is optimized by 2D or 3D echocardiography. The Clip is closed before advancing into the LV to avoid any interference or entanglement with chordae tendinae. The Clip is reopened in the LV. Fluoroscopy is helpful in positioning of a second MitraClip, as it should be aligned as parallel as possible to the first Clip. Entrapment of leaflet tissue between 2 MitraClips should be avoided, as this may cause uncorrectable residual MR.

ASSESSMENT OF COMPLICATIONS

The MitraClip is a safe procedure with low morbidity and mortality.[46,48,49] The most frequent complications are listed in **Table 8**.

PARAVALVULAR MITRAL LEAKS

The development of a PVL following cardiac valve surgery is one of the most frequent causes for reoperation.[66] It is generally due to a dehisced

suture or a complication of infected endocarditis. Sixty percent of PVLs occur in the first year after surgery,[67] with subsequent risk decreasing to between 0.06% and 5.4%.[68–72]

PVLs can be isolated, or multiple, and can occur in association with any valve type.[44,73–82] Most of the leaks remain small and asymptomatic[83] and even spontaneous closure of PVLs has been described, induced by fibrosis of the valve annulus.[84]

Clinically significant PVLs after surgical valve replacement are reported to occur in 1% to 5% of patients.[85–88] Clinically relevant PVMLs occur most frequently in association with mechanical mitral prostheses, and they are located most frequently in the mitral commissural areas (76%).[83,89,90]

TEE for localizing and closing PVLs is critical. 3D TEE is the optimal way to assess a PVL preprocedure, intraprocedure, and postprocedure.[91–94]

3D assessment in real-time provides en face views of the cardiac valves, allowing complete and adequate evaluation of the 3D character of PVLs in a single view. The size of the defects and location with respect to surrounding cardiac structures can usually be identified. This information is crucial for determining the approach, as well as device size and shape for closure. 3D TEE evaluation of such leaks often demonstrates

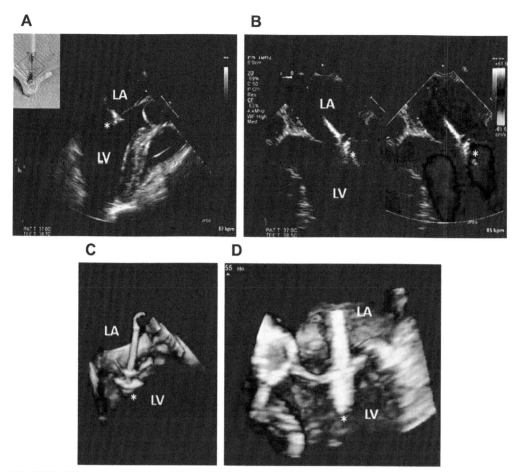

Fig. 19. (A) 2D TEE long axis view and (B) 4-chamber view during grasping of the mitral valve leaflets. The posterior leaflet insertion is well seen in (A and B), and the anterior leaflet insertion is better seen in the 4-chamber view. The 3D images (C, D) also confirm insertion of both leaflets. LA, left atrium; LV, left ventricle. A photo example of an open MitraClip is shown in the left upper box in (A). *Asterisks* represent the tip of the MitraClip in the LV.

oval or slitlike lesions and a larger extent of the defect than is seen by conventional 2D TEE.

Surgical repair of PVLs had been the standard treatment. However, as shown in **Table 9**, there is substantial increase in mortality and recurrence of PVLs with each reoperation.[95,96]

The first successfully performed percutaneous PVL closure was reported in 1992 by Hourihan and colleagues.[97] They used a double-umbrella Rashkind occluder device in 7 patients.

Case reports and small series that used a broad spectrum of different devices (the most frequently used are listed in **Table 10**) documented variable clinical outcomes (54%–100%) and technical success rates in a range from 63% to 100%.[85,98–106]

PARAVALVULAR MITRAL LEAK CLOSURE
Preprocedural Assessment

TEE is mandatory to identify the PVLs and to characterize the location, number, and shape of the PVLs, as paravalvular MR may be missed on TTE because of artifacts and reverberations caused by MV prosthesis. The leaks typically have an irregular shape.[107–109] An assessment in multiple angles including off-axis views is crucial to determine the exact location and severity of the regurgitation. The characteristic feature of a PVL is a color Doppler flow jet outside of the sewing ring of the implanted valve. To define the severity of a PVML, the MR jet width at its origin is measured. Vitarelli and colleagues[110] suggested 1 to 2 mm

A   **B**

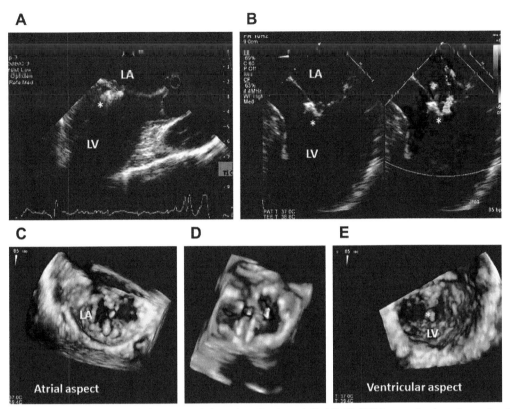

C   **D**   **E**

Atrial aspect   Ventricular aspect

Fig. 20. Images obtained postdeployment of the MitraClip (*asterisk*). (*A*) 2D TEE long axis view shows the Clip connecting the anterior and posterior mitral leaflets, also seen in the (*B*) 5-chamber view. (*C–E*) 3D TEE showing the Clip from the (*C, D*) atrial aspect and minimal mitral regurgitation and (*E*) showing the double orifice after the Clip deployment. LA, left atrium; LV, left ventricle.

for mild, 3 to 6 mm for moderate and greater than 6 mm to define a severe PVL. A multimodal approach including semiquantitative and quantitative parameters similar to those used for the evaluation of native valves[10,11,50] is also used, but the jets are frequently eccentric, thus, complicating assessment and quantification.

3D TEE improves the detection, location, and assessment of shape and size of PVMLs as well as guidance for PVML closure.[111–113] TEE plays an essential role during PVML closure by guiding the preferred TS puncture site, facilitating passage of wires and catheters across the PVML, providing navigation of catheters and guides in the LA or LV to approach the PVMLs, verifying correct canalization of the target lesions, sizing the defect, and positioning of the devices before deployment. A comprehensive evaluation of the procedural outcome includes the confirmation of normal mechanical valve function after device placement, the assessment of residual PV leakage, and the prompt detection of complications. The additional information rendered by 3D TEE (more precise evaluation of location and extent of the defects; facilitated wire, catheter, and device maneuvering and positioning; and a more comprehensive assessment of PVML severity postprocedure) may help avoiding complications such as suboptimal occluder alignment, malpositioning, or interference with neighboring structures and may shorten procedure times.

Box 4
Major steps for MitraClip implantation

1. TS puncture

2. Introduction of the steerable guide catheter into the LA

3. Advancement of the Clip delivery system into the LA

4. Steering and positioning of the MitraClip above the mitral valve

5. Advancing the MitraClip into the LV

6. Grasping of the leaflets and assessment of proper leaflet insertion

7. Clip detachment

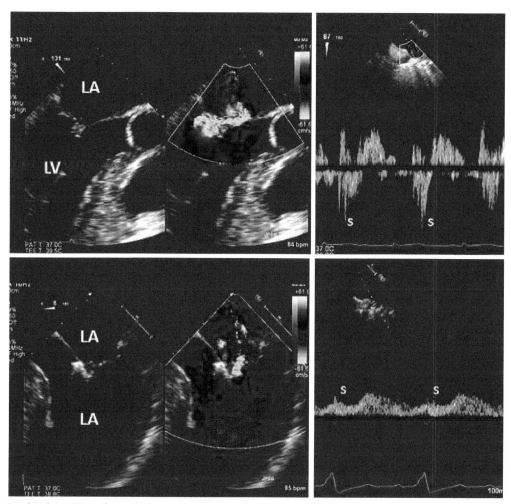

Fig. 21. (*Top*) Pre-MitraClip and (*Bottom*) post-MitraClip 2D TEE images showing (*top left*) severe mitral regurgitation with pulmonary vein systolic flow reversal (*top right*, S). After MitraClip deployment, the severe MR and flow reversal resolved (*bottom left and right*, respectively). LA, left atrium; LV, left ventricle.

The 3D TEE in **Fig. 22** illustrates the surgical view of the MV prostheses from an LA aspect. Communication between the echocardiologist and interventionalist is facilitated by referring to the MV prosthesis as a clock face, as seen in **Fig. 22**. In the surgical view, the aorta (at 12-o'clock position, anterior), the IAS, the fossa ovalis (at 3-o'clock position, medial), and the ostium of the LA appendage (at 9-o'clock position, lateral) serve as landmarks. Posterior is defined to be opposite of anterior (6-o'clock position), and the segments in between are defined as anterolateral, anteromedial, posterolateral, and posteromedial. The shape and the extent of the PVML in the anteromedial position can be assessed in detail.

TEE also helps to evaluate contraindications to percutaneous PVML closure. Patients with a mechanical instability of the prosthetic mitral valve causing a movement of the valve during the cardiac cycle ("rocking valve") (**Fig. 23**), patients in whom the PVML is too large to be percutaneously repaired (the authors do not recommend closing leaks >30% of the valve circumference), or patients with signs of active endocarditis or an intracardiac thrombus should not be considered as candidates for a percutaneous closure procedure. The morphologic evaluation of PV mitral leakages in a posterior location is shown in **Fig. 24**.

Intraprocedural Guidance

To date, there are no guidelines or randomized trials to indicate best practice for PVML closure. Consequently, the technical approach and results

Table 8
Complications that can result from the MitraClip procedure

Complication	Etiology	Treatment/Prevention
Pericardial effusion/tamponade	Transseptal puncture, guidewire or catheter perforation of the LA and LV	Pericardial drainage
Air embolism	Presence of large sheaths that allows air into the venous circulation	Aspiration and flushing of catheter as well as keeping catheter hub lower than the level of heart during catheter insertion or removal
Thrombus formation on the catheter	Presence of foreign objects that predispose to thrombus formation	Maintain ACT of between 250 and 300 s.
Partial Clip detachment	Inappropriate positioning or device malfunction	Appropriate echo guidance, careful assessment of leaflet insertion
Atrial and ventricular arrhythmias	Guidewire or catheter mechanical stimulation	Routine ECG monitoring during the procedure
Entrapment of chordae tendinae by the MitraClip	Inappropriate positioning	Use TEE to carefully monitor catheter and MitraClip position in the LV
Persistent ASD	Iatrogenic due to large size of MitraClip system	Most small and require no treatment; however, if there is SPo_2 desaturation due to left-to-right shunting, the defect should be closed at time of the procedure

Abbreviation: ACT, activated clotting time.

of each procedure are case dependent and may even vary for different lesions in the same patient.

During the procedure, continuous hemodynamic and electrocardiographic (ECG) monitoring is important, as wires or catheters that are advanced through a mechanical prosthesis may cause hemodynamic compromise or ventricular tachycardia once introduced into the left ventricle. The procedures are also guided by fluoroscopy (planes that show the valve in orthogonal projections are the most useful for device implantation)

in combination with continuous 2D and 3D TEE monitoring. If available, preacquired computed tomographic angiographic images (4D reconstructions) are displayed in the catheterization laboratory adjacent to the fluoroscopic images to help with probing of the defects and guiding LV puncture when a transapical approach is used.[106] To guide the procedure adequately, knowledge of the different approaches to mitral PVL closure is needed. The different access ways are illustrated in **Fig. 25**.

In most cases, the defect is probed antegradely (see **Fig. 25**A) using a femoral vein access and standard TS puncture techniques to gain entrance into the LA. Alternatively, a TS approach via an internal jugular vein may be preferable in case the leak is located close to the IAS (medial) (see **Fig. 25**A, dashed arrow). The PVML is probed with an end-hole diagnostic right or left Judkins coronary catheter and a hydrophilic 0.035-in wire (occasionally a narrower gauge wire may be helpful). Once across the lesion, a stiffer exchange length guidewire replaces the hydrophilic wire, and a delivery sheath of appropriate size is

Table 9
Recurrence and mortality rates associated with each reoperation for paravalvular leak

Reoperation	Recurrence Rate (%)	Mortality (%)
1st	8	13
2nd	20	15
3rd	42	37

Table 10
Most often used devices for paravalvular mitral leak closure (all used off-label)

Device	Shape of Device	Device Deployment
Amplatzer devices (AGA Medical, MN, USA):		
Septal occluder	Round	Either antegrade or retrograde
Muscular VSD occluder	Round	Either antegrade or retrograde
Duct occluder	Round	Only antegrade
Vascular plugs	Round	Either antegrade or retrograde
Amplatzer vascular plug III (AVP III) occluder	Oval	Either antegrade or retrograde
Vascular coils	Round	Either antegrade or retrograde

Abbreviation: VSD, ventricular septal defect.

advanced into the left ventricle. The proximal disc of the device is opened in the left ventricle; then, the device is pulled back to the ventricular side of the prosthetic valve ring. Once TEE (2D and 3D) and fluoroscopic imaging confirm proper position and orientation of the ventricular aspect of the device, the LA disc is deployed. In cases in which greater stability is needed during the delivery sheath advancement, a circuit is created by snaring the wire in the LA from the LV side via the

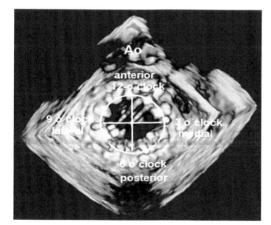

Fig. 22. En face surgical view from the left atrium of a prosthetic mitral valve (RT 3DTEE). The aorta (Ao) is seen at the 12-o'clock position (anterior), at the 3-o'clock position the fossa ovalis (medial) can be seen, the 6-o'clock position is posterior, and the 9-o'clock position (where the left atrial appendage is located) is lateral. The segments in between can be described as anteromedial, anterolateral, posteromedial, and posterolateral. An oval PVML can be seen in the anteromedial position adjacent to the ring of the prosthetic St. Jude Medical valve. ant.lat., anterolateral; ant.med., anteromedial; IAS, intraatrial septum; post.lat., posterolateral; post.med., posteromedial.

femoral artery, thus, creating an arteriovenous loop. The device is then deployed in the way described earlier.

If a retrograde approach is used (see **Fig. 25**B) (eg, in cases in which severe paravalvular regurgitation prevents defect crossing via an antegrade approach), femoral artery access allows a guidewire and support catheter (eg, right coronary Judkins 4.0 or multipurpose catheter) to be advanced across the aortic valve. The PVML is then probed with a long hydrophilic wire. In the next step, the guidewire is snared in the left atrium via TS access and externalized via a femoral vein to provide better support. A delivery sheath is then advanced over the wire through the defect, and the LA disc of the selected device is deployed first. Subsequently, the device is pulled back to the prosthetic valve ring, and if it permits proper device placement and orientation, the LV disc is deployed. With retrograde access, meticulous care is needed not to damage structures located in the left ventricle such as trabeculae, papillary muscles, or chordae. Transapical access (see **Fig. 25**C) is used for defects that cannot be crossed by an antegrade or retrograde approach.[114] Ruiz and colleagues[106] described transapical access as being preferable for patients with PVMLs located along the IAS.

The 2D and 3D TEE monitoring of the procedural steps are illustrated in **Fig. 26**.

Postprocedural Assessment

Immediately after device placement, 2D and 3D TEE are used to assess device position, device stability, and interaction with adjacent structures (eg, mechanical valve leaflet obstruction).

A residual leak and the degree of residual regurgitation should be assessed using a multimodal imaging approach according to current

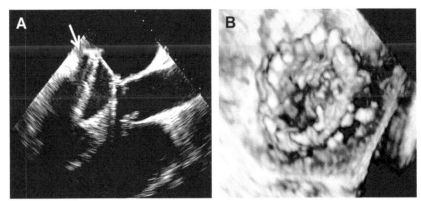

Fig. 23. Example of a nonsuitable patient for PVML closure: (*A*) A long axis view (100°) reveals a large dehiscence between the mitral annulus and the prosthetic mitral valve (*white arrow*) in the posterior location. (*B*) The 3D view from the LA confirms a large PVML, nearly half the circumference is ruptured, thus indicating that this is not a candidate for PVML closure.

guidelines.[10,11,50] Quantification of the paravalvular regurgitation can be achieved by using a volumetric assessment of regurgitation volumes and regurgitant fraction.[61] Complications have to be detected promptly. In **Table 11**, the most frequent complications occurring during PVML closure, their causes, and their prevention/treatment are summarized.

Postprocedural follow-up studies should include ECG, TTE, TEE, and assessment for hemolysis.

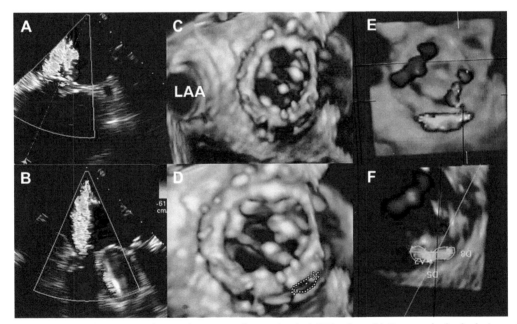

Fig. 24. Evaluation of a patient after implantation of a mechanical SJM valve with 3 paravalvular leaks in posterior location with 2D TEE and 3D TEE modalities (Philips iE33 including QLAB analysis). In (*A*), an intercommissural 2D TEE view (65°) is shown, and in (*B*), the corresponding long axis x-plane view (155°) showing a color flow jet posteriorly next to the prosthetic valve ring. In (*C*), the posterior leaks are presented in an en face view from the LA side, thus allowing a more detailed analysis and clarifying that 3 leaks separated by small tissue bridges are present; in (*D*), the direct delineation of one of the defects in an RT 3D TEE still frame image is shown. A full volume acquisition with color Doppler demonstrates the extension of the color jet adjacent to the prosthetic ring in (*E*), and in (*F*) the QLAB analysis of the regurgitant area is seen. LA, left atrium; LAA, left atrial appendage.

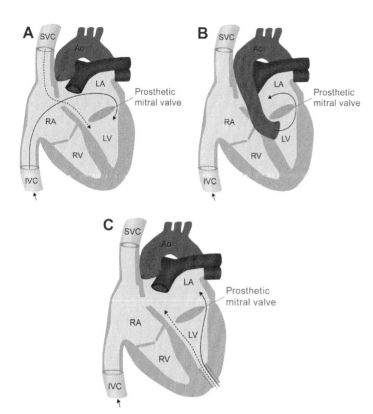

Fig. 25. Different approaches to PVML closure. (*A*) Antegrade approach via a transseptal access either from the femoral vein (*black arrow*) or from the jugular vein (*dashed black arrow*). (*B*) Retrograde access via a femoral artery and the aorta into the LV and through the PVML into the LA (the wire can be snared in the LA to create an arteriovenous loop). (*C*) Transapical access. Ao, aorta; IVC, inferior vena cava; LA, left atrium; LV, left ventricle; RA, right atrium; RV, right ventricle; SVC, superior vena cava.

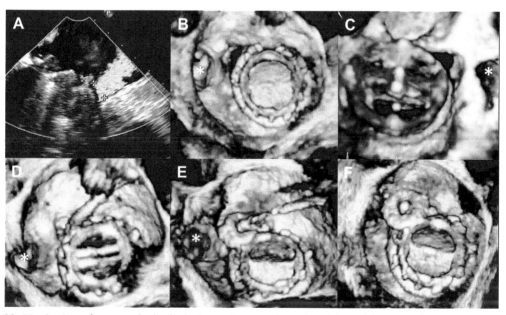

Fig. 26. Monitoring of a paravalvular leak closure in anterolateral position with a muscular ventricular septal defect occluder using an antegrade approach (the entrance of the LAA is marked with a white star). (*A*) 2D TEE (125°): The measurement of the width of the color jet through the defect is shown; (*B*) left atrial aspect of the defect in an en face view; (*C*) left ventricular aspect of the defect in an en face view; (*D*) the delivery catheter is advanced antegradely through the defect (LA aspect); (*E*) (LA aspect) both occluder discs are deliberated, and the LA disc can be identified. The device is still attached to the delivery cable (*F*) left atrial en face view showing the final device position. LA, left atrium; LAA, left atrial appendage.

Table 11
Complications that can occur from paravalvular mitral leak closure

Complication	Etiology	Treatment/Prevention
Pericardial effusion/ tamponade	Transseptal puncture, guidewire or catheter perforation of LA and LV	Pericardial drainage, surgery if needed
Air embolism	Presence of large sheaths that allow air into the circulation	Aspiration and flushing of catheter as well as keeping catheter hub lower than the level of heart during catheter insertion or removal
Thrombus formation either intracardiac or attached to wires/catheters	Presence of foreign material, which predispose to thrombus formation	Maintain ACT of between 250 and 300 s
Failure to cross the leak with the delivery sheath	Severe friction	Usage of hydrophilic sheaths, change of wire
Difficulty to probe the lesions	Difficult 3-dimensional navigation in large cardiac chambers	Usage of a steerable (eg, Agilis, St. Jude Medical) sheath that can be orientated toward the defect under real-time 3D TEE imaging guidance
Atrial and ventricular arrhythmias	Guidewire or catheter mechanical stimulation	Routine ECG monitoring during the procedure
Interference with valve leaflets	Deployed occluder constrains the valve mechanically	Appropriate echo guidance; repositioning of the device leads occasionally to satisfactory results; if this is not the case, surgery should be considered
Wire entrapment	Inappropriate positioning	Use TEE to carefully monitor catheter and wire position
Persistent residual leak	Due to mismatch of the device and defect shapes, additional leaks or delayed or even absent endothelialization[115]	An additional PVML closure procedure may be considered, alternatively surgery
Mitral leaflet erosion	Described by frame fractures of the device[116]	Surgical repair
Device-related infection	Any implanted foreign body is associated with the risk of device-related infection	Prevention: periinterventional administration of antibiotics If an infection occurs, in most cases the surgical device removal and valvular replacement or repair is necessary
Hemolysis	Occurs most likely shortly after the procedure (multiple and smaller wholes are more frequently associated with hemolysis)	Blood transfusion if necessary, monitoring; with ongoing endothelialization hemolysis may decrease over time. If it persists, a second closure procedure or surgical repair should be considered
Persistent ASD	Iatrogenic due to transseptal sheath	Most remain small and require no treatment
Device embolization	Unsecure position of the device due to a mismatch of the device size and the defect	Snares with large loop diameters (25–40 mm) should be close at hand to capture and retrieve the occluder (eg, Amplatz Goose Neck, eV3, MN, USA, or Lassos, Dr. Osypka, Germany). Rarely surgical removal may be necessary

Abbreviation: ACT, activated clotting time.

SUMMARY

As the mitral leaflets cannot be assessed by fluoroscopy, preprocedural assessment, procedural guidance, and postprocedural assessment of percutaneous mitral interventions for MS, MR, and MV PVLs rely heavily on echocardiography. Although 2D TEE has played a major role in guidance of the procedures, 3D TEE provides more detailed information on the MV anatomy and catheter and device position. Thus, combining 2D and 3D TEE improves results and reduces procedure time. Consequently, there is an increasing reliance on 3D TEE for mitral interventions.[57,117] A newly developed EchoNavigator system (Philips Healthcare, Andover, MA) may further facilitate procedural guidance by matching echocardiographic and fluoroscopic images. The EchoNavigator system is based upon technology that automatically recognizes and tracks the position of the TEE probe. Although only limited clinical data are available at this time, these new features of the Echo-Navigator system may facilitate guidance of the procedure by supporting the understanding of the spatial relation between the echo and x-ray image, thus making the interpretation and understanding of anatomic structures rendered by TEE easier. Echocardiography during percutaneous mitral valve procedures has evolved from transthoracic 2D echo guidance of PBMV to more complex procedures such as MitraClip and repair of PVLs. Imaging technology is continuing to evolve and improve. At present, 3D TEE and fluoroscopy are essential for the optimal guidance and outcomes of transcatheter MV procedures.

REFERENCES

1. Iung B, Cormier B, Ducimetiere P, et al. Immediate results of percutaneous mitral commissurotomy. A predictive model on a series of 1514 patients. Circulation 1996;94:2124–30.
2. Palacios IF. Farewell to surgical mitral commissurotomy for many patients. Circulation 1998;97:223–6.
3. Hung JS, Chern MS, Wu JJ, et al. Short and long-term results of catheter balloon percutaneous transvenous mitral commissurotomy. Am J Cardiol 1991;67:854–62.
4. Dean LS, Mickel M, Bonan R, et al. Four-year follow-up of patients undergoing percutaneous balloon mitral commissurotomy: a report from the National Heart, Lung, and Blood Institute Balloon Valvuloplasty Registry. J Am Coll Cardiol 1996;28:1452–7.
5. Abascal VM, Wilkins GT, Choong CY, et al. Echocardiographic evaluation of mitral valve structure and function in patients followed for at least 6 months after percutaneous balloon mitral valvuloplasty. J Am Coll Cardiol 1988;12:606–15.
6. Post JR, Feldman T, Isner J, et al. Inoue balloon mitral valvotomy in patients with severe valvular and subvalvular deformity. J Am Coll Cardiol 1995;25:1129–36.
7. Hernandez R, Banuelos C, Alfonso F, et al. Long-term clinical and echocardiographic follow-up after percutaneous mitral valvuloplasty with the Inoue balloon. Circulation 1999;99:1580–6.
8. Iung BL, Garbarz E, Michaud P, et al. Late results of percutaneous mitral commissurotomy in a series of 1024 patients: analysis of late clinical deterioration: frequency, anatomic findings and predictive factors. Circulation 1999;99:3272–8.
9. Chen CR, Cheng TO, Chen JY, et al. Long-term results of percutaneous balloon mitral valvuloplasty for mitral stenosis: a follow-up study to 11 years in 202 patients. Cathet Cardiovasc Diagn 1998;43:132–9.
10. Borger MA, Carrel TP, DeBonis M, et al. Guidelines on the management of valvular heart disease (version 2012) the Joint Task Force on the Management of Valvular Heart Disease of the European Society of Cardiology (ESC) and the European Association for Cardio-Thoracic Surgery (EACTS). Eur Heart J 2012;33:2451–96. http://dx.doi.org/10.1093/eurheartj/ehs109.
11. Bonow RO, Carabello BA, Chatterjee K, et al. American College of Cardiology/American Heart Association Task Force on Practice Guidelines. 2008 focused update incorporated into the ACC/ACC 2006 guidelines for the management of patients with valvular heart disease: a report of the American College of Cardiology/American Heart Association Task Force on Practice Guidelines/Writing Committee to revise the 1998 guidelines for the management of patients with valvular heart disease). Endorsed by the Society of Cardiovascular Anesthesiologists, Society for Cardiovascular Angiography and Interventions and Society of Thoracic Surgeons. J Am Coll Cardiol 2008;52(13):e1–142.
12. Vahanian A, Baumgartner H, Bax J, et al. Guidelines on the management of valvular heart disease of the European Society of Cardiology. Eur Heart J 2007;28:230–68.
13. Wood P. An appreciation of mitral stenosis. I: Clinical features. Br Med J 1954;4870:1051.
14. Rowe JC, Bland EF, Sprague HB, et al. The course of mitral stenosis without surgery: ten- and twenty-year perspectives. Ann Intern Med 1960;52:741–9.
15. Baumgartner H, Hung J, Bermejo J, et al. Echocardiographic assessment of valve stenosis: EAE/ASE recommendations for clinical practice. J Am Soc Echocardiogr 2009;22(1):1–23.
16. Faletra F, Pezzano A Jr, Fusco R, et al. Measurement of mitral valve area in mitral stenosis: four

echocardiographic measurements compared with direct measurements of anatomic orifices. J Am Coll Cardiol 1996;28:1190–7.

17. Min SY, Song JM, Kim YJ, et al. Discrepancy between mitral valve areas measured by two-dimensional planimetry and three dimensional transesophageal echocardiography in patients with mitral stenosis. Heart 2013;99(4):253–8.

18. Schlosshan D, Aggarwal G, Mathur G, et al. Real-time 3D transesophageal echocardiography for the evaluation of rheumatic mitral valve stenosis. J Am Coll Cardiol 2011;4(6):580–8.

19. Sugeng L, Weinert L, Lammertin G, et al. Accuracy of mitral valve area measurements using transthoracic rapid freehand 3-dimensional scanning: comparison with noninvasive and invasive measurements. J Am Soc Echocardiogr 2003;16(12):1292–300.

20. Thomas JD, Newell JB, Choong CY, et al. Physical and physiological determinants of transmitral velocity: numerical analysis. Am J Physiol 1991; 260(5 Pt 2):H1718–31.

21. Nishimura RA, Rihal CS, Tajik AJ, et al. Accurate measurement of the transmitral gradient in patients with mitral stenosis: a simultaneous catheterization and Doppler echocardiographic study. J Am Coll Cardiol 1994;24:152–8.

22. Gorlin R, Gorlin SG. Hydraulic formula for calculation of the area of the stenotic mitral valve, other cardiac valves, and central circulatory shunts. Am Heart J 1951;41:1–29.

23. Wilkins GT, Weyman AE, Abascal VM, et al. Percutaneous balloon dilatation of the mitral valve: an analysis of echocardiographic variables related to outcome and the mechanism of dilatation. Br Heart J 1988; 60:299–308.

24. Chen CG, Wang X, Wang Y, et al. Value of two-dimensional echocardiography in selecting patients and balloon sizes for percutaneous balloon mitral valvuloplasty. J Am Coll Cardiol 1989;14(7):1651–8.

25. Reid CL, Chandraratna PA, Kawanishi DT, et al. Influence of mitral valve morphology on double-balloon catheter balloon valvuloplasty in patients with mitral stenosis. Analysis of factors predicting immediate and 3-month results. Circulation 1989; 80(3):515–24.

26. Nobuyoshi M, Hamasaki N, Kimura T, et al. Indications, complications, and short-term clinical outcome of percutaneous transvenous mitral commissurotomy. Circulation 1989;80(4):782–92.

27. Cannan CR, Nishimura RA, Reeder GS, et al. Echocardiographic assessment of commissural calcium: a simple predictor of outcome after percutaneous mitral balloon valvotomy. J Am Coll Cardiol 1997; 29:175–80.

28. Sutaria N, Northridge DB, Shaw TR. Significance of commissural calcification on outcome of mitral balloon valvotomy. Heart 2000;84:398–402.

29. Padial LR, Freitas N, Sagie A, et al. Echocardiography can predict which patients will develop severe mitral regurgitation after percutaneous mitral valvotomy. J Am Coll Cardiol 1996;27:1225–31.

30. Iung B, Cormier B, Ducimetiere P, et al. Functional results 5 years after successful percutaneous mitral commissurotomy in a series of 528 patients and analysis of predictive factors. J Am Coll Cardiol 1996;27:407–14.

31. Anwar AM, Attia WM, Nosir YF, et al. Validation of a new score for the assessment of mitral stenosis using real-time three-dimensional echocardiography. J Am Soc Echocardiogr 2010;23(1):13–22.

32. Palacios IF, Sanchez PL, Harrell LC, et al. Which patients benefit from percutaneous mitral balloon valvuloplasty? Prevalvuloplasty and postvalvuloplasty variables that predict long term outcome. Circulation 2002;105:1465–71.

33. Chen CR, Cheng TO. Percutaneous balloon mitral valvuloplasty by the Inoue technique: a multicenter study of 4832 patients in China. Am Heart J 1995; 129:1197–203.

34. Thomas JD, Wilkins GT, Choong CY, et al. Inaccuracy of mitral pressure half-time immediately after percutaneous mitral valvotomy. Dependence on transmitral gradient and left atrial and ventricular compliance. Circulation 1988;78:980–93.

35. Otto CM, Davis KB, Holmes DR, et al. Methodologic issues in clinical evaluation of stenosis severity in adults undergoing aortic or mitral balloon valvuloplasty. Am J Cardiol 1992;69: 1607–16.

36. Reid CL, Rahimtoola SH. The role of echocardiography/Doppler in catheter balloon treatment of adults with aortic and mitral stenosis. Circulation 1991;84:240–9.

37. Vahanian A, Michel PL, Cormier B, et al. Results of percutaneous mitral commissurotomy in 200 patients. Am J Cardiol 1989;63:847–52.

38. Zamorano J, Perez de Isal L, Sugeng L, et al. Noninvasive assessment of mitral valve area during percutaneous balloon mitral valvuloplasty: role of real-time 3D echocardiography. Eur Heart J 2004; 25:2086–91.

39. Messika-Zeitoun D, Blanc J, Lung B, et al. Impact of degree of commissural opening after percutaneous mitral commissurotomy on long-term outcome. JACC Cardiovasc Imaging 2009;2:1–7.

40. Pan M, Medina A, Suarez de Lezo J, et al. Factors determining late success after mitral balloon valvulotomy. Am J Cardiol 1993;71(13):1181–5.

41. Zhang HP, Yen GS, Allen JW, et al. Comparison of late results of balloon valvotomy in mitral stenosis with versus without mitral regurgitation. Am J Cardiol 1998;81:51–5.

42. Jorge E, Baptista R, Faria H, et al. Mean pulmonary arterial pressure after percutaneous mitral

valvuloplasty predicts long-term adverse out-comes. Rev Port Cardiol 2012;31(1):19–25.

43. Jneid H, Cruz-Gonzalez I, Sanchez-Ledesma M, et al. Impact of pre- and postprocedural mitral regurgitation on outcomes after percutaneous mitral valvuloplasty for mitral stenosis. Am J Cardiol 2009;104(8):1122–7.

44. Conte J, Weissman N, Dearani JA, et al. A North American, prospective, multicenter assessment of the Mitroflow aortic pericardial prosthesis. Ann Thorac Surg 2010;90(1):144–152.e1–3.

45. Alfieri O, Maisano F, DeBonis M, et al. The edge-to-edge technique in mitral valve repair: a simple solution for complex problems. J Thorac Cardiovasc Surg 2001;122:674–81.

46. Feldman T, Wasserman HS, Herrmann HC, et al. Percutaneous mitral valve repair using the edge-to-edge technique. Six-month results of the EVEREST Phase I Clinical Trial. J Am Coll Cardiol 2005; 46(11):2134–40.

47. Feldman T, Kar S, Rinaldi M, et al, EVEREST Investigators. Percutaneous mitral repair with the Mitra-Clip system: safety and midterm durability in the initial EVEREST (Endovascular Valve Edge-to-Edge Repair Study) cohort. J Am Coll Cardiol 2009;54(8):686–94.

48. Franzen O, Baldus S, Rudolph V, et al. Acute outcomes of MitraClip therapy for mitral regurgitation in high-surgical-risk patients: emphasis on adverse valve morphology and severe left ventricular dysfunction. Eur Heart J 2010;31:1373–81.

49. Feldman T, Foster E, Glower DD, et al, EVEREST II Investigators. Percutaneous repair or surgery for mitral regurgitation. N Engl J Med 2011;364(15): 1395–406.

50. Lancelotti P, Moura L, Pierard LA, et al. European Association of Echocardiography recommendations for the assessment of valvular regurgitation. Part 2: mitral and tricuspid regurgitation (native valve disease). Eur J Echocardiogr 2010;11: 307–32.

51. Nguyen C, Lee E, Luo H, et al. Echocardiographic guidance for diagnostic and therapeutic procedures. Cardiovasc Diag Ther 2011;1:11–36.

52. La Canna G, Arendar I, Maisano F, et al. Real-time three-dimensional transesophageal echocardiography for assessment of mitral valve functional anatomy in patients with prolapse-related regurgitation. Am J Cardiol 2011;107(9):1365–74.

53. Grewal J, Mankad S, Freeman WK, et al. Real-time three-dimensional transesophageal echocardiography in the intraoperative assessment of mitral valve disease. J Am Soc Echocardiogr 2009; 22(1):34–41.

54. Ben Zekry S, Nagueh SF, Little SH, et al. Comparative accuracy of two- and three-dimensional transthoracic and transesophageal echocardiography in identifying mitral valve pathology in patients undergoing mitral valve repair: initial observations. J Am Soc Echocardiogr 2011;24(10):1079–85.

55. Thompson KA, Shiota T, Tolstrup K, et al. Utility of three-dimensional transesophageal echocardiography in the diagnosis of valvular perforations. Am J Cardiol 2011;107(1):100–2.

56. Salcedo EE, Quaife RA, Seres T, et al. A framework for systematic characterization of the mitral valve by real-time three-dimensional transesophageal echocardiography. J Am Soc Echocardiogr 2009; 22(10):1087–99.

57. Lang RM, Badano LP, Tsang W, et al. EAE/ASE recommendations for image acquisition and display using three-dimensional echocardiography. J Am Soc Echocardiogr 2012;25:3–46.

58. Biner S, Perk G, Kar S, et al. Utility of combined two-dimensional and three-dimensional transesophageal imaging for catheter-based mitral valve clip repair of mitral regurgitation. J Am Soc Echocardiogr 2011;24(6):611–7.

59. Slipczuk L, Siegel RJ, Jilaihawi H, et al. Optimizing procedural outcome in percutaneous mitral valve therapy using transesophageal imaging: a stepwise analysis. Expert Rev Cardiovasc Ther 2012; 10:901–6.

60. Lin BA, Forouhar AS, Pahlevan NM, et al. Color Doppler jet area overestimates regurgitant volume when multiple jets are present. J Am Soc Echocardiogr 2010;23(9):993–1000.

61. Blumlein S, Bouchard A, Schiller NB, et al. Quantitation of mitral regurgitation by Doppler echocardiography. Circulation 1986;74:306–14.

62. Kahlert P, Pflicht B, Schenk IM, et al. Direct measurement of size and shape of non-circular vena contracta in functional versus organic mitral regurgitation using real time 3-dimensional echocardiography. J Am Soc Echocardiogr 2008;21:912–21.

63. Chaim Y, Hung J, Chua S, et al. Direct measurement of vena contracta area by real-time 3-dimensional echocardiography for assessing severity of mitral regurgitation. Am J Cardiol 2009;104:978–83.

64. Herrmann HC, Rohatgi S, Wasserman HS, et al. Mitral valve hemodynamic effects of percutaneous edge-to-edge repair with the MitraClip™ device for mitral regurgitation. Catheter Cardiovasc Interv 2006;68:821–8.

65. Herrmann HC, Kar S, Siegel R, et al. Effect of percutaneous mitral repair with the MitraClip device on mitral valve area and gradient. EuroIntervention 2008;4:437–42.

66. Bernal J, Rabasa J, Gutuerrez-Garcia F, et al. The CarboMedics valve: experience with 1.049 implants. Ann Thorac Surg 1998;65:137–43.

67. Orzulak TA, Schaff HV, Danielson GK, et al. Results of reoperation for periprosthetic leakage. Ann Thorac Surg 1983;35:584–9.

68. Nakano K, Koyanagi H, Hashimoto A, et al. Twelve years experience with St. Jude Medical prosthesis. Ann Thorac Surg 1994;57:697–703.

69. Arom KV, Nicoloff DM, Kersten TE, et al. Ten years experience with St. Jude Medical valve prosthesis. Ann Thorac Surg 1989;47:831–7.

70. Rutledge R, Kim J, Appelbaum R. Actuarial analysis of prosthetic valve endocarditis in 1.598 patients with mechanical and bioprosthetic valves. Arch Surg 1985;120:469–72.

71. Ivert TS, Dismukes WE, Cobbs CG. Prosthetic valve endocarditis. Circulation 1984;69:223–32.

72. Arvay A, Lengyel M. Incidence and risk factors of prosthetic valve endocarditis. Eur J Cardiothorac Surg 1988;2:340–6.

73. Lehmann S, Walther T, Leontyev S, et al. Eight-year follow-up after prospectively randomized implantation of different mechanical aortic valves. Clin Res Cardiol 2008;97(6):376–82.

74. Englberger L, Schaff HV, Jamieson WR, et al. Importance of implant technique on risk of major paravalvular leak (PVL) after St. Jude mechanical heart valve replacement: a report from the Artificial Valve Endocarditis Reduction Trial (AVERT). Eur J Cardiothorac Surg 2005;28(6):838–43.

75. Emery RW, Krogh CC, Arom KV, et al. The St. Jude Medical cardiac valve prosthesis: a 25-year experience with single valve replacement. Ann Thorac Surg 2005;79(3):776–82 [discussion: 782–3].

76. Nitter-Hauge S, Abdelnoor M. Ten-year experience with the Medtronic Hall valvular prosthesis. A study of 1,104 patients. Circulation 1989;80(3 Pt 1):I43–8.

77. Li HH, Hahn J, Urbanski P, et al. Intermediate-term results with 1,019 CarboMedics aortic valves. Ann Thorac Surg 2001;71(4):1181–7 [discussion: 1187–8].

78. Spiliopoulos K, Haschemi A, Parasiris P, et al. Sorin Bicarbon bileaflet valve: a 9.8-year experience. Clinical performance of the prosthesis after heart valve replacement in 587 patients. Interact Cardiovasc Thorac Surg 2009;8(2):252–9.

79. Al-Khaja N, Belboul A, Larsson S, et al. Eleven years' experience with Carpentier-Edwards biological valves in relation to survival and complications. Eur J Cardiothorac Surg 1989;3(4):305–11.

80. Folliguet TA, Dibie A, Czitrom D, et al. Ten-years' clinical experience with the Sorin Pericarbon valve. J Heart Valve Dis 2000;9(3):423–8.

81. Riess FC, Cramer E, Hansen L, et al. Clinical results of the Medtronic Mosaic porcine bioprosthesis up to 13 years. Eur J Cardiothorac Surg 2010;37(1):145–53.

82. Bottio T, Rizzoli G, Thiene G, et al. Hemodynamic and clinical outcomes with the Biocor valve in the aortic position: an 8-year experience. J Thorac Cardiovasc Surg 2004;127(6):1616–23.

83. Ionescu A, Fraser AG, Butchart EG. Prevalence and clinical significance of incidental paraprosthetic valvar regurgitation: a prospective study using transesophageal echocardiography. Heart 2003; 89:1316–21.

84. Duvernoy WF, Gonzalez Lavin L, Anbe DT. Spontaneous closure of paravalvular leak after mitral valve replacement. Chest 1975;68:102–4.

85. Pate GE, Zubaidi A, Chandavimol M, et al. Percutaneous closure of prosthetic paravalvular leaks: case series and review. Catheter Cardiovasc Interv 2006;68:528–33.

86. Rallidis LS, Moyssakis IE, Ikonomidis I, et al. Natural history of early aortic paraprosthetic regurgitation: a five-year follow-up. Am Heart J 1999;138:351–7.

87. Miller DL, Morris JJ, Schaff HV, et al. Reoperation for aortic valve periprosthetic leakage: identification of patients at risk and results of operation. J Heart Valve Dis 1995;4:160–5.

88. Jindani A, Neville EM, Venn G, et al. Paraprosthetic leak: a complication of cardiac valve replacement. J Cardiovasc Surg (Torino) 1991;32:503–8.

89. Safi AM, Kwan T, Afflu E, et al. Paravalvular regurgitation: a rare complication following valve replacement surgery. Angiology 2000;51:479–87.

90. Genoni M, Franzen D, Tavakoli R, et al. Does the morphology of mitral paravalvular leaks influence symptoms and hemolysis? J Heart Valve Dis 2001;10(4):426–30.

91. Pate G, Webb J, Thompson C, et al. Percutaneous closure of a complex prosthetic mitral paravalvular leak using transesophageal echocardiographic guidance. Can J Cardiol 2004;20:452–5.

92. Chen YT, Kan MN, Chen JS, et al. Detection of prosthetic mitral valve leak: a comparative study using transesophageal echocardiography, transthoracic echocardiography and auscultation. J Clin Ultrasound 1990;18:557–61.

93. Sinha DP, Biswas S, Kumar S, et al. Studies on prosthetic valve function. A transesophageal echocardiographic assessment. J Assoc Physicians India 1996;44:525–8.

94. Faletra F, De Chiara F, Corno R, et al. Additional diagnostic value of multiplane echocardiography over biplane imaging in assessment of mitral prosthetic valves. Heart 1996;75:609–13.

95. Echevarria JR, Bernal JM, Rabasa JM, et al. Reoperation for bioprosthetic valve dysfunction. A decade of clinical experience. Eur J Cardiothorac Surg 1991;5:523–6 [discussion: 527].

96. ExpÓsito V, Garcia-Camarero T, Bernal JM, et al. Repeat mitral valve replacement: 30-years experience. Rev Esp Cardiol 2009;62(8):929–32.

97. Hourihan M, Perry SB, Mandell VS, et al. Transcatheter umbrella closure of valvular and paravalvular leaks. J Am Coll Cardiol 1992;20(6):1371–7.

98. Hein R, Wunderlich N, Robertson G, et al. Catheter closure of paravalvular leak. EuroIntervention 2006; 3:318–25.

99. Del Valle-Fernandez R, Martinez C, Jelnin V, et al. Paravalvular leak closure: single-center experience. Eur Heart J 2009;30(Abstract Suppl):920.

100. Pate GE, Thomson CR, Munt BI, et al. Techniques for percutaneous closure of prosthetic paravalvular leaks. Catheter Cardiovasc Interv 2006;67:158–66.

101. Shapira Y, Hirsch R, Kornowski R, et al. Percutaneous closure of perivalvular leaks with Amplatzer occluders: feasibility, safety, and short term results. J Heart Valve Dis 2007;16:305–13.

102. Sorajja P, Cabalka AK, Hagler DJ, et al. Successful percutaneous repair of perivalvular prosthetic regurgitation. Catheter Cardiovasc Interv 2007;70: 815–23.

103. Cortes M, Garcia E, Garcia-Fernandez MA, et al. Usefulness of transesophageal echocardiography in percutaneous transcatheter repair of paravalvular mitral regurgitation. Am J Cardiol 2008;101: 382–6.

104. Garcia Borbolla Fernandez R, Sanch Jaldon M, Calle Perez G, et al. Percutaneous treatment of mitral valve periprosthetic leakage. An alternative to high-risk surgery? Rev Esp Cardiol 2009;62: 438–41.

105. Nietlispach F, Johnson M, Moss RR, et al. Transcatheter closure of paravalvular defects using a purpose specific occluder. JACC Cardiovasc Interv 2010;3:759–65.

106. Ruiz C, Jelnin V, Kronzon I, et al. Clinical outcomes in patients undergoing percutaneous closure of periprosthetic paravalvular leaks. J Am Coll Cardiol 2011;58:2210–7.

107. Foster GP, Isselbacher EM, Rose GA, et al. Accurate localization of mitral regurgitant defects using multiplane transesophageal echocardiography. Ann Thorac Surg 1998;65(4):1025–31.

108. Chambers J, Monaghan M, Jackson G. Colour flow Doppler mapping in the assessment of prosthetic valve regurgitation. Br Heart J 1989;62:1–8

109. Kapur KK, Fan P, Nanda NC, et al. Doppler color flow mapping in the evaluation of prosthetic mitral and aortic valve function. J Am Coll Cardiol 1989; 13:1561–71.

110. Vitarelli A, Conde Y, Cimino E, et al. Assessment of severity of mechanical prosthetic mitral regurgitation by transesophageal echocardiography. Heart 2004;90:539–44.

111. Kronzon I, Sugeng L, Perk G, et al. Real-time 3-dimensional transesophageal echocardiography in the evaluation of post-operative mitral annuloplasty ring and prosthetic valve dehiscence. J Am Coll Cardiol 2009;53:1543–7.

112. Garcia-Fernandez MA, Cortes M, Garcia-Robles JA, et al. Utility of real-time three-dimensional echocardiography in evaluating the success of percutaneous transcatheter closure of mitral paravalvular leaks. J Am Soc Echocardiogr 2010;23:26–32.

113. Biner S, Kar S, Siegel RJ, et al. Value of colour Doppler three-dimensional transesophageal echocardiography in the percutaneous closure of mitral prosthesis paravalvular leak. Am J Cardiol 2010; 105:984–9.

114. Swaans MJ, Post MC, van der Ven J, et al. Transapical treatment of paravalvular leaks in patients with a logistic EuroSCORE of more than 15%: acute and 3-months outcomes of a "proof of concept" study. Catheter Cardiovasc Interv 2012;79:741–7.

115. Özkan M, Astargioglu MA, Gürcoy O. Evaluation of endothelialisation after percutaneous closure of paravalvular leaks. J Invasive Cardiol 2012;24(4): E72–4.

116. Rogers JH, Morris AS, Takeda PA, et al. Bioprosthetic leaflet erosion after percutaneous mitral paravalvular leak closure. J Am Coll Cardiol 2010; 3(1):122–3.

117. Wunderlich N, Franke J, Wilson N, et al. 3D echoguidance for structural heart interventions. Intervent Cardiol 2009;4(1):16–20.

APPENDIX A: ASSESSMENT OF MS SEVERITY

The MV area can be also be derived from Doppler echocardiography using the diastolic pressure half-time ($T_{1/2}$) method. $T_{1/2}$ is obtained by tracing the deceleration slope of the E-wave on Doppler spectral display of transmitral inflow. The MV area can be calculated from the following formula: $220/(T_{1/2})$. Limitations of this method include abnormal LA or LV compliance, associated aortic regurgitation, ASD, and patients who have previously had mitral valvuloplasty.

In case additional measurements are needed, the continuity equation and PISA methods can be used. The calculation of the MVA using the continuity equation is based on the assumption that the filling volume of diastolic mitral flow is equal to aortic stroke volume. The following formula is used:

$$MVA = \pi \left(\frac{D2}{4}\right) \left(\frac{VTI \ Aorta \ (cm)}{VTI \ mitral \ (cm)}\right)$$

D = LVOT diameter

The accuracy and reproducibility of the method are limited in that the number of measurements needed for this calculation increases the probability that measurement errors occur. In case atrial fibrillation or relevant mitral or aortic regurgitation is present, the continuity equation cannot be used.

The PISA method permits the assessment of mitral flow based on the hemispheric shape of the convergence zone of mitral flow in diastole on the LA side as seen by color Doppler. Subsequently, the MVA is calculated by dividing mitral volume flow by the maximum velocity of mitral flow in diastole as assessed by color CW Doppler:

$$MVA = \pi \, (r^2)(V_{alias})/\text{Peak } V_{mitral} \times \alpha/180°$$

r = radius of the hemispheric convergence zone (cm)

V_{alias} = aliasing velocity (cm/s)

Peak V_{mitral} = peak velocity of mitral inflow assessed with CW Doppler (cm/s)

α = opening angle of mitral leaflets relative to flow direction

This method is technically demanding but can be used in the presence of relevant MR.

3-Dimensional Echocardiography and Its Role in Preoperative Mitral Valve Evaluation

Michael N. Andrawes, MD*, Jared W. Feinman, MD

KEYWORDS

- 3D echocardiography • Mitral valve • Mitral regurgitation • Mitral stenosis
- Perioperative echocardiography

KEY POINTS

- The mitral valve (MV) is a complex structure, consisting of 2 leaflets with multiple scallops, a saddle-shaped annulus, numerous chords, and 2 papillary muscles.
- Three-dimensional echocardiography (3DE) allows simultaneous imaging of the entire MV apparatus from any acoustic window. Images can be displayed from any perspective.
- Our understanding of normal and diseased MV dynamics has been greatly enhanced by 3DE.
- The severity and mechanism of MV disease is more accurately assessed by 3DE with less interobserver and intraobserver variability.
- 3DE provides detailed information about valve morphology in both stenotic and regurgitant lesions of the MV, improving patient selection for surgical and nonsurgical treatment.
- Advanced analysis software allows quantification of the MV that can aid in surgical planning.

 Videos of a rheumatic mitral valve, P1 and P2 prolapse, and ischemic mitral regurgitation accompany this article at http://www.cardiology.theclinics.com/

INTRODUCTION

The mitral valve (MV) is a complex structure, consisting of 2 leaflets with multiple scallops, a saddle-shaped annulus, numerous chords, and 2 papillary muscles. This anatomy is reviewed in greater detail elsewhere in this issue of *Cardiology Clinics*. A comprehensive 2-dimensional transthoracic echocardiographic (2DTTE) examination of the MV necessitates that at least 4 different views be obtained, whereas a 2-dimensional transesophageal (2DTEE) examination requires 4 midesophageal and 2 transgastric views,[1,2] none of which allows for visualization of the MV and its supporting structures in their entirety. Using 3-dimensional echocardiography (3DE), all aspects of the MV apparatus, including individual leaflet scallops, the saddle-shaped annulus, and subvalvular structures, can be visualized simultaneously and from any angle (**Table 1**).[3] For this reason, evaluation of the mitral valve was one of the earliest applications of 3DE technology, and continues to be one of the most common indications for its use.[4]

THREE-DIMENSIONAL ECHOCARDIOGRAPHY TECHNOLOGY

The first 3DE techniques used standard 2DE transducers and a variety of methods to reconstruct multiple 2DE images into a 3D dataset. This was

Disclosures: None.
Department of Anesthesia, Critical Care, and Pain Medicine, Massachusetts General Hospital, 55 Fruit Street, Boston, MA 02114, USA
* Corresponding author.
E-mail address: mandrawes@parters.org

Cardiol Clin 31 (2013) 271–285
http://dx.doi.org/10.1016/j.ccl.2013.03.005
0733-8651/13/$ – see front matter © 2013 Elsevier Inc. All rights reserved.

Table 1
Echocardiographic views of the mitral valve

	Transthoracic	Transesophageal
2D	Parasternal short-axis	Midesophageal 4-chamber
		Midesophageal 2-chamber
	Parasternal long-axis	Midesophageal long-axis
		Midesophageal mitral commissural
	Apical 4-chamber	Transgastric basal short-axis
	Apical 2-chamber	Transgastric long-axis
3D	Parasternal long-axis	Any midesophageal view
	Apical 4-chamber	

cumbersome, time consuming, and often limited by reconstruction artifacts. Many of these limitations were overcome with the creation of a fully sampled matrix-array transducer, which allows the acquisition of real-time 3D echocardiographic images (RT3DE). Initially, postprocessing of these 3DE datasets was very time consuming, limiting their usefulness, but advances in computer processing power and software now allow rapid and in-depth analysis, both on-line and off-line. All of this has helped move 3DE out of its origins in the research laboratory and into routine clinical practice.

There are several modes for acquiring 3DE data, which are outlined in detail in the American Society of Echocardiography Recommendations for Image Acquisition and Display Using Three-Dimensional Echocardiography.[5] The 3DE data obtained using any of these modes may be displayed as either a 3D volume or surface rendering. The 3D dataset may also be broken down into multiple simultaneous 2D slices selected from the 3D dataset through multiplanar reconstruction (MPR). Measurements are generally made using these 2D slices, which may or may not correspond to standard 2DE imaging planes.

An additional function made possible by the matrix-array transducer is biplane 2DE imaging, in which a second imaging plane can be created at 90° from any point on the primary image. This biplane technology is occasionally referred to as "3D-guided" in the literature.

ADVANTAGES AND LIMITATIONS OF THREE-DIMENSIONAL ECHOCARDIOGRAPHY

In general, any 3D imaging technique offers a variety of advantages over 2D imaging. Most importantly, it is no longer necessary to make geometric, alignment, or anatomic assumptions. In many cases, it is possible to perform a more efficient examination, because a single 3D image displays data that would normally only be visualized across several 2D images. In addition, it is much easier to understand the spatial relationships between structures because they are no longer being seen in discrete 2D slices. Furthermore, 3D imaging can improve communication with surgeons and interventional cardiologists or radiologists by creating lifelike images that can be viewed from the perspective with which the operator is most comfortable.

Concerns over the time required to acquire and analyze 3D datasets have plagued evaluations of 3DE from the beginning, but advances in processing power and software interfaces, in conjunction with greater experience, have significantly enhanced the efficiency of these methods. Before the advent of the matrix-array transducer, it took approximately 10 minutes to acquire a dataset and an additional 60 minutes for analysis.[6] Matrix-array transducers allow real-time imaging, greatly reducing acquisition time to just 1 to 7 cardiac cycles. Meanwhile, advances in computing power and user interface have allowed for more efficient data analysis. Early studies with RT3DE reported 16 to 30 minutes to acquire and analyze datasets,[7] but this has been cut down to 1 to 3 minutes in the latest study reporting this metric.[8]

MITRAL STENOSIS

Although rheumatic heart disease is quite rare in developed countries, it remains a major problem worldwide, with an estimated prevalence of 15.6 million cases and 233,000 deaths each year.[9] The mitral valve is most frequently affected, resulting in mitral stenosis (MS) caused by leaflet thickening, leaflet calcification, commissural fusion, and/or chordal fusion, the net result of which is a funnel-shaped mitral opening. Echocardiography is the tool of choice to assess mitral stenosis at initial diagnosis and follow-up and is a key determinant of suitability for percutaneous mitral balloon valvotomy (PMBV) or surgical intervention.[10]

Three-Dimensional Echocardiography Planimetry of Mitral Valve Area

Mitral valve area (MVA) is the primary determinant of MS severity and is a key branch point in the management of these patients.[10,11] Planimetry by echocardiography provides a direct measure of MVA that does not rely on assumptions about flow, chamber compliance, or other valvular lesions, and is considered the reference measure of MVA.[11] Unfortunately, this measurement is also greatly dependent on operator skill and experience because of the need to precisely align the imaging plane with the narrowest orifice within the MV apparatus. The 3DE allows the capture of a data set that includes the entire MV orifice, from which the optimal imaging plane can be selected. In addition, 3DE allows this plane to be generated from any imaging window that allows good visualization of the MV orifice, whereas planimetry by 2DE is limited to transthoracic parasternal views.

Early studies demonstrated that planimetry of MVA by 3DE was feasible, but the rotational technique used was cumbersome and remained limited primarily to the research realm.[6,12] The advent of RT3DE made the assessment of MVA not only feasible, but rapid and increasingly accurate (**Fig. 1**; see also Video 1, available at http://www.cardiology.theclinics.com/). Binder and colleagues[13] demonstrated that being off-axis in a 2D image by just 6° resulted in an overestimation of MVA by 63%, and this error increased to 88% when combined with a 2-mm parallel shift in the imaging plane. Not surprisingly, interobserver variability was much smaller with 3DE and the MVA was obtained more easily and quickly using 3DE, despite the need to crop the 3D data set (**Fig. 2**). RT3DE assessment of MVA has also compared favorably with catheter-based measurements made using the Gorlin equation, often considered the gold standard in MS evaluation, more closely mirroring these values than MVA measured by 2DE planimetry.[7] This is especially true following PMBV.[14] Despite its widespread acceptance, the Gorlin equation is still dependent on several hemodynamic assumptions, leading some to argue that planimetry by 3DE should in fact be the new gold standard measurement of MVA.[15,16]

The superiority of 3DE to 2DE in determining MVA is much more significant for inexperienced echocardiographers. A prospective study by Messika-Zeitoun and colleagues[17] demonstrated that although highly experienced users were able to obtain accurate measurements of MVA using either 2DE or 3DE, 2DE assessments by less experienced echocardiographers varied widely. When these same users assessed MVA with 3DE, they achieved accuracy levels similar to the highly experienced echocardiographers. This increased accuracy in MVA assessment holds true with both 3DTTE and 3DTEE.[8,18]

An alternate method for assessing MVA that does not require cropping of a 3D dataset but takes advantage of the matrix-array transducer, is the so-called "3D-guided" approach. This method uses biplane imaging through the narrowest portion of the mitral orifice, as seen in the 2D parasternal long-axis view, to create an ideal MV short-axis view, eliminating much of the alignment error that accompanies pure 2DE (**Fig. 3**). This method reduces the overestimation of MVA seen with standard 2DE, more closely matches catheter-derived measures of MVA, and reduces interobserver and intraobserver variability. Perhaps more importantly, in one study by Sebag and colleagues[19] it increased the clinical grade of MS in 11 of 24 patients, which can have significant implications on patient care. This method may be more time efficient compared with off-line processing of 3D datasets, although differences in speed have not been formally evaluated.

Although much of the work on MVA has focused primarily on rheumatic MS, the measurement of MVA in calcific MS poses its own set of challenges. The mitral orifice takes on a more tubular shape, as opposed to the funnel shape seen in rheumatic disease, and the narrowest orifice is not located at the leaflet tips, making selection of an imaging plane for planimetry more difficult.

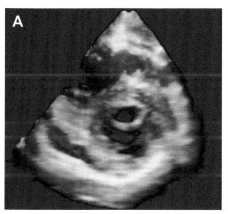
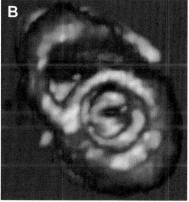

Fig. 1. A 3DTTE en face view of a rheumatic mitral valve from the LV perspective. (*A*) Parasternal window. (*B*) Apical window.

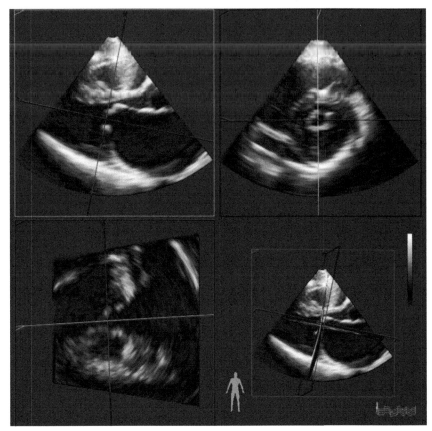

Fig. 2. Multiplanar reconstruction of a parasternal 3DTTE dataset showing precisely aligned long-axis (*upper left*) and short-axis (*upper right*) 2D cuts.

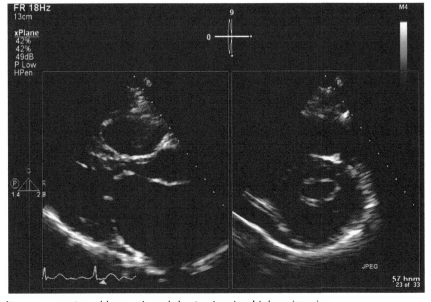

Fig. 3. Simultaneous parasternal long-axis and short-axis using biplane imaging.

These patients also often have concomitant coronary artery disease and left ventricular hypertrophy with associated diastolic dysfunction, which limits the validity of MVA by pressure half-time (PHT).[11] Chu and colleagues[20] demonstrated that 3D color Doppler could be used to determine the level of the mitral orifice at which planimetry should be performed, producing an MVA similar to that calculated using the continuity equation. The ability to accurately perform MV planimetry in these patients is particularly useful, as PHT tends to overestimate the MVA, consistent with the expected changes in left ventricular compliance.

Three-Dimensional Echocardiography Proximal Isovelocity Surface Area Measurement of Mitral Valve Area

The American Society of Echocardiography gives the proximal isovelocity surface area (PISA) calculation of MVA a level 2 recommendation, suggesting that its use be limited to situations in which planimetry and PHT are inconclusive because it is technically challenging to perform.[11] Additionally, this method assumes hemispherical convergence of flow and a circular orifice, both of which may not be true for the mitral valve where the orifice tends to be elliptical. An important advantage of 3DE is the ability to avoid such geometric assumptions.

Most of the work on 3DE PISA has been in the assessment of mitral regurgitation (MR), as discussed later in this article. However, Cobey and colleagues[21] described a novel method for the analysis of MVA by 3DE PISA in a recent case report of a patient undergoing mitral valve replacement (MVR) for MS. Using intraoperative 3DTEE with color Doppler, the 3D dataset was broken down into a series of 2D slices and the PISA arc length was measured in each slice. From these data, they were able to manually calculate a 3D PISA. They then automated this process with custom software. It is difficult to draw firm conclusions from this single report, but it does demonstrate the feasibility of such a technique.

Three-Dimensional Echocardiography and Patient Selection for Balloon Valvotomy

Modern percutaneous mitral balloon valvotomy (PMBV) was first described in 1984 by Inoue and colleagues[22] and has since become the preferred treatment, when available, in symptomatic patients and select asymptomatic patients with suitable anatomy.[10] Appropriate patient selection is essential for success and is determined by a variety of patient factors. Valve morphology is perhaps the most

important of these and is well assessed by echocardiography.[23] As a result, several scoring systems have emerged to assess these factors and predict success, the most popular of which by Wilkins and colleagues[24] assesses leaflet mobility, thickening, and calcification, as well as subvalvular thickening. Given the superiority of 3DE as compared with 2DE in assessing MV anatomy and structure, it is not surprising that interobserver variability is reduced when Wilkins score is applied to 3DE.[7]

Recently, a new RT3DE-based scoring system was compared with the Wilkins score in 74 patients before and after PMBV.[25] In this system, each leaflet is divided into individual scallops and each scallop is scored separately for thickness, mobility, and calcification. The subvalvular apparatus is also divided into 3 levels (proximal, middle, and distal) and scored at each level for thickness and separation. The degree of calcification by RT3DE was better able to predict mitral regurgitation after PMBV, whereas the degree of subvalvular involvement by RT3DE better predicted recurrence of symptoms at 1 year follow-up after PMBV. The RT3DE score also showed less interobserver and intraobserver variability.

Patient outcome after PMBV is largely determined by the degree of commissural splitting,[24,26] which is better visualized by 3DE.[17,27,28] In addition, the degree of MR after this procedure may be affected by leaflet tears that are also better visualized by 3DE.[27] The early detection of a leaflet tear using 3DE may allow for the avoidance of further balloon inflation, possibly preventing even worse postprocedure MR.

MITRAL REGURGITATION

MR is the most common valvular heart disease in the United States, affecting 2.5% of the population.[29] Echocardiography plays a vital role in the diagnosis and management of MR in that it allows for the determination of both MR severity, which dictates disease prognosis and the need for surgical referral,[30] and the structural etiology of MR, which affects the complexity and overall feasibility of potential mitral valve repair. Because of its improved spatial resolution and ability to capture all aspects of the mitral apparatus simultaneously, 3DE offers advantages over 2DE when examining the MV, making preoperative evaluation of MR one of the most common applications of 3DE.[5]

Three-Dimensional Echocardiography Color Doppler Assessment of MR Severity

The establishment of the degree of MR is an important first step in determining whether surgical referral is necessary. Surgical repair or replacement of the MV is recommended (Class I indication) or reasonable (Class IIa) in cases of severe MR with any of the following. (1) symptoms, (2) left ventricular (LV) dysfunction, (3) LV enlargement, (4) new-onset atrial fibrillation, or (5) pulmonary hypertension.[10] There is some debate as to the need for surgical referral in patients with severe MR alone, as the American College of Cardiology/American Heart Association guidelines call this a class IIa indication as long as MV repair can be performed with a greater than 90% likelihood of success, whereas the European Society of Cardiology guidelines consider it a class IIb indication.[31]

Traditionally, the assessment of MR severity has been based on measurements made using 2DE and color Doppler to estimate the effective regurgitant orifice area (EROA). The most straightforward of these surrogate measurements is the vena contracta width (VCW),[32] although the vena contracta area (VCA) can also be estimated using geometric assumptions or directly traced via planimetry of a short-axis view of the MR jet.[33] With the incorporation of color Doppler into 3DE, a 3D image of the MR jet can be obtained and reformatted, either off-line or in real-time, to create an en face view of the VCA, which can then be traced using planimetry (**Fig. 4**). The use of 3DE to measure VCA has been shown in numerous studies to grade MR severity more accurately than 2DE,[34] and compares favorably with results obtained using cardiac magnetic resonance imaging (CMR).[35] One study, by Zeng and colleagues,[36] used a VCA cutoff of 0.41 cm^2 to differentiate between moderate and severe MR with a sensitivity and specificity of 82% and 97%, respectively. A significant benefit of using 3DE VCA to assess MR is that the measurement is free from hemodynamic or geometric assumptions, which may make this technique more accurate than 2DE in patients with ischemic MR or an asymmetric or complex regurgitant orifice.

The other commonly used modality for grading MR severity using 2DE is the calculation of EROA using PISA. One benefit of 3DE over 2DE in PISA

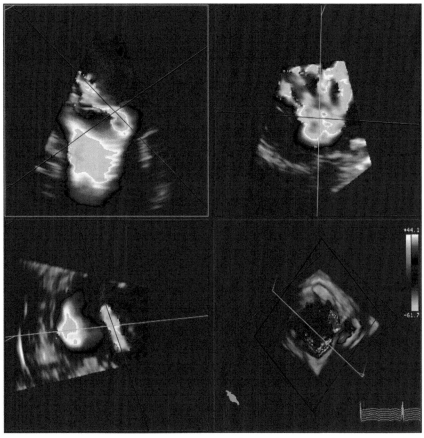

Fig. 4. A 3DTEE color multiplanar reconstruction of P1/P2 prolapse. The lower left panel is used to measure the VCA. Note the hemielliptical shape of the PISA in the upper left and upper right panels.

assessment is the ability to examine the jet from multiple angles to obtain the maximum radius of the PISA hemisphere, which has shown good correlation with EROA as measured by CMR.[37]

The problem with this methodology, whether 2DE or 3DE is used, is the inherent assumption that the PISA has a hemispheric shape. In reality, the PISA in most regurgitant valves is closer to a hemielliptic geometry (see **Fig. 4**). The 3DE with color Doppler allows for the measurement of the multiple axes necessary to calculate the EROA using a hemielliptic model, which more accurately grades MR severity than the 2DE PISA calculation.[38,39] A few studies have been done that attempt to eliminate geometric assumptions regarding the PISA altogether. Some use 3DE with color Doppler to directly measure the surface area of the region of flow convergence, either manually or via an automated program,[40,41] whereas others apply third-party software to directly calculate an anatomic regurgitant orifice area (AROA) after the construction of a 3D MV model.[42] These nongeometric methods have shown promise but are still in their early stages of development, and have not as yet been widely adopted for the quantification of MR severity.

Three-Dimensional Echocardiography Assessment of MV Structure and MR Etiology

Once the severity of MR is established, it is necessary to determine the etiology. The primary cause of MR in developed nations is degenerative mitral valve disease (DMVD), which can be further broken down into fibroelastic deficiency (FED) and Barlow disease (BD). The former is characterized primarily by thin, normal-appearing leaflets without excess tissue and the involvement of a single scallop of the MV, with or without accompanying chordal rupture, leading to prolapse and regurgitation. Valves with BD, on the other hand, contain thickened leaflets with excess tissue, multiple areas of prolapse and/or leaflet billowing, and chordal structures that may be calcified, thickened, elongated, or restricted. Accurately differentiating between these 2 entities and localizing the leaflet pathology with echocardiography is of paramount importance when evaluating a patient with MR, as it guides surgical decision making.[43]

The 3DE allows all aspects of the mitral apparatus to be visualized simultaneously from any perspective. This is possible with 3DTTE or 3DTEE, although 3DTEE allows for comparatively greater spatial resolution in determining mitral valve anatomy.[44] The 3D moving image can then be rotated to create an en face, or "surgeon's view," of the valve to aid in surgical decision making and communication among the surgeon, cardiologist, and anesthesiologist, as well as undergo further quantitative or image-based analysis using built-in tools or off-line software. Multiple studies have been performed comparing 2DE and 3DE for localizing leaflet pathology in MR and have consistently shown that 3DE more reliably identifies the correct prolapsing scallop(s) with reduced interobserver variability.[44–50] In one study by Chandra and colleagues,[51] 2DTEE identified the prolapsing scallop correctly in only 76% of patients compared with 92% of patients when 3DTEE was used (surgical inspection was the gold standard). This holds true for 3DTTE versus 2DTTE as well, but there is also evidence that 3DTTE is superior at detecting most prolapsing lesions when compared with 2DTEE.[47] This is important, in that 3DTTE may save some patients from undergoing an invasive preoperative TEE for MV repair planning.

The superiority of 3DE in accurately capturing leaflet segment pathology is especially true when the lesion is more complex than an isolated P2 prolapse; for example, cases with multileaflet prolapse, BD, commissural involvement, or a cleft (**Figs. 5** and **6**; movies of **Figs. 5** and **6** also can be seen in Videos 2 and 3, respectively, which are available at available at http://www.cardiology. theclinics.com/).[46,52] These patients often need a more complicated MV repair, using advanced techniques, such as a sliding plasty, neochord creation, chordal transfer, or commisuroplasty, to adequately repair the valve, while minimizing the risk of systolic anterior motion (SAM) of the MV.[53,54] The use of 3DE to correctly identify and describe complex MV pathology can aid in deciding which patients should be referred to a surgeon with greater experience performing complex MV repair and help the surgeon decide the type of repair that is necessary.

Three-Dimensional Quantitative Assessment of the MV

In addition to allowing views of the MV and its apparatus that are unattainable with 2DE, the proliferation of 3D MV analysis software has allowed for quantitative assessments of leaflet and annulus morphology that were previously impossible. The 2 most commonly used software systems for MV analysis are Philips' Mitral Valve Quantification (MVQ) program (Philips Healthcare, Inc, Andover, MA) and the 4D MV-Assessment software from TomTec (TomTec Imaging Systems GmbH, Munich, Germany). Both programs ask the user to mark key points along the MV annulus and leaflets (**Fig. 7**) and use these points to create a 3D model

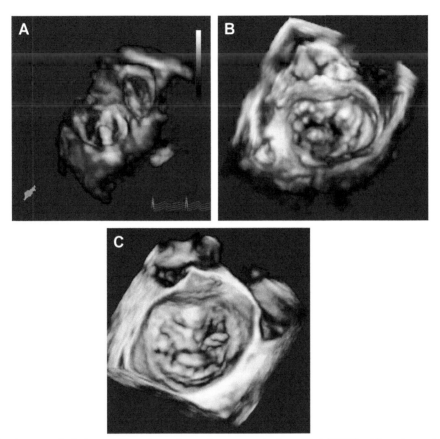

Fig. 5. (*A*) A 3DTTE apical view of P2 prolapse from the surgeon's view. (*B*) A 3DTEE midesophageal view of P1 and P2 prolapse from the surgeon's view. (*C*) A 3DTEE midesophageal view of prolapsing commissural leaflet.

(**Fig. 8**) of the valve with automated measurements of select parameters, including annulus circumference and diameter, leaflet diameter and area, tenting and billowing height, and aorto-mitral and leaflet angles (**Fig. 9**). The creation of the 3D MV model can be completed in as little as 5 to 7 minutes by experienced users with good interobserver reliability.[55] The clinical impact of these

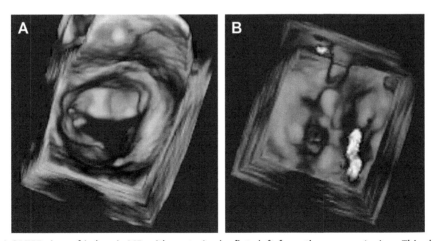

Fig. 6. (*A*) A 3DTEE view of ischemic MR with posterior leaflet cleft from the surgeon's view. This cleft was not seen on preoperative 2DTTE or intraoperative 2DTEE. The presence of this structural defect changed the surgical plan from a CABG to a CABG with MV repair. (*B*) Same with color Doppler, confirming the etiology of the MR is the cleft. Note stitch artifact.

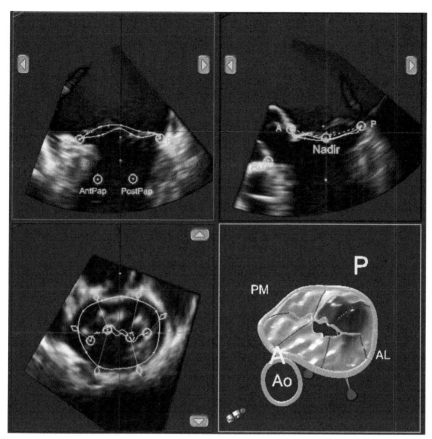

Fig. 7. Building the MV model in MVQ. A, anterior; AL, aneterolateral commissure; Ao, aortic valve; P, posterior; PM, posteromedial commissure.

measurements is still being evaluated, but they have so far offered new insights into the remodeling of the MV that occurs in various disease states and after surgical repair.

In DMVD, quantitative differences in MV structure have been uncovered between FED and BD, providing additional help in differentiating between the 2 entities. In the normal MV, the annulus has a saddle shape, which deepens further during systole, reducing leaflet stress.[56] In both FED and BD, the diameter, circumference, and area of the MV annulus are increased compared with controls. In FED, the annular height and annular height to commissural width ratio (AHCWR) are both reduced, indicating a flattening of the saddle-shaped annulus. Chordal rupture and

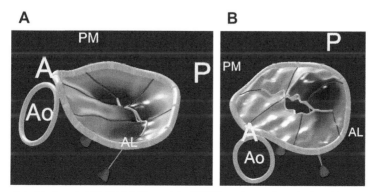

Fig. 8. (A) MVQ model of ischemic MR. (B) MVQ model of P1/P2 prolapse. A, anterior; AL, aneterolateral commissure; Ao, aortic valve; P, posterior; PM, posteromedial commissure.

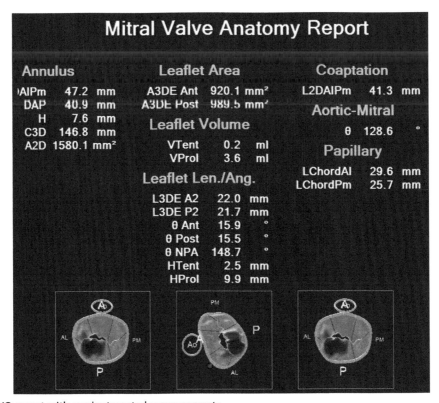

Fig. 9. MVQ report with semiautomated measurements.

severe MR are associated with more significant reductions in annular height and greater increases in annular diameter and area.[57] This may be because leaflet stress rises dramatically once AHCWR falls below 0.15, placing additional mechanical strain on leaflets and chordae that are already abnormal in structure.[58] Annular deepening during systole is also blunted in FED. In BD, on the other hand, the annular height and AHCWR are increased compared with controls.[59] Quantitative measurements based on leaflet length and volume are also helpful when evaluating DMVD. A leaflet billowing height of greater than 1 mm with a billowing volume of less than 1.15 mL is characteristic of FED, whereas those with BD have a billowing volume of greater than 1.15 mL.[51] Total leaflet area is also increased in both forms of DMVD, but to a lesser extent than the annular area, indicating a reduction in surplus leaflet tissue compared with a normal valve.[57]

Although DMVD is the most common cause of MR, ischemic MR (IMR) is also frequently encountered by cardiologists, anesthesiologists, and cardiac surgeons. The 3DE has allowed for a better understanding of the geometric changes that occur in IMR, and may even help predict which patients would benefit from MV repair. In IMR, the subvalvular apparatus and leaflets remain intact,

but dilation of the ventricle and mitral annulus leads to distortion of the valve, leaflet tethering, and incomplete closure and regurgitation. In IMR, unlike DMVD, the annulus does not dilate uniformly. Instead, dilation along the anterior-posterior and anterolateral-posteromedial directions is greater than that in other planes, leading to a distorted and flattened annular shape.[60] The angles between the annular plane and the anterior (ALA) and posterior leaflet (PLA) are indicative of the degree of tethering and regurgitation, and are more quickly and accurately assessed using 3DE than 2DE.[61] Normal values for the ALA and PLA are between 20 and 34°,[62] and a PLA greater than 45° is associated with an increased risk of recurrent MR and poor outcome after a restrictive annuloplasty,[63] which is the most common method of repair for IMR. Tenting height and tenting volume are also more easily and accurately assessed using 3DE, further clarifying the extent of IMR and remodeling.

Three-Dimensional Echocardiography and Surgical Planning

Many patients with severe MR will eventually be referred for surgical evaluation. Although replacement of the regurgitant MV with a mechanical or bioprosthetic valve is still an option, MV repair has become the preferred surgical approach since its adoption in the 1970s. Valve repair offers patients lower intraoperative mortality, improved long-term survival, a lower risk of thromboembolic events or hemorrhage, and improved postoperative LV function when compared with valve replacement.[64–66] Preoperative and intraoperative 3DE play key roles in determining the feasibility of MV repair, the level of complexity of the repair, and what techniques should be used to ensure a successful repair.

When considering a patient for MV repair, it is helpful to classify the lesion, using the information gleaned from 2DE and 3DE, according to a system originally developed by Carpentier (**Table 2**).[67] In a type I lesion, the surgeon will often repair the dilated annulus using only an annuloplasty ring, assuming annular dilation is the sole cause of MR. The 3DE can be useful in patients with Type I MR to both exclude a more complicated etiology for the regurgitation (eg, leaflet perforation or cleft), as well as to obtain quantitative measurements of the annulus itself that can be helpful in the repair. Although 2DE has been unable to consistently measure appropriate ring size for MV repair, the early data with 3DE, and particularly 3DTEE, has been promising.[68,69] The 3DE-derived ring sizing will likely become more accurate and commonly used as noninvasive methods for MV repair (which do not allow for direct surgical sizing) are adopted.

Type II lesions are the most commonly encountered and are where 3DE has the greatest role. Much was said earlier in this article regarding the effectiveness of 3DE versus 2DE in determining the prolapsing segment and differentiating between FED and BD using both structural and quantitative methods. We will instead focus on the utility of 3DE in determining repair type. Several different methods of repairing the MV exist, and the decision as to which method or methods to use in any given case is based upon the anatomy of the prolapsing valve, which is best seen using 3DE. If 3DE reveals FED with only a prolapsing, tall P2 segment, then a simple triangular or quadrangular resection with annuloplasty ring may be all that is needed to repair the valve. If echocardiography shows that all of the posterior segments appear long and thin (1.0–1.5 cm), then resection may not leave enough posterior leaflet for successful coaptation, so neochord creation or chordal transfer may be a better approach. Prolapse of the anterior leaflet alone may be treated by triangular resection, chordal transfer, or neochord creation.

If 3DE demonstrates a valve more consistent with BD with multiple tall, prolapsing segments, then a repair using several techniques is likely to be necessary. This may include a posterior leaflet sliding plasty to reduce the risk of SAM by reducing the posterior leaflet area and height of P2.[55] Although triangular and quadrangular resections are now widely practiced, some of the other, more complex, repair methods are best left to surgeons who specialize in MV repair. By using 3DE to better map out the anatomy of the valve pathology, patient disease can be more accurately matched to surgical skill set when making referrals.[70]

Type IIIa lesions, seen most commonly in rheumatic heart disease, are the least amenable to successful repair. Therefore, it is important to differentiate this type of lesion from the others. If the anterior leaflet appears thin and mobile, then mitral repair may be feasible via division of affected chords and patch augmentation of the restricted leaflet(s). If, on the other hand, the anterior leaflet appears thick, calcified, and immobile on echocardiography, then repair is unlikely to be successful.[53] The 3DE can be helpful in these cases to get an accurate sense of the anatomy and motion of both leaflets

Table 2
Carpentier classification of mitral regurgitation

Classification	Leaflet Motion	Jet Direction	Etiology
Type I	Normal motion	Central	Annular dilation Leaflet perforation Mitral cleft
Type II	Excessive motion	Eccentric (*directed away from prolapsed leaflet*)	Leaflet prolapse or flail from FED or BD
Type IIIa	Restricted motion in systole and diastole	Eccentric (*directed toward restricted leaflet*) or Central	Rheumatic disease
Type IIIb	Restricted motion in systole only	Eccentric (*directed toward restricted leaflet*) or Central	Ischemic heart disease Dilated cardiomyopathy

in their entirety, and 3D quantitative measurements of the degree of leaflet tethering may also be made.

Type IIIb lesions are seen most commonly in ischemic MR and are often associated with papillary muscle dysfunction. The primary repair for a type IIIb valve is a downsizing ring annuloplasty. It is important to first determine if advanced signs of ischemic remodeling are present, as these will make the repair less likely to succeed and may warrant valve replacement instead. These markers include LV end-diastolic diameter greater than 65 mm, a tenting height greater than 15 mm, or a PLA greater than 45°,[63,71] and 3DE may be helpful in more quickly and accurately making these measurements when compared with 2DE.[61]

SUMMARY

The 3DE technology continues to evolve and remains an area of active research, but has already proven to be of significant benefit in our understanding of the mitral apparatus and its accompanying disease states. Several of the applications mentioned here are both clinically relevant and practical for daily use. The full potential of 3DE, however, remains to be realized.

SUPPLEMENTARY DATA

Supplementary data related to this article can be found online at http://dx.doi.org/10.1016/j.ccl.2013.03.005.

REFERENCES

1. Lancellotti P, Moura L, Pierard LA, et al. European Association of Echocardiography recommendations for the assessment of valvular regurgitation. Part 2: mitral and tricuspid regurgitation (native valve disease). Eur J Echocardiogr 2010;11(4): 307–32.

2. Shanewise JS, Cheung AT, Aronson S, et al. ASE/SCA guidelines for performing a comprehensive intraoperative multiplane transesophageal echocardiography examination: recommendations of the American Society of Echocardiography Council for Intraoperative Echocardiography and the Society of Cardiovascular Anesthesiologists Task Force for Certification in Perioperative Transesophageal Echocardiography. Anesth Analg 1999;89(4):870–84.

3. Sugeng L, Shernan SK, Salgo IS, et al. Live 3-dimensional transesophageal echocardiography initial experience using the fully-sampled matrix array probe. J Am Coll Cardiol 2008;52(6):446–9.

4. Binder T, Globits S, Zangeneh M, et al. Value of three-dimensional echocardiography as an adjunct to conventional transesophageal echocardiography. Cardiology 1996;87(4):335–42.

5. Lang RM, Badano LP, Tsang W, et al. EAE/ASE recommendations for image acquisition and display using three-dimensional echocardiography. J Am Soc Echocardiogr 2012;25(1):3–40.

6. Chen Q, Nosir YF, Vletter WB, et al. Accurate assessment of mitral valve area in patients with mitral stenosis by three-dimensional echocardiography. J Am Soc Echocardiogr 1997;10(2):133–40.

7. Zamorano J, Cordeiro P, Sugeng L, et al. Real-time three-dimensional echocardiography for rheumatic mitral valve stenosis evaluation: an accurate and novel approach. J Am Coll Cardiol 2004;43(11): 2091–6.

8. Dreyfus J, Brochet E, Lepage L, et al. Real-time 3D transoesophageal measurement of the mitral valve area in patients with mitral stenosis. Eur J Echocardiogr 2011;12(10):750–5.

9. Carapetis JR, Steer AC, Mulholland EK, et al. The global burden of group A streptococcal diseases. Lancet Infect Dis 2005;5(11):685–94.

10. Bonow RO, Carabello BA, Chatterjee K, et al. 2008 Focused update incorporated into the ACC/AHA 2006 guidelines for the management of patients with valvular heart disease: a report of the American College of Cardiology/American Heart Association Task Force on Practice Guidelines (Writing Committee to Revise the 1998 Guidelines for the Management of Patients with Valvular Heart Disease): endorsed by the Society of Cardiovascular Anesthesiologists, Society for Cardiovascular Angiography and Interventions, and Society of Thoracic Surgeons. Circulation 2008;118(15):e523–661.

11. Baumgartner H, Hung J, Bermejo J, et al. Echocardiographic assessment of valve stenosis: EAE/ASE recommendations for clinical practice. J Am Soc Echocardiogr 2009;22(1):1–23 [quiz: 101–2].

12. Kupferwasser I, Mohr-Kahaly S, Menzel T, et al. Quantification of mitral valve stenosis by three-dimensional transesophageal echocardiography. Int J Card Imaging 1996;12(4):241–7.

13. Binder TM, Rosenhek R, Porenta G, et al. Improved assessment of mitral valve stenosis by volumetric real-time three-dimensional echocardiography. J Am Coll Cardiol 2000;36(4):1355–61.

14. Zamorano J, Perez de Isla L, Sugeng L, et al. Non-invasive assessment of mitral valve area during percutaneous balloon mitral valvuloplasty: role of real-time 3D echocardiography. Eur Heart J 2004; 25(23):2086–91.

15. Mannaerts HF, Kamp O, Visser CA. Should mitral valve area assessment in patients with mitral stenosis be based on anatomical or on functional evaluation? A plea for 3D echocardiography as the new clinical standard. Eur Heart J 2004; 25(23):2073–4.

16. Perez de Isla L, Casanova C, Almeria C, et al. Which method should be the reference method to

evaluate the severity of rheumatic mitral stenosis? Gorlin's method versus 3D-echo. Eur J Echocardiogr 2007;8(6):470–3.

17. Messika-Zeitoun D, Brochet E, Holmin C, et al. Three-dimensional evaluation of the mitral valve area and commissural opening before and after percutaneous mitral commissurotomy in patients with mitral stenosis. Eur Heart J 2007;28(1):72–9.

18. Schlosshan D, Aggarwal G, Mathur G, et al. Real-time 3D transesophageal echocardiography for the evaluation of rheumatic mitral stenosis. JACC Cardiovasc Imaging 2011;4(6):580–8.

19. Sebag IA, Morgan JG, Handschumacher MD, et al. Usefulness of three-dimensionally guided assessment of mitral stenosis using matrix-array ultrasound. Am J Cardiol 2005;96(8):1151–6.

20. Chu JW, Levine RA, Chua S, et al. Assessing mitral valve area and orifice geometry in calcific mitral stenosis: a new solution by real-time three-dimensional echocardiography. J Am Soc Echocardiogr 2008;21(9):1006–9.

21. Cobey FC, McInnis JA, Gelfand BJ, et al. A method for automating 3-dimensional proximal isovelocity surface area measurement. J Cardiothorac Vasc Anesth 2012;26(3):507–11.

22. Inoue K, Owaki T, Nakamura T, et al. Clinical application of transvenous mitral commissurotomy by a new balloon catheter. J Thorac Cardiovasc Surg 1984;87(3):394–402.

23. Pan M, Medina A, Suarez de Lezo J, et al. Factors determining late success after mitral balloon valvulotomy. Am J Cardiol 1993;71(13):1181–5.

24. Wilkins GT, Weyman AE, Abascal VM, et al. Percutaneous balloon dilatation of the mitral valve: an analysis of echocardiographic variables related to outcome and the mechanism of dilatation. Br Heart J 1988;60(4):299–308.

25. Anwar AM, Attia WM, Nosir YF, et al. Validation of a new score for the assessment of mitral stenosis using real-time three-dimensional echocardiography. J Am Soc Echocardiogr 2010;23(1):13–22.

26. Messika-Zeitoun D, Blanc J, Iung B, et al. Impact of degree of commissural opening after percutaneous mitral commissurotomy on long-term outcome. JACC Cardiovasc Imaging 2009;2(1):1–7.

27. Applebaum RM, Kasliwal RR, Kanojia A, et al. Utility of three-dimensional echocardiography during balloon mitral valvuloplasty. J Am Coll Cardiol 1998;32(5):1405–9.

28. Langerveld J, Valocik G, Plokker HW, et al. Additional value of three-dimensional transesophageal echocardiography for patients with mitral valve stenosis undergoing balloon valvuloplasty. J Am Soc Echocardiogr 2003;16(8):841–9.

29. Nkomo VT, Gardin JM, Skelton TN, et al. Burden of valvular heart diseases: a population-based study. Lancet 2006;368(9540):1005–11.

30. Enriquez-Sarano M, Avierinos JF, Messika-Zeitoun D, et al. Quantitative determinants of the outcome of asymptomatic mitral regurgitation. N Engl J Med 2005;352(9):875–83.

31. Vahanian A, Alfieri O, Andreotti F, et al. Guidelines on the management of valvular heart disease (version 2012). Eur Heart J 2012;33(19):2451–96.

32. Tribouilloy C, Shen WF, Quere JP, et al. Assessment of severity of mitral regurgitation by measuring regurgitant jet width at its origin with transesophageal Doppler color flow imaging. Circulation 1992;85(4):1248–53.

33. Mele D, Vandervoort P, Palacios I, et al. Proximal jet size by Doppler color flow mapping predicts severity of mitral regurgitation. Clinical studies. Circulation 1995;91(3):746–54.

34. Thavendiranathan P, Phelan D, Thomas JD, et al. Quantitative assessment of mitral regurgitation: validation of new methods. J Am Coll Cardiol 2012;60(16):1470–83.

35. Marsan NA, Westenberg JJ, Ypenburg C, et al. Quantification of functional mitral regurgitation by real-time 3D echocardiography: comparison with 3D velocity-encoded cardiac magnetic resonance. JACC Cardiovasc Imaging 2009;2(11):1245–52.

36. Zeng X, Levine RA, Hua L, et al. Diagnostic value of vena contracta area in the quantification of mitral regurgitation severity by color Doppler 3D echocardiography. Circ Cardiovasc Imaging 2011;4(5):506–13.

37. Sitges M, Jones M, Shiota T, et al. Real-time three-dimensional color Doppler evaluation of the flow convergence zone for quantification of mitral regurgitation: validation experimental animal study and initial clinical experience. J Am Soc Echocardiogr 2003;16(1):38–45.

38. Yosefy C, Hung J, Chua S, et al. Direct measurement of vena contracta area by real-time 3-dimensional echocardiography for assessing severity of mitral regurgitation. Am J Cardiol 2009;104(7):978–83.

39. Matsumura Y, Fukuda S, Tran H, et al. Geometry of the proximal isovelocity surface area in mitral regurgitation by 3-dimensional color Doppler echocardiography: difference between functional mitral regurgitation and prolapse regurgitation. Am Heart J 2008;155(2):231–8.

40. Little SH, Igo SR, Pirat B, et al. In vitro validation of real-time three-dimensional color Doppler echocardiography for direct measurement of proximal isovelocity surface area in mitral regurgitation. Am J Cardiol 2007;99(10):1440–7.

41. Grady L, Datta S, Kutter O, et al. Regurgitation quantification using 3D PISA in volume echocardiography. Med Image Comput Comput Assist Interv 2011;14(Pt 3):512–9.

42. Chandra S, Salgo IS, Sugeng L, et al. A three-dimensional insight into the complexity of flow convergence in mitral regurgitation: adjunctive benefit of anatomic regurgitant orifice area. Am J Physiol Heart Circ Physiol 2011;301(3):H1015–24.

43. Adams DH, Anyanwu AC. The cardiologist's role in increasing the rate of mitral valve repair in degenerative disease. Curr Opin Cardiol 2008;23(2): 105–10.

44. Flachskampf FA, Badano L, Daniel WG, et al. Recommendations for transoesophageal echocardiography: update 2010. Eur J Echocardiogr 2010; 11(7):557–76.

45. Chen X, Sun D, Yang J, et al. Preoperative assessment of mitral valve prolapse and chordae rupture using real time three-dimensional transesophageal echocardiography. Echocardiography 2011;28(9): 1003–10.

46. Pepi M, Tamborini G, Maltagliati A, et al. Head-to-head comparison of two- and three-dimensional transthoracic and transesophageal echocardiography in the localization of mitral valve prolapse. J Am Coll Cardiol 2006;48(12):2524–30.

47. Tamborini G, Muratori M, Maltagliati A, et al. Preoperative transthoracic real-time three-dimensional echocardiography in patients undergoing mitral valve repair: accuracy in cases with simple vs. complex prolapse lesions. Eur J Echocardiogr 2010;11(9):778–85.

48. Manda J, Kesanolla SK, Hsuing MC, et al. Comparison of real time two-dimensional with live/real time three-dimensional transesophageal echocardiography in the evaluation of mitral valve prolapse and chordae rupture. Echocardiography 2008; 25(10):1131–7.

49. Grewal J, Mankad S, Freeman WK, et al. Real-time three-dimensional transesophageal echocardiography in the intraoperative assessment of mitral valve disease. J Am Soc Echocardiogr 2009; 22(1):34–41.

50. Ben Zekry S, Nagueh SF, Little SH, et al. Comparative accuracy of two- and three-dimensional transthoracic and transesophageal echocardiography in identifying mitral valve pathology in patients undergoing mitral valve repair: initial observations. J Am Soc Echocardiogr 2011; 24(10):1079–85.

51. Chandra S, Salgo IS, Sugeng L, et al. Characterization of degenerative mitral valve disease using morphologic analysis of real-time three-dimensional echocardiographic images: objective insight into complexity and planning of mitral valve repair. Circ Cardiovasc Imaging 2011;4(1):24–32.

52. Biaggi P, Greutmann M, Crean A. Utility of three-dimensional transesophageal echocardiography: anatomy, mechanism, and severity of regurgitation in a patient with an isolated cleft posterior mitral valve. J Am Soc Echocardiogr 2010; 23(10):1114.e1–4.

53. Fischer GW, Anyanwu AC, Adams DH. Intraoperative classification of mitral valve dysfunction: the role of the anesthesiologist in mitral valve reconstruction. J Cardiothorac Vasc Anesth 2009;23(4): 531–43.

54. Jebara VA, Mihaileanu S, Acar C, et al. Left ventricular outflow tract obstruction after mitral valve repair. Results of the sliding leaflet technique. Circulation 1993;88(5 Pt 2):II30–4.

55. Maffessanti F, Marsan NA, Tamborini G, et al. Quantitative analysis of mitral valve apparatus in mitral valve prolapse before and after annuloplasty: a three-dimensional intraoperative transesophageal study. J Am Soc Echocardiogr 2011;24(4): 405–13.

56. Grewal J, Suri R, Mankad S, et al. Mitral annular dynamics in myxomatous valve disease: new insights with real-time 3-dimensional echocardiography. Circulation 2010;121(12):1423–31.

57. Lee AP, Hsiung MC, Salgo IS, et al. Quantitative analysis of mitral valve morphology in mitral valve prolapse using real-time three-dimensional echocardiography: importance of annular saddle-shape in pathogenesis of mitral regurgitation. Circulation 2013;127(7):832–41.

58. Salgo IS, Gorman JH 3rd, Gorman RC, et al. Effect of annular shape on leaflet curvature in reducing mitral leaflet stress. Circulation 2002; 106(6):711–7.

59. Kovalova S, Necas J. RT-3D TEE: characteristics of mitral annulus using mitral valve quantification (MVQ) program. Echocardiography 2011;28(4): 461–7.

60. Daimon M, Saracino G, Gillinov AM, et al. Local dysfunction and asymmetrical deformation of mitral annular geometry in ischemic mitral regurgitation: a novel computerized 3D echocardiographic analysis. Echocardiography 2008;25(4):414–23.

61. Fattouch K, Castrovinci S, Murana G, et al. Multiplane two-dimensional versus real time three-dimensional transesophageal echocardiography in ischemic mitral regurgitation. Echocardiography 2011;28(10):1125–32.

62. Shakil O, Jainandunsing JS, Ilic R, et al. Ischemic mitral regurgitation: an intraoperative echocardiographic perspective. J Cardiothorac Vasc Anesth 2012. [Epub ahead of print].

63. Magne J, Pibarot P, Dagenais F, et al. Preoperative posterior leaflet angle accurately predicts outcome after restrictive mitral valve annuloplasty for ischemic mitral regurgitation. Circulation 2007; 115(6):782–91.

64. Lee EM, Shapiro LM, Wells FC. Superiority of mitral valve repair in surgery for degenerative mitral regurgitation. Eur Heart J 1997;18(4):655–63.

65. Enriquez-Sarano M, Schaff HV, Orszulak TA, et al. Valve repair improves the outcome of surgery for mitral regurgitation. A multivariate analysis. Circulation 1995;91(4):1022–8.

66. Akins CW, Hilgenberg AD, Buckley MJ, et al. Mitral valve reconstruction versus replacement for degenerative or ischemic mitral regurgitation. Ann Thorac Surg 1994;58(3):668–75 [discussion: 675–6].

67. Carpentier A. Cardiac valve surgery—the "French correction". J Thorac Cardiovasc Surg 1983;86(3): 323 37.

68. Cook RC, Nifong LW, Lashley GG, et al. Echocardiographic measurements alone do not provide accurate non-invasive selection of annuloplasty band size for robotic mitral valve repair. J Heart Valve Dis 2006;15(4):524–7 [discussion: 527].

69. Ender J, Koncar-Zeh J, Mukherjee C, et al. Value of augmented reality-enhanced transesophageal echocardiography (TEE) for determining optimal annuloplasty ring size during mitral valve repair. Ann Thorac Surg 2008;86(5):1473–8.

70. Chikwe J, Adams DH, Su KN, et al. Can three-dimensional echocardiography accurately predict complexity of mitral valve repair? Eur J Cardiothorac Surg 2012;41(3):518–24.

71. Braun J, van de Veire NR, Klautz RJ, et al. Restrictive mitral annuloplasty cures ischemic mitral regurgitation and heart failure. Ann Thorac Surg 2008; 85(2):430–6 [discussion: 436–7].

Mitral Prosthetic Valve Assessment by Echocardiographic Guidelines

Rebecca T. Hahn, MD, FACC, FASE

KEYWORDS

- Mitral valve replacement • Echocardiography • Prosthetic heart valves • Effective orifice area

KEY POINTS

- Echocardiography with Doppler is the most widely used imaging modality for the assessment of prosthetic valve function.
- Compared with a native valve, the prosthetic valve is inherently obstructive, and the type and size of prosthesis determines what is considered normal function.
- Assessing prosthetic valve function is an integrative process, requiring knowledge of clinical information as well assessment of multiple echocardiographic parameters. These parameters include: two dimensional and three dimensional imaging of the prosthesis, and a comprehensive Doppler evaluation.

The assessment of mitral prosthetic valve function requires an integrative process using 2-dimensional (2D), 3-dimensional (3D), and Doppler echocardiographic modalities. In addition, because of acoustic shadowing of important cardiac anatomy, transesophageal echocardiography (TEE) is frequently required as an adjunct to transthoracic echocardiography (TTE). American and European guidelines for the management of valvular heart disease have been recently published, and address the choice and initial evaluation of prosthetic heart valves.[1–3] In addition, the American Society of Echocardiography has published guidelines on the echocardiographic assessment of prosthetic valve function[4] and the utility of 3D echocardiography.[5] This review discusses the echocardiographic assessment of prosthetic mitral valve (MV) function based on current guidelines.

PROSTHETIC HEART VALVES

A complete assessment of prosthetic valve function requires an understanding of the appearance and normal function of each type of prosthetic valve currently being implanted in the MV position. As newer valves are developed, functional assessments may change.

Mechanical Valves

Prior mechanical valve types no longer implanted include the caged ball and caged disc valve; the former may still be seen in patients given the extreme long-term durability of the valve (**Fig. 1**). The caged ball valve, designed by Charles Hufnagel, was first implanted in 1952. The Starr-Edwards valve soon followed in 1961 and became one of the longest-lasting manufactured valves to date, with production ending in 2007. This valve consists of a silicone ball enclosed in a wire cage composed of 3 or 4 wire arches. The orifice for blood flow is a ring, around the poppet, which exhibits an excursion of 1 to 2 cm and on closure results in minimal regurgitation. Because of this unusual orifice, calculations of effective orifice area (EOA) are difficult, peak velocities are high, and large pressure drops are seen in the wake of the ball. These low-pressure regions increase the

Columbia University Medical Center, New York-Presbyterian Hospital, 161 Fort Washington Avenue, HIP6-623, New York, NY 10032, USA
E-mail address: rth2@columbia.edu

Cardiol Clin 31 (2013) 287–309
http://dx.doi.org/10.1016/j.ccl.2013.03.004
0733-8651/13/$ – see front matter © 2013 Elsevier Inc. All rights reserved.

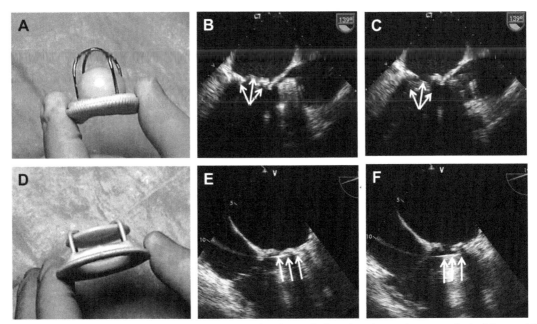

Fig. 1. The Starr-Edwards prosthesis (*A*) is composed of a silicone ball enclosed in a wire cage. The ball (*arrows*) is seated in the sewing ring when closed (*B*) and moves forward into the cage when open (*C*). The caged disc valve (*D*) has a similar design, with the disc (*arrows*) seating at the sewing ring when closed (*E*) and moving forward into the cage when open (*F*).

thrombogenicity of the valve. High shear forces around the ball also increase the risk of hemolysis. A variant of this design, the caged disc (Beall-Surgitool or Cross-Jones), was not as popular because of poor durability, and production was stopped in the 1970s.

Key Features of the Ball-in-Cage Valve:

- Little or no leak (low velocity backflow of 2–5 mL/beat)
- Large pressure drops secondary to wake (significant pressure-recovery), hence
- Higher peak velocities

Two primary forms of mechanical heart valves are currently being implanted, the bileaflet valve and the monoleaflet valve. There are several manufacturers of the bileaflet mechanical valve (**Fig. 2**), which was first released in 1977 (St Jude and CarboMedics); they are currently the most commonly implanted valves in the modern era. Two semilunar discs are attached to a rigid sewing ring by hinges. Differences between manufacturers and models exist with respect to the sewing cuff, opening angle, valve profile, and leaflet hinge mechanism. The discs have a closing angle of between 110° and 130° and an opening angle of 75° to 90°. In the open position there are 3 orifices which, because of the position of the hinges, create a small central slit-like

orifice and 2 larger lateral semicircular orifices. Because of this design, they have the largest EOA of all the mechanical valves (2.4–3.2 cm^2), with little intrinsic mitral regurgitation (MR). These intrinsic "washing" jets may prevent thrombus formation at the sites of closure. The jets are of short duration, narrow, and typically symmetric, with low (nonaliasing) velocities[6,7] and regurgitant fraction of less than 10% to 15%. These jets represent real, albeit small, regurgitant jets, which should be distinguished from jets created by motion or closing of the occluder.

Key Features of the Bileaflet Mechanical Valve:

- Both leaflets are typically visualized; however, acoustic noise is common
- For the St Jude Medical
  - Opening angle = 75° to 90°
  - Closing position = 120° for valves ≤25 mm and 130° for valves ≥27 mm
- Three orifices are seen in diastole with highest velocity from central orifice
- Intrinsic, small, flame-shaped washing jets of MR are seen
- Note: CarboMedics valve with recessed pivots may have larger regurgitant jets

The monoleaflet valves (**Fig. 3**) have a single disc secured to the sewing ring by either lateral or central metal struts. The disc has a closing angle of

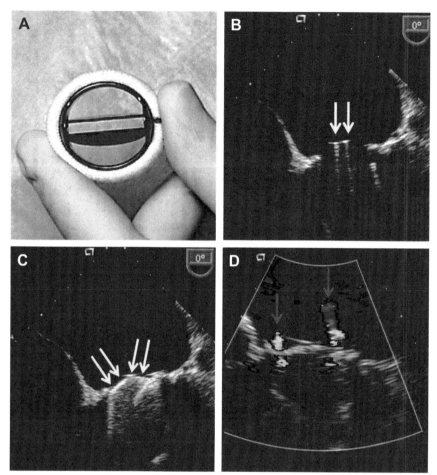

Fig. 2. The bileaflet mechanical valve (*A*) is composed of 2 semilunar discs attached to a rigid sewing ring by hinges. The opening angle of the 2 discs ranges from 75° to 90°. Echocardiographically the discs commonly create a "comet-tail" reverberation artifact (*B, yellow arrows*). The closing angle of the 2 discs ranges between 110° and 130° (*C*) as indicated by the *yellow arrows*. Intrinsic "washing" jets are seen around the moving parts of the valve (*D, red arrows*).

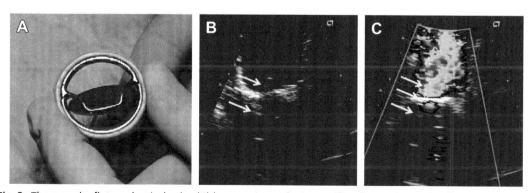

Fig. 3. The monoleaflet mechanical valve (*A*) has a major and minor orifice disc angle ranging from 60° to 80° (*B*) as indicated by the *yellow arrows*. In these images from the apical long-axis view, the major orifice faces the left ventricular outflow tract, creating marked turbulence.

between 110° and 130°, and an opening angle of 60° to 80°. The orifices for these valves are asymmetric, with a major orifice at the site of forward disc excursion (in the direction of flow) and a minor orifice at the site of retrograde disc excursion. There is significant shear stress in the wake of the disc and struts. The EOA of these valves ranges from 1.5 to 2.1 cm^2.

Key Features of the Monoleaflet Mechanical Valve:

- Major and minor orifice disc angle ranging from 60° to 80°
- Normal backflow = 5 to 9 mL/beat
- For MV regurgitation, the major orifice should be toward the free wall

○ Marked turbulence is created if the major orifice faces the left ventricular outflow tract (LVOT)

Bioprosthetic Heart Valves

Biological valves contain leaflets made from living material whether porcine or bovine tissue, homografts or autografts, mounted on a stent (**Fig. 4**). There are no commercially available stentless valves for the mitral position at this time.

The stented porcine bioprosthesis (see **Fig. 4**A, B) was first released in 1970 (Hancock and Carpentier-Edwards), and is a xenograft of a pig aortic valve mounted on a stent. The commissures of the valve must be supported for the valve to function, creating the classic "crown" appearance of the

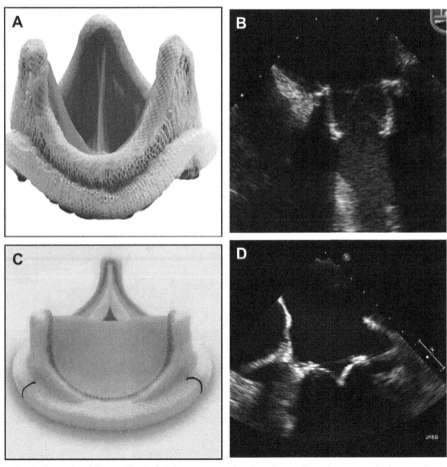

Fig. 4. The stented porcine bioprosthesis (A) is a xenograft of a pig aortic valve, mounted on a stent. The commissures of the valve must be supported for the valve to function, creating the classic "crown" appearance of the 3 struts. Echocardiographically, the lowest borders of the cusps (the sinuses of Valsalva) align with the lower edge of the stent (B). The stented pericardial prostheses (C) contain bovine or equine pericardial cusps mounted on struts. The profile of these valves is typically lower than the porcine xenograft. Echocardiographically the leaflets are centered in the valve frame (D).

3 struts. The height of the valve is the height of the sinus of Valsalva, and thus typically 1.7 to 2.0 cm. Because this is a biological aortic valve, the lowest borders of the cusps (the sinuses of Valsalva) align with the lower edge of the stent, and leaflet coaptation occurs just distal to this point. Backflow is uncommon (10% of normally functioning valves).

The stented pericardial prostheses contain bovine (Carpentier-Edwards, released in 1982) or equine pericardial cusps, sterilized and mounted on struts. The profile of these valves is typically lower than that of the porcine xenograft, and the leaflets are centered in the valve frame. A small central or commissural jet is common, and cusp design allows for valve shrinkage. Thus small central jets are more common with this type of stented valve.

Key Features of the Biological Prosthetic Valve:

- Radiographically the Carpentier-Edwards valves appear as a crown (in contrast to the Hancock valve, which appears as a circular ring)
- Porcine forward flow has higher turbulence (peaked flow profile) than the pericardial valve (flat flow profile)
  - Backflow is less common, seen in only 10% of normally functioning valves
  - High pressure drop secondary to stents, hence obligatory stenosis
- Pericardial valve
  - Very small central or commissural jets common
  - Advantages over porcine bioprosthesis include better hemodynamics, greater durability (high number of collagen cross-links), and extra tissue to allow for shrinkage

Although the first successful implantation of a stentless MV prosthesis was performed in 1960, further development has been hindered by the extreme individual variability of the MV apparatus, the lack of durability and the lack of hemodynamic superiority of these valves over the currently available bioprosthetic valves.[8] Homografts,[9] xenografts,[10] tubular sleeves,[11] bileaflet/chordal bioprosthesis,[12-14] and even partial replacement[13] have been investigated; however, defining their clinical utility remains challenging.

ASSESSING PROSTHETIC MITRAL VALVE FUNCTION
General Recommendations

Echocardiography with Doppler is the most widely used imaging modality for the assessment of prosthetic valve function. Compared with a native valve the prosthetic valve is inherently obstructive, and the type and size of prosthesis determines what is considered normal function. Therefore gradients, EOA, and degree of physiologic regurgitation will vary based on valve type, manufacturer, and valve size, and the echocardiographic interpretation of function will depend on knowledge of the exact type, size, and even the date of implantation. **Table 1** is a summary of reported EOAs, calculated by the continuity equation, for a variety of valve types and sizes reported by recent studies.[15-18] Valve types and other hemodynamic characteristics not listed can be found in previously published reviews.[4,19]

General recommendations outlined in prior guidelines[2-4] and reviews[20] for the evaluation of prosthetic valves should be followed (**Table 2**), including first the acquisition of pertinent patient information such as valve type, size, and implantation date. Comparison with baseline or follow-up studies is particularly useful in deciding valvular dysfunction. Follow-up recommendations vary by guideline, with the Canadian guidelines recommending that an initial echocardiogram be performed at discharge or within 30 days of implant.[21] The European guidelines[3] recommend that the initial baseline study be performed ideally 6 to 12 weeks following surgery. The American College of Cardiology guidelines[1] recommend that the first postoperative assessment be performed 4 to 6 weeks after, if not before, hospital discharge. Annual routine follow-up echocardiograms are not recommended for mechanical valves or within the first 5 years following bioprosthetic valve replacement. Annual follow-up is recommended after 5 years in patients with a bioprosthesis.[1,21] New Appropriate Use Criteria for Echocardiography[22] give yet another recommendation: routine surveillance is inappropriate less than 3 years following valve implantation in the absence of known or suspected valve dysfunction, but is appropriate from 3 years following implantation (for either mechanical or bioprosthetic valves). Routine surveillance TEE was also deemed appropriate from 3 years following implantation in the absence of known or suspected valve dysfunction.

Heart rate and blood pressure should be recorded with each study. Transvalvular gradients vary depending on heart rate and blood pressure. Because diastolic filling time varies significantly with heart rate, recording the value at the time of Doppler evaluation is particularly important when assessing prosthetic MV function. Finally, height, weight, and body surface area are necessary to determine the presence of prosthesis-patient mismatch (PPM).

Prosthetic material causes numerous ultrasound artifacts, including acoustic shadowing,

Table 1
Common prosthetic mitral valves types and sizes, with reported effective orifice areas

	Prosthetic Valve Size (mm)					
	25	27	29	31	33	Reference
Stented Bioprostheses						
Medtronic Mosaic	1.42 ± 0.29	1.62 ± 0.47	1.83 ± 0.68	1.70 ± 0.41	2.71 ± 0.77	Blauwet et al,[18] 2010
Medtronic Hancock II	1.44 ± 0.59	1.51 ± 0.32	1.80 ± 0.69	1.58 ± 0.31[a]	—	Blauwet et al,[18] 2010
Carpentier-Edwards Perimount	1.75 ± 0.53	1.88 + 0.52	2.02 ± 0.57	2.09 ± 0.48	2.24 ± 0.97	Blauwet et al,[18] 2010
Carpentier-Edwards Duraflex	—	1.44 ± 0.4	1.53 ± 0.5	1.67 ± 0.6	1.65 ± 0.7	Blauwet et al,[16] 2009
Mechanical Prostheses						
St Jude Medical Standard	1.5 ± 0.3	1.7 ± 0.4	1.8 ± 0.4	2.0 ± 0.5	2.0 ± 0.5	Magne et al,[15] 2007
MCRI On-X[b]	2.2 ± 0.9	2.2 ± 0.9	2.2 ± 0.9	2.2 ± 0.9	2.2 ± 0.9	Magne et al,[15] 2007
Sorin CarboMedics	1.88 ± 0.43	2.12 ± 0.50	2.31 ± 0.54	2.21 ± 0.52	2.19 ± 0.46	Blauwet et al,[17] 2012

Effective orifice area is expressed as mean values available in the literature calculated by continuity equation.
[a] Small number of patients; data may be unreliable.
[b] The strut and leaflets of the MCRI On-X valve are identical for all sizes (25–33 mm).

reverberation, refraction, and mirror artifacts. Assessing the function of the prosthetic MV is thus particularly challenging from TTE windows. Imaging from multiple and sometimes off-axis views are required (**Fig. 5**). Whereas diastolic flow into the left ventricle and the flow on the left ventricular (LV) side of the prosthesis can be imaged, the left atrium is far-field in every TTE view, making color Doppler imaging of prosthetic regurgitation problematic. The imaging window for TEE is ideal for visualizing the left atrium and pulmonary veins and the left atrial (LA) side of the prosthesis, while Doppler interrogation of these same structures can also be optimized. Imaging of the left ventricle and subvalvular apparatus is more limited. Therefore, a complete TTE and TEE may be necessary for accurate assessment of prosthetic MV function.

Utility of TTE Versus TEE for Mitral Prosthetic Valve Evaluation:

- TEE superior to TTE:
  - MR assessment
  - Structural valve failure
  - Thrombus
  - Endocarditis: vegetations, abscess
- TEE equal to TTE:
  - MV gradient/area by Doppler
- TTE superior to TEE
  - Left ventricular function and subvalvular apparatus

A comprehensive Doppler evaluation follows the same principles as for native valve stenosis and regurgitation assessment.[23,24] Pulsed-wave (PW) Doppler and continuous-wave (CW) Doppler should be performed from multiple windows to minimize insonation angle, optimize imaging, and accurately assess flow. High sweep speeds (100 mm/s) may increase the accuracy of Doppler measurements. In addition, averaging values from 1 to 3 cycles in sinus rhythm and 5 to 15 cycles in atrial fibrillation is recommended. For calculations of EOA or Doppler velocity index (DVI), which require measurement of stroke volumes from different cardiac cycles, and measurement of peak transvalvular velocity-time integral (VTI), matching the respective cycles lengths to within 10% is advised.[4] For the mitral prosthesis, the cycle length of mitral inflow should be matched with the preceding interval of LV or right ventricular (RV) outflow velocity.

Although it is important to record the pressure half-time, it is not appropriate to use the pressure half-time formula to calculate EOA for prosthetic valves. This concept is an extremely important one to remember. The pressure half-time method of calculating MV area was validated for native mitral valves[25]; however, flow characteristics of prosthetic valves, as well as compliance characteristics of the post-surgical atrium and ventricle, limit the utility of the pressure half-time method. Early studies of

Table 2
Essential parameters in the comprehensive evaluation of prosthetic valve function

Parameter	Feature
Clinical information	Symptoms and related clinical findings Date of valve replacement Type and size of the prosthetic valve Height/weight/body surface area Blood pressure and heart rate
Indirect echo signs of mitral valve dysfunction	Left and right ventricular size, function, and hypertrophy Left and right atrial size Concomitant valvular disease Estimation of pulmonary artery pressure
Previous postoperative study(ies) (if available)	Comparison of above parameters is particularly helpful in suspected prosthetic valvular dysfunction
Imaging of the valve	Motion of leaflets or occluder Presence of calcification on the leaflets or abnormal echo density(ies) on the various components of the prosthesis Valve sewing-ring integrity and motion
Doppler echo of the valve	Contour of the jet velocity signal Peak velocity and gradient Mean pressure gradient Velocity-time integral of the jet Doppler velocity index Pressure half-time in mitral valve and tricuspid valve Effective orifice area Presence, location, and severity of regurgitation

Modified from Zoghbi WA, Chambers JB, Dumesnil JG, et al. Recommendations for evaluation of prosthetic valves with echocardiography and Doppler ultrasound: a report From the American Society of Echocardiography's Guidelines and Standards Committee and the Task Force on Prosthetic Valves, developed in conjunction with the American College of Cardiology Cardiovascular Imaging Committee, Cardiac Imaging Committee of the American Heart Association, the European Association of Echocardiography, a registered branch of the European Society of Cardiology, the Japanese Society of Echocardiography and the Canadian Society of Echocardiography, endorsed by the American College of Cardiology Foundation, American Heart Association, European Association of Echocardiography, a registered branch of the European Society of Cardiology, the Japanese Society of Echocardiography, and Canadian Society of Echocardiography. J Am Soc Echocardiogr 2009;22:975–1014; with permission.

bioprosthetic[26,27] and mechanical[28] mitral prostheses showed that areas by the pressure half-time method varied significantly and failed to correlate with the actual area of the prosthetic valve. Bitar and colleagues[28] showed that mechanical prosthetic valve areas calculated using the continuity equation method yielded smaller EOAs than provided by the manufacturer, but were more accurate

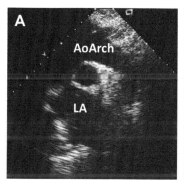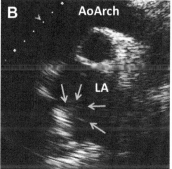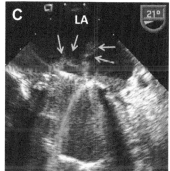

Fig. 5. Transthoracic imaging of prosthetic mitral valve morphology and function is limited by acoustic shadowing of the left atrium. Suprasternal notch imaging (*A*) of the left atrium may circumvent the acoustic shadowing and allow imaging of vegetations (see zoomed TTE image *B*, *arrows*). These vegetations were easily imaged on subsequent transesophageal imaging (*C*, *arrows*). AoArch, aortic arch; LA, left atrium.

in differentiating various valve sizes ($P = .0002$) compared with mean gradient ($P = .013$) or pressure half-time (P not significant). Although the absolute values of EOA calculated by the continuity equation may underestimate the true geometric valve area, these investigators suggest that use of the continuity equation–derived valve area for assessing longitudinal valve function in a given patient may be more accurate than the pressure half-time method. Subsequent large studies of normal mechanical and bioprosthetic valve hemodynamics confirm these earlier findings.[16–18] Pressure half-time measurements of greater than 200 milliseconds can be used as a semiquantitative assessment of prosthetic stenosis; however, because this parameter is very dependent on chronotropy, atrial compliance, and ventricular compliance, it can be normal in the setting of significant prosthetic valve dysfunction.

Double-envelope spectral Doppler profiles (**Fig. 6**) may often be seen in the setting of mechanical prostheses.[29] This profile is related to different flow characteristics of the mechanical orifices. In the setting of a single tilting disc, a large major and small minor orifice may create a dense and typically lower velocity jet arising from the major orifice, and a faint, higher velocity jet from the minor orifice. Similarly, the bileaflet disc mechanical valve generates a dense, lower-velocity jet arising from the lateral orifices, with a faint, higher-velocity jet arising from the central orifice. Because peak early diastolic velocity may be a better measure of mechanic mitral stenosis than pressure half-time[30] for either valve, the dense, lower-velocity jet should be used to assess function and calculate EOA using the continuity equation.

Transthoracic Imaging and Doppler Evaluation of the Prosthetic Mitral Valve

Because of the limitations of TTE described earlier, indirect signs of MV dysfunction, including LV and LA size, concomitant valvular disease, and estimation of pulmonary artery pressures, must be assessed (see **Table 2**). When imaging the valve, the following assessments should always be included: motion of leaflets or occluder, presence of calcification or abnormal echo-densities, and valve sewing-ring integrity and motion. When performing Doppler imaging of the valve, the following parameters should be recorded: contour of the jet velocity signals, transvalvular velocities and gradients, VTI, DVI, pressure half-time, EOA (by continuity equation), and presence/location/severity of regurgitation.

Parasternal long-axis views can be particularly useful in assessing the mitral prosthesis, and this is usually the first image for evaluation of the thickness and motion of leaflets or occluders as well as integrity and morphology of the valve sewing ring. Mechanical valves create significant reverberation and shadowing artifacts, making an assessment from this view difficult. Nonetheless, depending on the orientation of the mechanical occluders, the number of discs and excursion can be assessed. Shadowing is typically less with bioprosthetic valves, and leaflet morphology and function can frequently be imaged. Because of the dynamic narrowing and motion of the mitral annulus, some prosthetic valve motion may be normal.

The parasternal long-axis view also allows an assessment of LV size and function as well as the LV outflow tract (OT). Current surgical

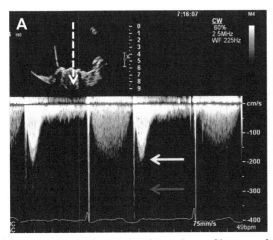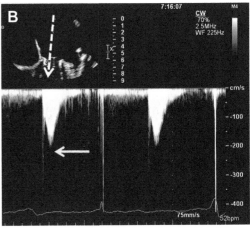

Fig. 6. Double-envelope spectral Doppler profiles may often be seen in the setting of mechanical prostheses. The bileaflet disc mechanical valve generates a dense, lower-velocity jet arising from the lateral orifices (*A and B, yellow arrow*), with a faint, higher-velocity jet from the central orifice (*A, red arrow*). The denser, lower-velocity jet should be used to assess function.

techniques attempt to retain native MV apparatus such as papillary muscles, chordae tendinae, and attached leaflets, which typically necessitates tilting the prosthetic valve frequently toward the ventricular septum to avoid these native structures. Particularly with high-profile valves such as the porcine xenograft, strut impingement of the LVOT and septum may lead to significant outflow gradients. In the setting of marked anterior prosthetic valve tilting, transmitral diastolic or regurgitant systolic flow from the parasternal view may be parallel to the insonation beam, allowing on-axis Doppler assessment of valve function. Both CW and color Doppler can thus be performed.

Parasternal inflow views are important in assessing the severity of tricuspid regurgitation and measuring right atrial–RV gradients for estimations of pulmonary artery pressures. Parasternal outflow views may also be important in assessing the severity of pulmonary hypertension, and are strongly recommended. Numerous recent reviews and guidelines discuss the echocardiographic evaluation of pulmonary hemodynamics.[31–34]

Parasternal short-axis views can also be extremely important for assessing prosthetic valve function. The orientation of the occluders or struts can be easily imaged and may be important in assessing function. The anatomic orientation of the occluders should mimic the native valve opening; this preserves the inflow pattern and intraventricular LV vortices that are important for filling. Pop and colleagues[35] found that when the single tilting disc major orifice directed flow anteriorly as opposed to posteriorly, the transvalvular gradients were higher. Orientation is less of an issue for the bileaflet valve, given its superior flow characteristics.

Apical views are essential for assessing the leaflets or occluders and the integrity of the sewing ring, and for performing accurate Doppler assessment of function. Not infrequently, the closing angle of occluders, particularly in the bileaflet mechanical valve, can be measured. Off-axis views may be necessary for the accurate Doppler assessment of valvular function; aligning the insonation beam parallel to flow is crucial. The transmitral peak velocity and peak or mean gradients are influenced by ventricular and atrial function, chamber compliances, and relative chamber pressures, as discussed earlier. Therefore although peak velocity and pressure half-time should be measured, these measures cannot, in isolation, be used to assess prosthetic valve function.

Transesophageal Imaging

TEE windows are ideal for assessing the morphology and flow of prosthetic valve and sewing ring within the left atrium and pulmonary veins. The most useful views include the mid-esophageal 4-chamber, commissural, 2-chamber, and 3-chamber views. However, transgastric views may be useful when assessing LV size and function or papillary muscle and chordal anatomy.

For mechanical valves, the occluder motion and the closing and opening angles should be assessed. In the setting of abnormal disc motion, the etiology should be determined. In addition, intrinsic regurgitant jets must be distinguished from pathologic regurgitant jets. Unlike intrinsic "washing" jets, pathologic regurgitant jets are usually holosystolic, wide, and asymmetric. These jets are frequently eccentric and wall-hugging, extending far into the receiving chamber and with mosaic or turbulent color Doppler jets.

Color Doppler Features of Physiologic Leakage:

- Short and narrow
- Typically symmetric (typically with bileaflet valve)
- Low velocity, nonaliasing

Features of Pathologic Regurgitation:

- Large, wide jet
- Asymmetric and eccentric (paravalvular)
- High velocity, aliasing

Three-Dimensional Imaging and Doppler

3D TEE has completely changed the imaging paradigm for evaluation of the MV apparatus. Its primary use is morphologic, allowing the echocardiographer to create a 3D en-face surgical view of the valve, which is extremely useful for determining prosthetic valve function and defining the extent and location of paravalvular regurgitation. The MV should be oriented with the aortic valve in the 12-o'clock position (**Fig. 7**), regardless of whether viewed from the LA or the LV perspective; this creates the standard "surgeon's view," which enhances communication of abnormal findings intraprocedurally. For a full discussion of 3D TEE, the reader is referred to the recently published American Society of Echocardiography recommendations.[5]

Multiple modes of 3D acquisition are available. Narrow-angle 3D mode allows real-time (single-beat) imaging of a narrow-angle pyramidal volume. Although this may be sufficient to visualize the native mitral apparatus, it is rarely adequate for imaging the entire prosthesis and sewing ring. Instead, the full-volume or user-defined acquisition modes have larger acquisition sectors, ideal for imaging the entire mitral prosthesis. The loss

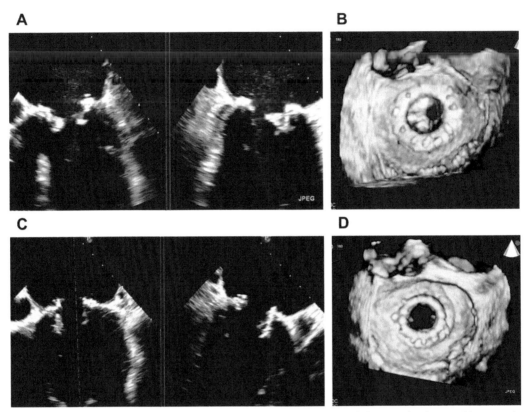

Fig. 7. Three-dimensional (3D) imaging enhances morphologic imaging of the mitral valve. In this example of bioprosthetic valve stenosis, simultaneous multiplane imaging (*A*) shows significant thickening of 2 of the cusps. User-defined real-time 3D (*B*) further enhances visualization of the 2 immobile cusps. Following transcatheter valve-in-valve procedure in the same patient, 3D imaging confirms the position and function of the new transcatheter valve (*C, D*). During real-time 3D imaging, the mitral valve should be oriented with the aortic valve in the 12 o'clock position, whether viewed from the left atrial or the left ventricular perspective.

of temporal resolution with larger volumes may be resolved by using a multibeat acquisition.

Multiple 3D TEE color-flow Doppler modes are also available as narrow-angle, full-volume, and user-defined modes. As with noncolor imaging, the trade-off between image size and temporal resolution is the primary challenge. Multibeat acquisition may solve the temporal resolution, but at the cost of splice artifacts that may affect accurate measurement of regurgitant jet size. During conscious sedation or in the operating room with an intubated patient, "breath holds" significantly reduce cardiac motion during multibeat acquisitions.

ASSESSING PROSTHETIC MITRAL VALVE COMPLICATIONS

Prosthetic valve dysfunction may be categorized as structural or nonstructural.[36] Structural valve dysfunction includes dysfunction or deterioration intrinsic to the valve, including calcification, leaflet

tear, or flail; this is more common in biological valves, and may occur earlier in younger patients. Other patient comorbidities such as renal failure may increase the risk of calcification. Nonstructural valve dysfunction characteristically occurs early following implantation, and is defined as any abnormality not intrinsic to the valve itself. These complications are usually related to technical issues and include suture dehiscence with associated paravalvular regurgitation, problems related to retained native mitral apparatus, and PPM. Other nonstructural problems such as pannus formation are late complications.

Structural Valve Dysfunction

Echocardiography is the primary imaging modality for determining the presence of pathologic prosthetic valve stenosis or regurgitation. **Table 3** lists the Doppler parameters used to assess prosthetic MV function. The typical peak velocity for a bileaflet mechanical valve is usually less than 1.9 m/s[19,30,37]

Table 3
Doppler parameters for the evaluation of prosthetic mitral valve stenosis

	Normal[a]	Possible Stenosis[b]	Suggests Significant Stenosis[a,b]
Peak velocity[c,d]	<1.9 m/s	1.9–2.5 m/s	≥2.5 m/s
Mean gradient[c,d]	≤5 mm Hg	6–10 mm Hg	>10 mm Hg
VTI$_{PrMV}$/VTI$_{LVOT}$[c,d]	<2.2	2.2–2.5	>2.5
Effective orifice area	≥2.0 cm^2	1–2 cm^2	<1 cm^2
PHT	<130 ms	130–200 ms	>200 ms

Abbreviations: PHT, pressure half-time; VTI$_{LVOT}$, velocity-time integral across the left ventricular outflow tract by pulsed-wave Doppler; VTI$_{PrMV}$, velocity-time integral across the mitral valve by continuous-wave Doppler.

[a] Best specificity for normality or abnormality is seen if the majority of the parameters listed are normal or abnormal, respectively.

[b] Values of the parameters should prompt a closer evaluation of valve function and/or other considerations such as increased flow, increased heart rate, or prosthesis-patient mismatch.

[c] These parameters are also abnormal in the presence of significant prosthetic mitral.

[d] Slightly higher cutoff values than shown may be seen in some bioprosthetic valves.

Modified from Zoghbi WA, Chambers JB, Dumesnil JG, et al. Recommendations for evaluation of prosthetic valves with echocardiography and Doppler ultrasound: a report From the American Society of Echocardiography's Guidelines and Standards Committee and the Task Force on Prosthetic Valves, developed in conjunction with the American College of Cardiology Cardiovascular Imaging Committee, Cardiac Imaging Committee of the American Heart Association, the European Association of Echocardiography, a registered branch of the European Society of Cardiology, the Japanese Society of Echocardiography and the Canadian Society of Echocardiography, endorsed by the American College of Cardiology Foundation, American Heart Association, European Association of Echocardiography, a registered branch of the European Society of Cardiology, the Japanese Society of Echocardiography, and Canadian Society of Echocardiography. J Am Soc Echocardiogr 2009;22:975–1014; with permission.

with a mean gradient of less than 5 to 6 mm Hg. However, ventricular systolic and diastolic function, as well as intraventricular pressures, must always be considered when using peak velocities and gradients to assess valvular function. Because some bioprosthetic valves have a smaller EOA for a given prosthetic valve size, normal peak velocities may be greater than 1.9 m/s. The differential diagnosis for a high-velocity or mean gradient includes hyperdynamic state, tachycardia, PPM, regurgitation, or stenosis. Prosthetic MV stenosis is usually associated with high velocities (≥2.5 m/s) and mean gradients (>10 mm Hg). The VTI across the MV by CW Doppler (VTI$_{PrMV}$) compared with the VTI across the LVOT by PW Doppler (VTI$_{LVOT}$) gives an assessment of relative flow. If this ratio is less than 2.2, relative flows are equal. If it is greater than 2.5, transmitral flow is greater than LV outflow, suggesting either stenosis or regurgitation. Calculating the EOA as well as the pressure half-time may help distinguish stenosis from regurgitation (see **Table 3**). Pseudonormalization of this parameter, however, may occur in the setting of tachycardia, altered atrial and ventricular compliance or relaxation, aortic regurgitation, and high peak-pressure difference at the beginning of diastole. Thus, normal (<130 milliseconds) or even intermediate (130–200 milliseconds) pressure half-time measurements should be interpreted with caution.

Qualitative assessment of prosthetic MV regurgitation uses many of the same parameters as for native valve regurgitation[23] as well as the parameters already outlined here. In addition, excessive motion of the sewing ring may be a clue to paravalvular dehiscence. A rocking motion of greater than 15° of sewing-ring excursion is abnormal (**Fig. 8**A, B). Although acoustic shadowing frequently prevents an accurate assessment of regurgitant jets, proximal flow convergence on the LV side of the sewing ring may be an indication of significant regurgitation (see **Fig. 8**C). In addition, turbulent color flow within the left atrium distal to the acoustic shadow may also be seen. Quantifying prosthetic MV regurgitation, however, is particularly problematic. Unlike with native MV regurgitation or even prosthetic aortic valve regurgitation whereby comparative flow measurements and transvalvular stroke volumes can be quantified, the only method for quantifying regurgitant volume for the mitral prosthesis is to subtract the Doppler-derived LV or RV stroke volume from the 2D-derived LV stroke volume. Using 3D-derived LV stroke volume may increase the accuracy of this method,[38,39] but systematically underestimates volumes compared with magnetic resonance imaging.[39] At present, integrating multiple qualitative and semiquantitative methods is still the recommended approach for assessing prosthetic MV regurgitation (**Tables 4** and **5**). 3D color Doppler, however, seems a promising method for assessing prosthetic valve function,[40,41] although studies are limited. Localization of the regurgitant

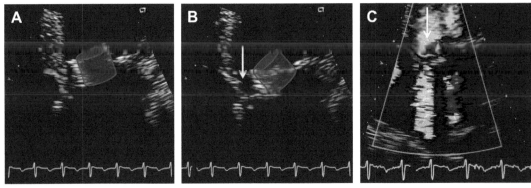

Fig. 8. Abnormal motion of the prosthetic sewing ring consistent with dehiscence can be detected by transthoracic imaging. In these apical 4-chamber views, the position of the bioprosthetic mitral valve in diastole (*A*) and systole (*B*) show greater than 15 of sewing-ring excursion suggestive of dehiscence of the medial sewing ring (*yellow arrow*). In addition, color flow Doppler shows a prominent proximal flow convergence (*C, yellow arrow*) on the left ventricular side of the sewing ring, indicating significant regurgitation.

jets, as well as measurement of the color Doppler vena contracta dimensions and area, is possible and highly useful, particularly when contemplating transcatheter closure.[42,43] In particular, the circumferential length of the jets may determine the size of the closure device, and is best visualized using 3D imaging.[43]

Using these parameters, a suggested algorithm for assessing mechanical prosthetic MV function is shown in **Fig. 9**. A case example of

Table 4
Transthoracic echocardiographic findings suggestive of significant prosthetic mitral regurgitation in mechanical valves with normal pressure half-time

Finding	Sn (%)	Sp (%)	Comments
Peak mitral velocity $\geq$1.9 m/s[a]	90	89	Also consider high flow, PPM
$VTI_{PrMV}/VTI_{LVOT} \geq$2.5[a]	89	91	Measurement errors $\uparrow$ in AFib; Also consider PPM
Mean gradient $\geq$5 mm Hg[a]	90	70	At physiologic HR; also consider high flow, PPM
Maximal TR jet velocity >3 m/s[a]	80	71	Consider residual postoperative pulmonary hypertension or other causes
LV stroke volume derived by 2D or 3D is >30% higher than systemic stroke volume by Doppler	Moderate Sn	Specific	Validation lacking; significant MR is suspected when LV function is nl to $\uparrow$'d and VTI_{LVOT} is <16 cm
Systolic flow convergence seen in the left ventricle toward the prosthesis	Low Sn	Specific	Validation lacking; technically challenging

Abbreviations: 2D, 2-dimensional; 3D, 3-dimensional; AFib, atrial fibrillation; HR, heart rate; LV, left ventricular; MR, mitral regurgitation; PPM, prosthesis-patient mismatch; Sn, sensitivity; Sp, specificity; TR, tricuspid regurgitation; VTI_{LVOT}, velocity-time integral across the left ventricular outflow tract by pulsed-wave Doppler; VTI_{PrMv}, velocity-time integral across the mitral valve by continuous-wave Doppler.
  [a] Data from Olmos et al. When both peak velocity and VTI ratio are elevated with a normal pressure half-time, specificity is close to 100%.
  Modified from Zoghbi WA, Chambers JB, Dumesnil JG, et al. Recommendations for evaluation of prosthetic valves with echocardiography and Doppler ultrasound: a report From the American Society of Echocardiography's Guidelines and Standards Committee and the Task Force on Prosthetic Valves, developed in conjunction with the American College of Cardiology Cardiovascular Imaging Committee, Cardiac Imaging Committee of the American Heart Association, the European Association of Echocardiography, a registered branch of the European Society of Cardiology, the Japanese Society of Echocardiography and the Canadian Society of Echocardiography, endorsed by the American College of Cardiology Foundation, American Heart Association, European Association of Echocardiography, a registered branch of the European Society of Cardiology, the Japanese Society of Echocardiography, and Canadian Society of Echocardiography. J Am Soc Echocardiogr 2009;22:975–1014; with permission.

Table 5
Doppler echocardiographic criteria for severity of prosthetic mitral valve regurgitation (central and paravalvular)

Echo Variable	Parameter	Mild	Moderate	Severe
Indirect signs	LV size[a]	Normal	Normal or dilated	Usually dilated
	Pulmonary hypertension (sPAP $\geq$50 mm Hg at rest and $\geq$60 mm Hg with exercise)	Generally absent	Variable	Generally present
	Valve structure and motion	Usually normal	Usually abnormal[b]	Usually abnormal[b]
Doppler parameters (qualitative)	Color flow jet area[c]	Small, central jet (usually <4 cm^2 or <20% of LA area)	Variable	Large central jet (usually $\geq$8 cm^2 or >40% of LA area); variable size wall impinging/jet swirling in LA
	Flow convergence	None or minimal	Intermediate	Large
	Jet density: CW Doppler	Incomplete or faint	Dense	Dense
	Jet contour: CW Doppler	Parabolic	Usually parabolic	Early peaking, triangular
	Pulmonary venous flow: PW Doppler	Systolic dominance	Systolic blunting	Systolic flow reversal
	VTI$_{PrMV}$/VTI$_{LVO}$: PW Doppler	<2.2	2.2–2.5	>2.5
Doppler parameters (quantitative)	Vena contracta width (mm)	1–2	3–6	>6
	Regurgitant volume (mL/best)	<30	30–59	$\geq$60
	Regurgitant fraction (%)	<30	30–49	$\geq$50
	Effective regurgitant orifice area (mm^2)[d]	<20–30	30–49	$\geq$50

Abbreviations: CW, continuous-wave; LA, left atrium; PW, pulsed-wave; sPAP, systolic pulmonary artery pressure.

[a] LV size applied only to chronic lesions.

[b] Abnormal mechanical valves: immobile occluder, dehiscence, or rocking (paravalvular regurgitation). Abnormal biological valves: leaflet thickening calcification or prolapse, dehiscence, or rocking (paravalvular regurgitation).

[c] Parameter applicable to central jets and is less accurate in eccentric jets.

[d] Because of the eccentric nature of many of these lesions, effective regurgitant orifice area is often overestimated; hence, the cut off used to detect severe MR is larger than for native valvular disease.

Modified from Zoghbi WA, Chambers JB, Dumesnil JG, et al. Recommendations for evaluation of prosthetic valves with echocardiography and Doppler ultrasound: a report From the American Society of Echocardiography's Guidelines and Standards Committee and the Task Force on Prosthetic Valves, developed in conjunction with the American College of Cardiology Cardiovascular Imaging Committee, Cardiac Imaging Committee of the American Heart Association, the European Association of Echocardiography, a registered branch of the European Society of Cardiology, the Japanese Society of Echocardiography and the Canadian Society of Echocardiography, endorsed by the American College of Cardiology Foundation, American Heart Association, European Association of Echocardiography, a registered branch of the European Society of Cardiology, the Japanese Society of Echocardiography, and Canadian Society of Echocardiography. J Am Soc Echocardiogr 2009;22:975–1014; with permission.

the Doppler measurements used to assess prosthetic valve function is shown in **Fig. 10**. Using the algorithm, the high peak velocity and mean gradient, high VTI$_{PrMv}$/VTI$_{LVO}$ ratio, but low pressure half-time is suggestive of significant prosthetic mitral regurgitation, which was confirmed by TEE (**Fig. 11**).

Stress Echo

Evaluating dyspnea in patients with prosthetic mitral regurgitation may require functional testing with stress echocardiography. The primary goal of the test is to record gradients across the mitral prosthesis and tricuspid valve. Although data for prosthetic valves is not available, it is reasonable to use a

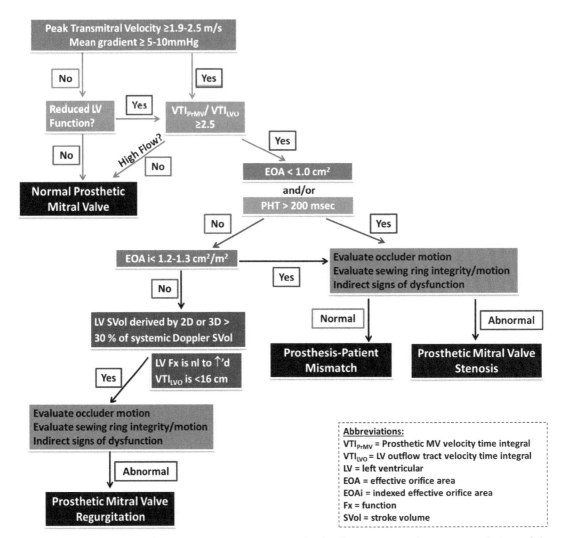

Fig. 9. Suggested algorithm for determining mechanic mitral valve function using the recommendations of the American Society of Echocardiography. (*From* Zoghbi WA, Chambers JB, Dumesnil JG, et al. Recommendations for evaluation of prosthetic valves with echocardiography and Doppler ultrasound: a report From the American Society of Echocardiography's Guidelines and Standards Committee and the Task Force on Prosthetic Valves, developed in conjunction with the American College of Cardiology Cardiovascular Imaging Committee, Cardiac Imaging Committee of the American Heart Association, the European Association of Echocardiography, a registered branch of the European Society of Cardiology, the Japanese Society of Echocardiography and the Canadian Society of Echocardiography, endorsed by the American College of Cardiology Foundation, American Heart Association, European Association of Echocardiography, a registered branch of the European Society of Cardiology, the Japanese Society of Echocardiography, and Canadian Society of Echocardiography. J Am Soc Echocardiogr 2009;22:975–1014; with permission.)

mean gradient of greater than 18 mm Hg to indicate obstruction.[44] High estimated pulmonary artery pressures during stress offers additional indirect evidence for significant prosthetic valve dysfunction.

Nonstructural Valve Dysfunction

Suture dehiscence and paravalvular regurgitation may present clinically as heart failure (if the regurgitant volume is large) or hemolysis. Hemolysis with paravalvular regurgitation has been ascribed to 3 basic mechanisms.[45] Fragmentation occurs when a jet is divided by the dehisced annular sewing ring. Collision of the jet with the ligament of Marshall or LA appendage wall causes rapid deceleration. Acceleration of the jet through a very small orifice, typically in the setting of high LV systolic pressures, may also cause hemolysis (**Fig. 12**).

A

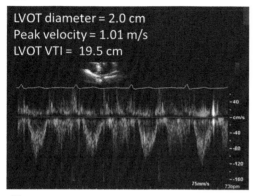

LVOT diameter = 2.0 cm
Peak velocity = 1.01 m/s
LVOT VTI = 19.5 cm

B

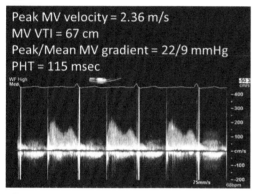

Peak MV velocity = 2.36 m/s
MV VTI = 67 cm
Peak/Mean MV gradient = 22/9 mmHg
PHT = 115 msec

C

Doppler Parameter	
Peak velocity	2.36 m/s
Mean gradient	9 mmHg
VTI$_{PrMv}$/VTI$_{LVO}$	3.4
PHT	115

Fig. 10. A case example of the Doppler measurements used to assess prosthetic valve function. *Panel A* is the spectral PW Doppler across the LVOT. *Panel B* is the spectral CW Doppler across the MV. *Panel C* is a summary of the important hemodynamic findings. See text for explanation and final assessment of MV function. LVOT, left ventricular outflow tract; MV, mitral valve; PHT, pressure halftime; VTI, velocity time integral; VTI$_{LVO}$, velocity time integral of the LVOT; VTI$_{PrMv}$ velocity time integral of the prosthetic MV.

Patients with paravalvular regurgitation without hemolysis had free jets or slow deceleration.

MV replacement is typically performed with preservation of native papillary muscle, chordae tendinae, and attached leaflets. Multiple studies have

suggested that this surgical technique prevents postoperative deterioration of ventricular function, and presumably diminishes the risk of myocardial rupture.[46–49] Numerous reports of LVOT obstruction by either retained anterior mitral leaflet[50,51] or high-profile prosthetic valve struts[52,53] suggest that this complication is not benign and may result in progressive symptoms. Changes to surgical technique have made this complication less frequent.

PPM, an indicator of the intrinsic relationship of the implanted valve to the cardiac output requirements of the patient, has been most extensively studied for prosthetic aortic valves[54] and occurs in the setting of a morphologically normal valve. Mitral PPM has been associated with postoperative pulmonary artery hypertension,[55] congestive heart failure,[56] and higher mortality.[15,56] There have been multiple suggested definitions of mitral PPM using the EOA indexed to body surface area (iEOA):

- Clinically insignificant if iEOA >1.2 cm²/m², moderate if >0.9 and ≤1.2 cm²/m², and severe if ≤0.9 cm²/m²[15]
- Present if iEOA ≤1.25 cm²/m²[56]
- Present if iEOA <1.3 cm²/m²[57]

Nonetheless, an accurate assessment of iEOA is essential in determining or predicting PPM. It is well known that manufacturer-quoted in vitro geometric orifice area (GOA) overestimates in vivo EOA and should not be used.[58,59] Instead, tables of expected EOA should be used when selecting the appropriate size of valve to ensure adequate indexed EOA. Recent use of transcatheter valves for treatment of bioprosthetic structural valve dysfunction (see **Fig. 8**) has led to the generation of more accurate tables sizing the internal diameters of the sewing rings.[60,61]

Thrombosis and Endocarditis

Both structural and nonstructural valve dysfunction categories are exclusive of prosthetic valve thrombosis or prosthetic valve endocarditis. Valve thrombosis is defined as any thrombus attached to or near an implanted valve that occludes part of the blood-flow path, interferes with valve function, or is sufficiently large to justify treatment. Distinguishing pannus from thrombus may be difficult.[4,62] Occurring almost exclusively on mechanical valves, thrombi are generally large, tissue-density masses that may interfere with occluder motion. For the MV, thrombi will not infrequently extend beyond the surgical ring onto the wall of the left atrium. The clinical history may give further clues, because a short duration of symptoms (typically dyspnea or

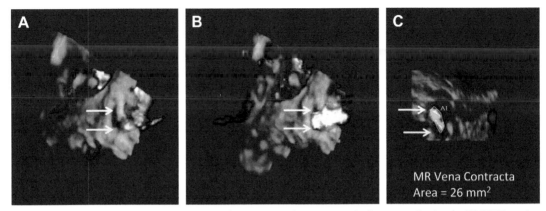

Fig. 11. Follow-up TEE for the case in **Fig. 10**, showing significant paravalvular regurgitation by 3D TEE imaging. *Panel A* is a diastolic frame with the defect clearly imaged (*between yellow arrows*). *Panel B* is the systolic frame with color regurgitant jet (*between yellow arrows*). *Panel C* is the measured vena contracta consistent with moderate mitral regurgitation.

an embolic event) and inadequate anticoagulation or cause for increased coagulability are commonly associated with thrombi.[4,63] The combination of tissue-density mass and inadequate anticoagulation has a positive and negative predictive value of 87% and 89%, respectively.[64,65] Lin and colleagues[65] formalized a grading scheme for predicting thrombus versus pannus. In this study of 53 patients with surgical confirmation, the TEE predictors of thrombus included mobile mass (tissue density), attachment to occluder, elevated gradient (peak transaortic prosthetic valve gradient $\geq$50 mm Hg, mean transmitral prosthetic valve gradient $\geq$10 mm Hg), and International Normalized Ratio (INR) of at least 2.5. The prevalence of thrombus was 14% with up to 1 predictor, 69% with 2 predictors, and 91% with 3 or more predictors.

Thrombolysis in high-risk patients with occlusive prosthetic valve thrombus has an overall success rate of 81%, but is associated with significant complications of systemic emboli (18%) and high mortality rate (15%–17%).[66] The International PRO-TEE Registry of 107 patients evaluated whether quantitation of thrombus burden with TEE could help risk-stratify patients undergoing thrombolysis of prosthetic valve thrombosis. Although the initial success rate of thrombolysis was 85%, the complication rate was 17.8% and deaths occurred in 5.6%. Multivariate predictors of complications included: thrombus area by TEE (odds ratio [OR] 2.41 per 1 cm^2 increment, 95% confidence interval [CI] 1.12–5.19) and prior history of stroke (OR 4.55, 95% CI 1.35–15.38). A thrombus area of less than 0.85 cm^2 was associated with a lower risk of embolic phenomenon or death from thrombolysis.[63] For nonobstructive prosthetic thrombus complicated by embolic events, surgical intervention may be warranted, particularly if the thrombus is large ($\geq$10 mm) or unresponsive to anticoagulation.[67]

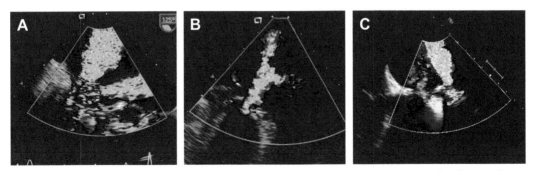

Fig. 12. Mechanisms of hemolysis in the setting of paravalvular regurgitation. Fragmentation (panel *A*) occurs when a jet is divided by the dehisced annular sewing ring. Collision (panel *B*) occurs when the jet rapidly decelerates by striking the ligament of Marshall or LA appendage wall, causes rapid deceleration. Acceleration (panel *C*) occurs when the regurgitant orifice is small, typically in the setting of high LV systolic pressures.

Predictors of Thrombus:

- Mobile mass of soft-tissue density
- Attachment to occluder and/or extension into left atrium (for MV prosthesis)
- Elevated gradient (peak AVR ≥50 mm Hg, mean MV regurgitation ≥10 mm Hg)
- INR ≤2.5
- Short duration of symptoms

Predictors of Pannus:

- Aortic position of prosthesis
- Higher video intensity ratio (more echo dense)

The risk of endocarditis increases significantly in the setting of a prosthetic valve, and prosthetic valve endocarditis accounts for up to 30% of cases of infective endocarditis.[68–71] Prosthetic valve endocarditis is an independent risk factor for in-hospital mortality.[72] The incidence of prosthetic valve endocarditis (0.1 to 2.3 per 100 patient-years) has a bimodal distribution pattern, with an early peak within 6 weeks of surgery (incidence of 3% within the first year) and late peak from 1 year onward following surgery.[73–75] The diagnosis of prosthetic valve endocarditis can be divided into "definite" and "probable" according to Durack and colleagues,[76] and is fully discussed in published guidelines.[71] Positive blood cultures are not required for the diagnosis, and culture-negative endocarditis should only refer to negative blood-culture results and not just the absence of any proof of infection. In addition to the standard Duke criteria, new prosthetic valve dehiscence may be considered major criteria.

Not all patients with prosthetic valve endocarditis require surgical intervention.[77] Studies have suggested that conservative management of prosthetic valve endocarditis is possible in the absence of "complicated" prosthetic valve endocarditis, defined as the presence of a new or changing heart murmur, new or worsening heart failure, new or progressive cardiac conduction abnormalities, or prolonged fever during therapy.[68,78] Although short-term outcomes of prosthetic valve endocarditis treated with surgery are worse than those for native valve endocarditis, long-term survival is not significantly different.[79] It is therefore important to recognize echocardiographic features of endocarditis that may suggest a need for surgical intervention (see Table 6), noting, however, that a recent review of observational studies suggests that further, rigorous investigations are required.[77]

Echocardiography is an integral tool for the diagnosis and management of prosthetic valve endocarditis. Vegetations, valve dysfunction, and periannular extension are the primary findings.

Five Echocardiographic Characteristics of Vegetations:

- Texture: gray-scale/reflectance of myocardium
- Location: upstream side of valve/in path of jet
- Characteristic motion: chaotic, orbiting, vibrations

Table 6
Echocardiographic features that suggest potential need for surgical intervention

Finding Consistent with Infective Endocarditis	Features that Suggest Potential Need for Surgical Intervention
Vegetation	Persistent vegetation after systemic embolization Anterior mitral leaflet vegetation, particularly with size 10 mm[a] One embolic event during first 2 wk of antimicrobial therapy[a] Increase in vegetation size despite appropriate antimicrobial therapy[a,b]
Valvular dysfunction	Acute aortic or mitral insufficiency with signs of ventricular failure[b] Heart failure unresponsive to medical therapy[b] Valve perforation or rupture[b]
Perivalvular extension	Valvular dehiscence, rupture, or fistula[b] New heart block[b] Large abscess or extension of abscess despite appropriate antimicrobial therapy[b]

[a] Risk of embolization.
[b] Risk of heart failure or failure of medical therapy.
Modified from Baddour LM, Wilson WR, Bayer AS, et al. Infective endocarditis: diagnosis, antimicrobial therapy, and management of complications: a statement for healthcare professionals from the Committee on Rheumatic Fever, Endocarditis, and Kawasaki Disease, Council on Cardiovascular Disease in the Young, and the Councils on Clinical Cardiology, Stroke, and Cardiovascular Surgery and Anesthesia, American Heart Association: endorsed by the Infectious Diseases Society of America. Circulation 2005;111(23):e394–434; with permission.

Table 7
Sensitivity and specificity of TTE and TEE in the diagnosis of prosthetic valve endocarditis

Authors,[Ref.] Year	N	Criteria	Valve Type	TTE Sensitivity (%)	TTE Specificity (%)	TEE Sensitivity (%)	TEE Specificity (%)
Vegetation Detection							
Shively et al,[81] 1991	61	Clinical or pathologic	3 PVE	44	98	94	100
Daniel et al,[82] 1993	126	Surgery or autopsy	Biological (n = 101)	65	78	87	91
			Mechanical (n = 23)	22	48	83	87
			Total	57	63	86	88
Kini et al,[83] 2010	114	TEE	NA	64		NA	NA
Range				22–65	48–98	83–94	87–100
Periannular Extension Detection							
Daniel et al,[84] 1991	46/118	Surgery or autopsy	12 PVE	28	99	87	95
Choussat et al,[85] 1999	233	Surgery (in 91%)	77 PVE	36	NA	80	NA
Hill et al,[86] 2007	44/115	Surgery	26 PVE	NA	NA	48	99
Range				28–36	99	48–87	95–99

Abbreviations: NA, no data available; PVE, prosthetic valve endocarditis.

Table 8
Use of echocardiography in infectious endocarditis

Diagnostic Test	Assessment
Diagnostic TTE[a] (at presentation)	Valvular function (regurgitation/stenosis, prosthetic valve stability) Ventricular function and hemodynamics (congestive heart failure) Vegetation characterization (size, location, mobility) Suspected complications of infectious endocarditis (periannular abscess, perforation, shunt)
TEE[b] (at presentation)	Clinical suspicion high in setting of negative or nondiagnostic TTE Prosthetic valve Suspected complications of infectious endocarditis (periannular abscess, perforation, shunt)
Repeat TTE or TEE	High suspicion of infectious endocarditis in setting of negative initial test (culture-negative incidence of subactue bacterial endocarditis ~10%) High risk patients Virulent organism (staphylococci or fungi) Clinical deterioration Persistent or recurrent fever or bacteremia New murmur

[a] Test of choice if clinical suspicion for infectious endocarditis is low.
[b] Test of choice if clinical suspicion for infectious endocarditis is high.

- Shape: lobulated, amorphous
  - Accompanying abnormalities: regurgitation, abscess, pseudoaneurysm, fistulas, prosthetic dehiscence, paravalvular leak

Diagnosis of Periannular Extension:

- Clinical characteristics: Persistent bacteremia or fever, recurrent emboli, heart block (88% positive predictive value, 45% sensitivity), congestive heart failure, new pathologic murmur while on therapy
- Echocardiographic characteristics: valvular dehiscence, rupture, or fistula
  - Location: periannular: 23% to 60% of aortic valve, 15% to 16% of MV
  - Nonhomogeneous
    - Echo-dense paravalvular mass
    - Echo-free cavities
  - Doppler may reveal no flow or fistula formation, and rupture into an adjacent cavity leaving a pseudoaneurysm

The diagnosis of a mitral-aortic pseudoaneurysm of the intervalvular fibrosa deserves special mention. Although most frequently a complication of aortic prosthetic valve endocarditis, it can be seen with mitral prosthetic valve endocarditis as well as in native valve endocarditis. The aortic root and mitral annulus are connected by a fibrous region called the subaortic curtain or intervalvular fibrosa. This site of infection is not an uncommon one following prosthetic valve implantation. The diagnosis of an abscess with fistula formation is made by visualization of an echo-free space in the mitral-aortic intervalvular fibrosa, with systolic expansion and diastolic collapse, and prominent pulsatility from a communication with the LVOT.[80] Further fistula formation between the pseudoaneurysm and the aorta or left atrium may reduce the pulsatility.

Because TTE is often limited in assessing prosthetic valve endocarditis and its complications, TEE is recommended for patients with prosthetic valves, rated at least "possible infectious endocarditis" by clinical criteria, or complicated infectious endocarditis (ie, paravalvular abscess).[71] **Table 7** is a summary of the sensitivity and specificity of TTE in comparison with TEE in the detection of prosthetic valve vegetations and periannular extension.[81-86] **Table 8** is a summary of the use of echocardiography in the diagnosis of infectious endocarditis based on the current guidelines.[1,71,87]

REFERENCES

1. Bonow RO, Carabello BA, Kanu C, et al. ACC/AHA 2006 guidelines for the management of patients with valvular heart disease: a report of the American College of Cardiology/American Heart Association Task Force on Practice Guidelines (Writing Committee to revise the 1998 Guidelines for the Management of Patients with Valvular Heart Disease): developed in collaboration with the Society of Cardiovascular Anesthesiologists: endorsed by the Society for Cardiovascular Angiography and Interventions and the Society of Thoracic Surgeons. Circulation 2006;114(5):e84–231.

2. Bonow RO, Carabello BA, Chatterjee K, et al. 2008 focused update incorporated into the ACC/AHA 2006 guidelines for the management of patients with valvular heart disease: a report of the American College of Cardiology/American Heart Association Task Force on Practice Guidelines (Writing Committee to revise the 1998 Guidelines for the Management of Patients with Valvular Heart Disease). Endorsed by the Society of Cardiovascular Anesthesiologists, Society for Cardiovascular Angiography and Interventions, and Society of Thoracic Surgeons. J Am Coll Cardiol 2008;52(13):e1–142.

3. Vahanian A, Alfieri O, Andreotti F, et al. Guidelines on the management of valvular heart disease (version 2012): the Joint Task Force on the Management of Valvular Heart Disease of the European Society of Cardiology (ESC) and the European Association for Cardio-Thoracic Surgery (EACTS). Eur J Cardiothorac Surg 2012;42(4):S1–44.

4. Zoghbi WA, Chambers JB, Dumesnil JG, et al. Recommendations for evaluation of prosthetic valves with echocardiography and Doppler ultrasound: a report from the American Society of Echocardiography's Guidelines and Standards Committee and the Task Force on Prosthetic Valves, developed in conjunction with the American College of Cardiology Cardiovascular Imaging Committee, Cardiac Imaging Committee of the American Heart Association, the European Association of Echocardiography, a registered branch of the European Society of Cardiology, the Japanese Society of Echocardiography and the Canadian Society of Echocardiography, endorsed by the American College of Cardiology Foundation, American Heart Association, European Association of Echocardiography, a registered branch of the European Society of Cardiology, the Japanese Society of Echocardiography, and Canadian Society of Echocardiography. J Am Soc Echocardiogr 2009;22(9):975–1014 [quiz: 82–4].

5. Lang RM, Badano LP, Tsang W, et al. EAE/ASE recommendations for image acquisition and display using three-dimensional echocardiography. J Am Soc Echocardiogr 2012;25(1):3–46.

6. Hixson CS, Smith MD, Mattson MD, et al. Comparison of transesophageal color flow Doppler imaging of normal mitral regurgitant jets in St. Jude

Medical and Medtronic Hall cardiac prostheses. J Am Soc Echocardiogr 1992;5(1):57–62.

7. Lange HW, Olson JD, Pedersen WR, et al. Transesophageal color Doppler echocardiography of the normal St. Jude Medical mitral valve prosthesis. Am Heart J 1991;122(2):489–94.

8. Frater RW. Stentless mitral valves. J Thorac Cardiovasc Surg 2007;133(4):861–4.

9. Chauvaud S, Waldmann T, d'Attellis N, et al. Homograft replacement of the mitral valve in young recipients: mid-term results. Eur J Cardiothorac Surg 2003;23(4):560–6.

10. Timek TA, Lai DT, Tibayan FA, et al. Hemodynamic performance of an unstented xenograft mitral valve substitute. J Thorac Cardiovasc Surg 2002;124(3):541–52.

11. Deac RF, Simionescu D, Deac D. New evolution in mitral physiology and surgery: mitral stentless pericardial valve. Ann Thorac Surg 1995;60(Suppl 2):S433–8.

12. Frater RW, Sussman M, Middlemost S, et al. Quattro valve trial at mid-term: December 1996 to November 2004. J Heart Valve Dis 2006;15(2):230–7 [discussion: 7].

13. Navia JL, Doi K, Atik FA, et al. Acute in vivo evaluation of a new stentless mitral valve. J Thorac Cardiovasc Surg 2007;133(4):986–94.

14. Kasegawa H, Iwasaki K, Kusunose S, et al. Assessment of a novel stentless mitral valve using a pulsatile mitral valve simulator. J Heart Valve Dis 2012;21(1):71–5.

15. Magne J, Mathieu P, Dumesnil JG, et al. Impact of prosthesis-patient mismatch on survival after mitral valve replacement. Circulation 2007;115(11):1417–25.

16. Blauwet LA, Malouf JF, Connolly HM, et al. Doppler echocardiography of 240 normal Carpentier-Edwards Duraflex porcine mitral bioprostheses: a comprehensive assessment including time velocity integral ratio and prosthesis performance index. J Am Soc Echocardiogr 2009;22(4):388–93.

17. Blauwet LA, Malouf JF, Connolly HM, et al. Comprehensive hemodynamic assessment of 305 normal CarboMedics mitral valve prostheses based on early postimplantation echocardiographic studies. J Am Soc Echocardiogr 2012;25(2):173–81.

18. Blauwet LA, Malouf JF, Connolly HM, et al. Comprehensive echocardiographic assessment of normal mitral Medtronic Hancock II, Medtronic Mosaic, and Carpentier-Edwards Perimount bioprostheses early after implantation. J Am Soc Echocardiogr 2010;23(6):656–66.

19. Rosenhek R, Binder T, Maurer G, et al. Normal values for Doppler echocardiographic assessment of heart valve prostheses. J Am Soc Echocardiogr 2003;16(11):1116–27.

20. Pibarot P, Dumesnil JG. Prosthetic heart valves: selection of the optimal prosthesis and long-term management. Circulation 2009;119(7):1034–48.

21. Jamieson WR, Cartier PC, Allard M, et al. Surgical management of valvular heart disease 2004. Can J Cardiol 2004;20(Suppl E):7E–120E.

22. Douglas PS, Garcia MJ, Haines DE, et al. ACCF/ASE/AHA/ASNC/HFSA/HRS/SCAI/SCCM/SCCT/SCMR 2011 appropriate use criteria for echocardiography. A report of the American College of Cardiology Foundation Appropriate Use Criteria Task Force, American Society of Echocardiography, American Heart Association, American Society of Nuclear Cardiology, Heart Failure Society of America, Heart Rhythm Society, Society for Cardiovascular Angiography and Interventions, Society of Critical Care Medicine, Society of Cardiovascular Computed Tomography, and Society for Cardiovascular Magnetic Resonance endorsed by the American College of Chest Physicians. J Am Coll Cardiol 2011;57(9):1126–66.

23. Zoghbi WA, Enriquez-Sarano M, Foster E, et al. Recommendations for evaluation of the severity of native valvular regurgitation with two-dimensional and Doppler echocardiography. J Am Soc Echocardiogr 2003;16(7):777–802.

24. Baumgartner H, Hung J, Bermejo J, et al. Echocardiographic assessment of valve stenosis: EAE/ASE recommendations for clinical practice. J Am Soc Echocardiogr 2009;22(1):1–23 [quiz: 101–2].

25. Hatle L, Angelsen B, Tromsdal A. Noninvasive assessment of atrioventricular pressure half-time by Doppler ultrasound. Circulation 1979;60(5):1096–104.

26. Dumesnil JG, Honos GN, Lemieux M, et al. Validation and applications of mitral prosthetic valvular areas calculated by Doppler echocardiography. Am J Cardiol 1990;65(22):1443–8.

27. Dumesnil JG, Yoganathan AP. Valve prosthesis hemodynamics and the problem of high transprosthetic pressure gradients. Eur J Cardiothorac Surg 1992;6(Suppl 1):S34–7 [discussion: S8].

28. Bitar JN, Lechin ME, Salazar G, et al. Doppler echocardiographic assessment with the continuity equation of St. Jude Medical mechanical prostheses in the mitral valve position. Am J Cardiol 1995;76(4):287–93.

29. Gadhinglajkar S, Namboodiri N, Pillai V, et al. Double-envelope continuous-wave Doppler flow profile across a tilting-disc mitral prosthesis: intraoperative significance. J Cardiothorac Vasc Anesth 2011;25(3):491–4.

30. Fernandes V, Olmos L, Nagueh SF, et al. Peak early diastolic velocity rather than pressure half-time is the best index of mechanical prosthetic mitral valve function. Am J Cardiol 2002;89(6):704–10.

31. Rudski LG, Lai WW, Afilalo J, et al. Guidelines for the echocardiographic assessment of the right heart in adults: a report from the American Society of Echocardiography endorsed by the European Association of Echocardiography, a registered branch of the European Society of Cardiology, and the Canadian Society of Echocardiography. J Am Soc Echocardiogr 2010;23(7):685–713 [quiz: 86–8].

32. Milan A, Magnino C, Veglio F. Echocardiographic indexes for the non-invasive evaluation of pulmonary hemodynamics. J Am Soc Echocardiogr 2010;23(3):225–39 [quiz: 332–4].

33. Aduen JF, Castello R, Daniels JT, et al. Accuracy and precision of three echocardiographic methods for estimating mean pulmonary artery pressure. Chest 2011;139(2):347–52.

34. Bossone E, D'Andrea A, D'Alto M, et al. Echocardiography in pulmonary arterial hypertension: from diagnosis to prognosis. J Am Soc Echocardiogr 2013;26(1):1–14.

35. Pop G, Sutherland GR, Roelandt J, et al. What is the ideal orientation of a mitral disc prosthesis? An in vivo haemodynamic study based on colour flow imaging and continuous wave Doppler. Eur Heart J 1989;10(4):346–53.

36. Akins CW, Miller DC, Turina MI, et al. Guidelines for reporting mortality and morbidity after cardiac valve interventions. J Thorac Cardiovasc Surg 2008;135(4):732–8.

37. Olmos L, Salazar G, Barbetseas J, et al. Usefulness of transthoracic echocardiography in detecting significant prosthetic mitral valve regurgitation. Am J Cardiol 1999;83(2):199–205.

38. Ruddox V, Mathisen M, Baekkevar M, et al. Is 3D echocardiography superior to 2D echocardiography in general practice?: a systematic review of studies published between 2007 and 2012. Int J Cardiol 2013. [Epub ahead of print].

39. Dorosz JL, Lezotte DC, Weitzenkamp DA, et al. Performance of 3-dimensional echocardiography in measuring left ventricular volumes and ejection fraction: a systematic review and meta-analysis. J Am Coll Cardiol 2012;59(20):1799–808.

40. Krim SR, Vivo RP, Patel A, et al. Direct assessment of normal mechanical mitral valve orifice area by real time 3D echocardiography. JACC Cardiovasc Imaging 2012;5(5):478–83.

41. Singh P, Manda J, Hsiung MC, et al. Live/real time three-dimensional transesophageal echocardiographic evaluation of mitral and aortic valve prosthetic paravalvular regurgitation. Echocardiography 2009;26(8):980–7.

42. Zamorano JL, Badano LP, Bruce C, et al. EAE/ASE recommendations for the use of echocardiography in new transcatheter interventions for valvular heart disease. J Am Soc Echocardiogr 2011;24(9):937–65.

43. Biner S, Kar S, Siegel RJ, et al. Value of color Doppler three-dimensional transesophageal echocardiography in the percutaneous closure of mitral prosthesis paravalvular leak. Am J Cardiol 2010;105(7):984–9.

44. Reis G, Motta MS, Barbosa MM, et al. Dobutamine stress echocardiography for noninvasive assessment and risk stratification of patients with rheumatic mitral stenosis. J Am Coll Cardiol 2004;43(3):393–401.

45. Garcia MJ, Vandervoort P, Stewart WJ, et al. Mechanisms of hemolysis with mitral prosthetic regurgitation. Study using transesophageal echocardiography and fluid dynamic simulation. J Am Coll Cardiol 1996;27(2):399–406.

46. David TE, Burns RJ, Bacchus CM, et al. Mitral valve replacement for mitral regurgitation with and without preservation of chordae tendineae. J Thorac Cardiovasc Surg 1984;88(5 Pt 1):718–25.

47. David TE. Mitral valve replacement with preservation of chordae tendinae: rationale and technical considerations. Ann Thorac Surg 1986;41(6):680–2.

48. Spencer FC, Galloway AC, Colvin SB. A clinical evaluation of the hypothesis that rupture of the left ventricle following mitral valve replacement can be prevented by preservation of the chordae of the mural leaflet. Ann Surg 1985;202(6):673–80.

49. Miki S, Kusuhara K, Ueda Y, et al. Mitral valve replacement with preservation of chordae tendineae and papillary muscles. Ann Thorac Surg 1988;45(1):28–34.

50. Come PC, Riley MF, Weintraub RM, et al. Dynamic left ventricular outflow tract obstruction when the anterior leaflet is retained at prosthetic mitral valve replacement. Ann Thorac Surg 1987;43(5):561–3.

51. Waggoner AD, Perez JE, Barzilai B, et al. Left ventricular outflow obstruction resulting from insertion of mitral prostheses leaving the native leaflets intact: adverse clinical outcome in seven patients. Am Heart J 1991;122(2):483–8.

52. Rosenzweig MS, Nanda NC. Two-dimensional echocardiographic detection of left ventricular wall impaction by mitral prosthesis. Am Heart J 1983;106(5 Pt 1):1069–76.

53. Freedberg RS, Kronzon I, Gindea AJ, et al. Noninvasive diagnosis of left ventricular outflow tract obstruction caused by a porcine mitral prosthesis. J Am Coll Cardiol 1987;9(3):698–700.

54. Head SJ, Mokhles MM, Osnabrugge RL, et al. The impact of prosthesis-patient mismatch on long-term survival after aortic valve replacement: a systematic review and meta-analysis of 34 observational studies comprising 27 186 patients with 133 141 patient-years. Eur Heart J 2012;33(12):1518–29.

55. Li M, Dumesnil JG, Mathieu P, et al. Impact of valve prosthesis-patient mismatch on pulmonary arterial

pressure after mitral valve replacement. J Am Coll Cardiol 2005;45(7):1034–40.

56. Lam BK, Chan V, Hendry P, et al. The impact of patient-prosthesis mismatch on late outcomes after mitral valve replacement. J Thorac Cardiovasc Surg 2007;133(6):1464–73.

57. Bouchard D, Vanden Eynden F, Demers P, et al. Patient-prosthesis mismatch in the mitral position affects midterm survival and functional status. Can J Cardiol 2010;26(10):532–6.

58. Bleiziffer S, Eichinger WB, Hettich I, et al. Prediction of valve prosthesis-patient mismatch prior to aortic valve replacement: which is the best method? Heart 2007;93(5):615–20.

59. Muneretto C, Bisleri G, Negri A, et al. The concept of patient-prosthesis mismatch. J Heart Valve Dis 2004;13(Suppl 1):S59–62.

60. Piazza N, Bleiziffer S, Brockmann G, et al. Transcatheter aortic valve implantation for failing surgical aortic bioprosthetic valve: from concept to clinical application and evaluation (part 1). JACC Cardiovasc Interv 2011;4(7):721–32.

61. Piazza N, Bleiziffer S, Brockmann G, et al. Transcatheter aortic valve implantation for failing surgical aortic bioprosthetic valve: from concept to clinical application and evaluation (part 2). JACC Cardiovasc Interv 2011;4(7):733–42.

62. Roudaut R, Serri K, Lafitte S. Thrombosis of prosthetic heart valves: diagnosis and therapeutic considerations. Heart 2007;93(1):137–42.

63. Tong AT, Roudaut R, Ozkan M, et al. Transesophageal echocardiography improves risk assessment of thrombolysis of prosthetic valve thrombosis: results of the international PRO-TEE registry. J Am Coll Cardiol 2004;43(1):77–84.

64. Barbetseas J, Nagueh SF, Pitsavos C, et al. Differentiating thrombus from pannus formation in obstructed mechanical prosthetic valves: an evaluation of clinical, transthoracic and transesophageal echocardiographic parameters. J Am Coll Cardiol 1998;32(5):1410–7.

65. Lin SS, Tiong IY, Asher CR, et al. Prediction of thrombus-related mechanical prosthetic valve dysfunction using transesophageal echocardiography. Am J Cardiol 2000;86(10):1097–101.

66. Zabalgoitia M. Echocardiographic assessment of prosthetic heart valves. Curr Probl Cardiol 2000;25(3):157–218.

67. Laplace G, Lafitte S, Labeque JN, et al. Clinical significance of early thrombosis after prosthetic mitral valve replacement: a postoperative monocentric study of 680 patients. J Am Coll Cardiol 2004;43(7):1283–90.

68. Calderwood SB, Swinski LA, Karchmer AW, et al. Prosthetic valve endocarditis. Analysis of factors affecting outcome of therapy. J Thorac Cardiovasc Surg 1986;92(4):776–83.

69. Habib G, Tribouilloy C, Thuny F, et al. Prosthetic valve endocarditis: who needs surgery? A multicentre study of 104 cases. Heart 2005;91(7):954–9.

70. Tornos P, Iung B, Permanyer-Miralda G, et al. Infective endocarditis in Europe: lessons from the Euro heart survey. Heart 2005;91(5):571–5.

71. Baddour LM, Wilson WR, Bayer AS, et al. Infective endocarditis: diagnosis, antimicrobial therapy, and management of complications: a statement for healthcare professionals from the Committee on Rheumatic Fever, Endocarditis, and Kawasaki Disease, Council on Cardiovascular Disease in the Young, and the Councils on Clinical Cardiology, Stroke, and Cardiovascular Surgery and Anesthesia, American Heart Association: endorsed by the Infectious Diseases Society of America. Circulation 2005;111(23):e394–434.

72. Murdoch DR, Corey GR, Hoen B, et al. Clinical presentation, etiology, and outcome of infective endocarditis in the 21st century: the International Collaboration on Endocarditis-Prospective Cohort Study. Arch Intern Med 2009;169(5):463–73.

73. Ivert TS, Dismukes WE, Cobbs CG, et al. Prosthetic valve endocarditis. Circulation 1984;69(2):223–32.

74. Lytle BW, Priest BP, Taylor PC, et al. Surgical treatment of prosthetic valve endocarditis. J Thorac Cardiovasc Surg 1996;111(1):198–207 [discussion: 10].

75. Vlessis AA, Khaki A, Grunkemeier GL, et al. Risk, diagnosis and management of prosthetic valve endocarditis: a review. J Heart Valve Dis 1997;6(5):443–65.

76. Durack DT, Lukes AS, Bright DK. New criteria for diagnosis of infective endocarditis: utilization of specific echocardiographic findings. Duke Endocarditis Service. Am J Med 1994;96(3):200–9.

77. Tleyjeh IM, Kashour T, Zimmerman V, et al. The role of valve surgery in infective endocarditis management: a systematic review of observational studies that included propensity score analysis. Am Heart J 2008;156(5):901–9.

78. Hill EE, Herregods MC, Vanderschueren S, et al. Management of prosthetic valve infective endocarditis. Am J Cardiol 2008;101(8):1174–8.

79. Manne MB, Shrestha NK, Lytle BW, et al. Outcomes after surgical treatment of native and prosthetic valve infective endocarditis. Ann Thorac Surg 2012;93(2):489–93.

80. Sudhakar S, Sewani A, Agrawal M, et al. Pseudoaneurysm of the mitral-aortic intervalvular fibrosa (MAIVF): a comprehensive review. J Am Soc Echocardiogr 2010;23(10):1009–18 [quiz: 112].

81. Shively BK, Gurule FT, Roldan CA, et al. Diagnostic value of transesophageal compared with transthoracic echocardiography in infective endocarditis. J Am Coll Cardiol 1991;18(2):391–7.

82. Daniel WG, Mugge A, Grote J, et al. Comparison of transthoracic and transesophageal echocardiography for detection of abnormalities of prosthetic and bioprosthetic valves in the mitral and aortic positions. Am J Cardiol 1993;71(2):210–5.

83. Kini V, Logani S, Ky B, et al. Transthoracic and transesophageal echocardiography for the indication of suspected infective endocarditis: vegetations, blood cultures and imaging. J Am Soc Echocardiogr 2010;23(4):396–402.

84. Daniel WG, Mugge A, Martin RP, et al. Improvement in the diagnosis of abscesses associated with endocarditis by transesophageal echocardiography. N Engl J Med 1991;324(12):795–800.

85. Choussat R, Thomas D, Isnard R, et al. Perivalvular abscesses associated with endocarditis; clinical features and prognostic factors of overall survival in a series of 233 cases. Perivalvular Abscesses French Multicentre Study. Eur Heart J 1999;20(3):232–41.

86. Hill EE, Herijgers P, Claus P, et al. Abscess in infective endocarditis: the value of transesophageal echocardiography and outcome: a 5-year study. Am Heart J 2007;154(5):923–8.

87. Cheitlin MD, Armstrong WF, Aurigemma GP, et al. ACC/AHA/ASE 2003 guideline update for the clinical application of echocardiography: summary article. A report of the American College of Cardiology/American Heart Association Task Force on Practice Guidelines (ACC/AHA/ASE Committee to Update the 1997 Guidelines for the Clinical Application of Echocardiography). J Am Soc Echocardiogr 2003; 16(10):1091–110.

Stress Echocardiography and Mitral Valvular Heart Disease

Julien Magne, PhD, Patrizio Lancellotti, MD, PhD*,
Luc A. Pierard, MD, PhD*

KEYWORDS

- Mitral valve • Exercise stress echocardiography • Mitral regurgitation • Mitral stenosis
- Systolic pulmonary arterial pressure

KEY POINTS

- The European Society of Cardiology's recently updated guidelines emphasize the usefulness of exercise stress echocardiography in patients with valvular heart disease. Exercise-induced changes in valve hemodynamics, particularly systolic pulmonary arterial pressure and left ventricular function, should be assessed in patients with mitral valve disease.
- In asymptomatic patients with moderate or severe mitral regurgitation (MR) without left ventricular dysfunction/dilatation, exercise stress echocardiography may identify a subset of patients with reduced cardiac event-free survival who are at a higher risk of developing symptoms.
- In secondary MR, dynamic changes in MR may play a role in the pathogenesis of pulmonary oedema and of reduced survival.
- In patients with mitral stenosis who are asymptomatic, the development of symptoms during exercise is strongly related to the kinetics of the changes in the systolic pulmonary arterial pressure.

INTRODUCTION

The European Society of Cardiology's (ESC) most recent guidelines highlight that exercise stress echocardiography *"may provide additional information to better identify the cardiac origin of dyspnea."*[1] There is a strong body of evidence supporting the usefulness of stress echocardiography in providing useful information that may guide the clinical management of patients with mitral valvular heart disease and risk stratification, specifically in the absence of symptoms or equivocal symptoms.

Both exercise and dobutamine stress echocardiography are widely accepted as important diagnostic and prognostic tools in the assessment of known or suspected coronary artery disease. However, in patients with mitral regurgitation

(MR), dobutamine infusion induces a decrease in the degree of MR in most cases; therefore, exercise stress echocardiography, being more physiologic, is preferred for the assessment of the dynamic behavior of MR. The most common variations of exercise stress echocardiography involve exercise on a treadmill or upright bicycle ergometry and immediate postexercise imaging.[2] However, the semisupine bicycle stress test has the benefit of continuous echocardiographic monitoring, which represents an important advantage for quantifying changes in regurgitant volumes and, more importantly, the measurement of peak exercise systolic pulmonary arterial pressure (SPAP), which tends to rapidly decrease after exercise cessation. In addition, the acquisition of echocardiographic images throughout the stress

Source of funding: Dr Magne is the research associate from the F.R.S-FNRS, Brussels, Belgium and received grants from the Fonds Léon Fredericq, Liège, Belgium.
Department of Cardiology, GIGA Cardiovascular Sciences, Heart Valve Clinic, University Hospital Sart Tilman, University of Liège, Liège 4000, Belgium
* Corresponding author. University of Liège, CHU Sart Tilman, Liège 4000, Belgium.
E-mail addresses: plancellotti@chu.ulg.ac.be; lpierard@chu.ulg.ac.be

Cardiol Clin 31 (2013) 311–321
http://dx.doi.org/10.1016/j.ccl.2013.03.008
0733-8651/13/$ – see front matter © 2013 Elsevier Inc. All rights reserved.

cardiology.theclinics.com

test may also help to characterize the hemody-namic and ventricular biphasic responses. There is now growing evidence suggesting that in both patients with MR (ie, primary and secondary MR) or mitral stenosis (MS), upstream repercussions of exercise-induced changes in mitral antegrade (ie, mitral inflow) or retrograde (regurgitation) flow can also be accurately appraised by the assessment of SPAP. Additionally, the presence of contractile reserve and inducible ischemia can also be easily identified at both low and high exercise levels.

EXERCISE STRESS ECHOCARDIOGRAPHY PROTOCOL

Exercise echocardiography (ie, imaging performed during exercise) requires training and experience and the use of an adequate stress table. In the case of mitral valve disease, image acquisition focuses on parameters related to mitral valve hemodynamics, the left ventricle (LV), and SPAP.

A symptom-limited graded exercise test is recommended, and at least 85% of the age-predicted heart rate should be the target in the absence of symptoms. The test should be adapted to the clinical condition of patients and should be performed under the supervision of an experienced person. The American College of Cardiology/American Heart Association's practice guidelines recommend using a Bruce modified protocol[3]; when combined with imaging during exercise, it should be performed on a dedicated tilting exercise table (**Fig. 1**). Typically, the initial workload of 25 W is maintained for 2 minutes and subsequently increased every 2 minutes by 25 W. However, increases of 10 W may be more appropriate in elderly patients or in sedentary patients. Blood pressure and a 12-lead electrocardiogram should be recorded at rest and at each step of the test. Patients should also be monitored and questioned for symptoms during the test. The exercise test may be terminated promptly when the target heart rate is achieved or in case of typical chest pain,

significantly limiting breathlessness, dizziness, muscular exhaustion, hypotension (drop in systolic blood pressure ≥20 mm Hg), a significant ventricular arrhythmia, or more than a 2 mm horizontal or downsloping ST depression. The following contraindications should be strictly respected[1]: physical or mental disability to adequately perform an exercise stress test,[2] high blood pressure (systolic arterial pressure >200 mm Hg or diastolic arterial pressure >110 mm Hg),[3] uncontrolled or symptomatic arrhythmias, and[4] systemic illness.

SEQUENCE OF EXERCISE IMAGING

Comprehensive resting echocardiography should be performed in the same position as the imaging during the exercise stress test. Throughout the stress test, mean pressure gradient (in patients with MS) or MR severity, and SPAP measurement can be obtained at the end of each stage of exercise. Based on the anticipated length of duration of exercise, LV function may be assessed 2 or 3 times during exercise. Because of the frequent biphasic hemodynamic and mechanical responses during exercise, image acquisition throughout the test may help to unmask this phenomenon assessment of LV function (ie, gray-scale images of 2-, 3- and 4-chamber apical views and parasternal short- and long-axis views) during the first stage of exercise, at an intermediate stage, and at peak exercise is recommended to characterize the pathophysiologic consequences of exercise on the LV (see **Fig. 1**). In this regard, at each step of exercise, the following sequence for imaging is recommended[1]: continuous-wave Doppler imaging of the tricuspid valve for assessment of tricuspid regurgitation (TR),[2] pulsed-wave Doppler imaging at the level of the mitral leaflet tips for the mitral inflow Doppler profile,[3] continuous-wave Doppler imaging of the MR jet,[4] color Doppler imaging of the mitral valve in the apical 4-chamber view, and[5] proximal isovelocity surface area-specific image acquisition. At peak exercise (ie, within the minute before and the minute after the end of exercise), the

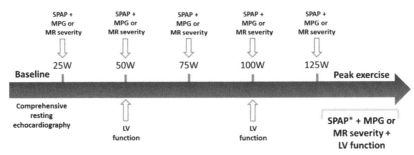

Fig. 1. Exercise stress echocardiography protocol including the sequence of acquisition. The asterisk indicates that special care should be taken to acquire SPAP at peak exercise. MPG, mean pressure gradient.

imaging sequence recommended is[1] gray-scale images in 2-, 3-, and 4-chamber apical, parasternal short- and long-axis views[2]; pulsed-wave Doppler imaging in the LV outflow tract[3]; pulsed-wave Doppler imaging of the mitral valve[4]; color Doppler imaging of the mitral valve in the apical 4-chamber view[5]; PISA-specific imaging; and[6] continuous-wave Doppler imaging of the MR. Special care should also be taken to obtain the continuous-wave Doppler profile of TR at peak exercise.

Change in the LV filling pressure estimation (ie, E/Ea ratio) should be obtained at low-level exercise (usually around 100 beats per minute [bpm]) to avoid E- and A-waves fusion and to ensure good tissue Doppler imaging quality and during recovery. A rapid increase in pressure gradients or in SPAP can indicate a more severe disease process or an absence of pulmonary vascular function adaptation, low pulmonary compliance, and markedly increased pulmonary resistance.

The assessment of exercise-induced changes in LV systolic function is also very useful. Worsening in wall motion from the baseline classically indicates an ischemic insult. The absence of LV contractile reserve is generally characterized by a change in LV ejection fraction less than 4%[4,5] or in myocardial long-axis function (derived from tissue Doppler imaging or 2-dimensional [2D] speckle tracking).[6,7]

PRIMARY MR

Primary MR, which is predominantly caused by rheumatic and degenerative mitral valve disease, is caused by an anatomic alteration of the valvular or subvalvular mitral apparatus that includes mitral leaflet prolapse and flail leaflet. The prognosis of patients with primary MR is highly variable. In symptomatic patients whereby the severity of MR is estimated to be only mild at rest, exercise echocardiography might be useful in elucidating the cause of symptoms by determining if the severity of MR increases or pulmonary arterial hypertension (PHT) develops during exercise.[8] The evaluation of patients at rest, as generally performed in routine clinical practice, may fail to detect the cause of the symptoms. Some patients may ignore or not report their symptoms or they may reduce their level of physical activity to avoid or minimize symptoms. It has been demonstrated that maximum exercise capacity is markedly reduced in approximately 20% of patients with asymptomatic primary MR, and these patients have a worse outcome, regardless MR severity.[9]

The ESC's recently updated guidelines state that *"exercise echocardiography is useful to quantify exercise induced changes in MR, in SPAP and*

in LV function."[1] In addition, the development of PHT during exercise (ie, SPAP >60 mm Hg) is now an indication for surgery in asymptomatic patients with severe MR and no LV dysfunction or dilatation (class IIb, evidence C).

Exercise-Induced Changes in MR Severity

In asymptomatic patients with primary mitral valve disease, the value of exercise echocardiography has recently been highlighted.[10,11] It was previously thought that primary MR, as opposed to secondary ischemic MR, is relatively stable during exercise. However, recent data demonstrating that the severity of MR changes significantly during exercise in a large proportion of patients with primary MR contradict this belief (**Fig. 2**). Stoddard and colleagues[8] were the first to examine 94 patients with mitral valve prolapse and no MR in basal conditions using exercise stress echocardiography. After symptom-limited exercise, 30 patients (32%) developed transient MR. These patients were also found to have higher left atrial sizes and volumes, LV end-diastolic volumes, and mitral valve prolapse scores. Moreover, an exercise-induced increase in MR was more frequently present in patients with prior syncopal episodes. During the follow-up period of 38 months, the patients with exercise-induced MR had a 6-fold greater incidence of cardiovascular morbid events, particularly syncope (43% vs 5%) and congestive heart failure (17% vs 0%).

In a larger cohort of asymptomatic patients with moderate to severe primary MR (mitral valve prolapse or flail leaflet) submitted to exercise echocardiography, the authors' group has shown that the mean effective regurgitant orifice area (EROA) and regurgitant volumes significantly increased in 32% of patients by 10 mm^2 or more and 15 mL or more, respectively.[10] Importantly, more than 50% of patients with moderate resting MR developed severe MR during exercise (**Table 1**). An exercise-induced marked increase in MR was also a powerful marker of reduced symptom-free survival. At the 2-year follow-up, only 30% of patients developing a higher degree of MR during exercise remained asymptomatic.

Exercise-Induced Pulmonary Hypertension

In many cardiac diseases, exercise-induced PHT is considered a predictor of resting PHT and an early marker of the consequences of the disease on pulmonary vascular function. In a series of 78 asymptomatic patients with primary MR and no LV dysfunction/dilatation, the authors' group reported a low incidence of PHT at rest (15%) but a much higher rate of exercise-induced PHT (46%). The

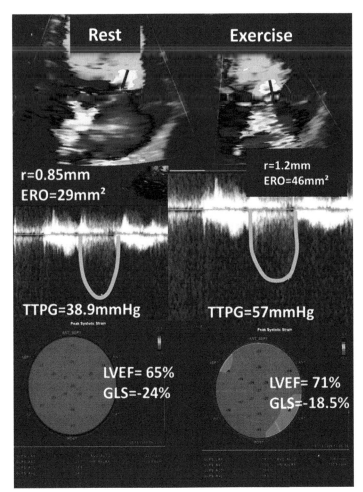

Fig. 2. Exercise-induced changes in primary MR. ERO, effective regurgitant orifice; GLS, global longitudinal strain; LVEF, LV ejection fraction; r, PISA radius; TTPG, transtricuspid pressure gradient.

Table 1
Exercise echocardiographic parameters useful for risk stratification

Parameters		References
Primary MR		
Exercise-induced increase in ERO area	>+10 mm²	Magne et al[10]
Exercise-induced increase in regurgitant volume	>+15 mL	Magne et al[10]
Exercise systolic pulmonary arterial pressure	>60 mm Hg	Magne et al[11]
LV contractile reserve		
Exercise-induced changes in LV ejection fraction	>+4%	Lee et al,[4] Lancellotti et al[6]
Exercise-induced changes in LV global long strain	>+2%	Lancellotti et al,[6] Magne et al[7]
Secondary MR		
Exercise-induced changes in ERO	>+13 mm²	Lancellotti et al[12,13]
MS		
Peak exercise transmitral mean pressure gradient	>18 mm Hg	Reis et al[14]
Increase in rest SPAP at 60 W	≥90%	Brochet et al[15]

Abbreviations: ERO, effective regurgitant orifice; long, longitudinal.

presence of PHT at rest seemed to be mainly related to age, LV end-systolic volume, and E/Ea ratio, with age and resting SPAP also independently associated with PHT during exercise. Nonetheless, the main determinant of both exercise-induced increases in SPAP and PHT was an exercise-induced increase in MR severity. Consequently, the main harmful consequence of the presence of dynamic MR is the development of exercise PHT. The follow-up of this cohort of patients after 2 years revealed that resting PHT was not associated with a significantly reduced symptom-free survival after an adjustment for age and sex. In contrast, exercise PHT was associated with significantly reduced symptom-free survival both in univariate (at 2 years: 75% ± 7% vs 35% ± 8%, P<.0001) and multivariate analysis, with a 3.4 increased risk of developing symptoms within the follow-up period. At the 3-year follow-up, only 20% of patients with exercise PHT at baseline remained free of symptoms. Recently, Marwick and his group reported similar results in a comparable cohort of 196 patients.[16] The results of their study revealed that exercise SPAP is also an independent predictor for the requirement of mitral valve surgery. They also reported that patients without exercise PHT and exercise-induced right ventricular (RV) dysfunction, have an intermediate outcome. More importantly, the concomitant presence of both exercise PHT and RV dysfunction identified patients with the worst outcome. In a multivariate analysis, RV function, exercise SPAP, and tricuspid annulus plane systolic excursion at peak exercise provided the best significant predictive model. These results suggest that the presence of PHT during exercise should also be considered with RV function during exercise and that the combination of progressive RV dysfunction and PHT herald the worst prognosis in asymptomatic patients with primary MR.

LV Contractile Reserve

LV contractile reserve, assessed during stress echocardiography, can reveal subclinical LV dysfunction and predict postoperative LV function after mitral valve surgery.[4,6] An inability to demonstrate an increase in the LV ejection fraction or a reduction in the end-systolic volume with exercise reflects the presence of impaired contractile reserve. An exercise end-systolic volume index greater than 25 cm^3/m^2 was shown to be the best predictor of developing postoperative LV dysfunction in minimally symptomatic patients with severe MR. In asymptomatic patients with chronic severe MR and normal LV function, an increase in ejection fraction with exercise of less than 4% predicts the development

of postoperative LV dysfunction and cardiac morbidity in surgically treated patients and progressive deterioration of LV function in medically treated patients.[4] Recent data suggest that a 2D strain obtained during exercise could be useful to identify the presence of latent LV dysfunction in these patients (see **Fig. 2**, **Table 1**). A less than 1.9% increase in global longitudinal strain during exercise had better sensitivity and specificity than an inadequate increase in LV ejection fraction in predicting postoperative LV dysfunction and the development of impairment in LV function in medically treated patients.[6] The authors' recent findings suggest that the absence of LV contractile reserve, as assessed with 2D speckle tracking analysis, is a strong independent predictor of elevated brain natriuretic peptide levels and of reduced cardiac event-free survival. In addition, LV the contractile reserve has been shown to provide incremental prognostic value for patients suitable for surgery.

Exercise Stress Echocardiography and Management

Exercise stress echocardiography allows the identification of the subset of patients prone to more frequent and rapid occurrence of symptoms along with a reduction in the cardiac event-free survival. In line with the current guidelines, patients who developed exercise PHT may be considered for early surgical intervention (ie, even in the absence of symptoms or LV dysfunction/dilatation). In addition, the absence of any LV contractile reserve may also be a trigger for surgery, particularly in a high-volume surgical center with excellent rates for mitral valve repair. Hence, all patients with asymptomatic severe MR and preserved LV function should be closely followed up. At peak exercise, blood sample and exercise BNP measurement had incremental prognostic value and may add an objective marker of early and latent LV dysfunction.[17]

SECONDARY MR

The prevalence and incidence of secondary MR is high and on the increase because of the epidemiologic burden of pro-atherosclerotic factors, coronary artery disease, and of metabolic disorders and obesity. Secondary MR is a frequent complication of heart failure, which results from LV remodeling and dysfunction.[18] Secondary MR develops despite a structurally normal mitral valve. It results from the apical and outward displacement of one or both papillary muscles tethering the mitral leaflets and from decreased LV-generated forces required to close them. The clinical importance of secondary ischemic MR is underestimated.

In the ESC's current guidelines, the dynamic component of secondary MR is emphasized, with exercise testing having a role in its evaluation. The main role of stress echocardiography in secondary ischemic MR is to determine the extent of dysfunctional but viable myocardium. The identification of viable myocardium with pharmacologic stress echocardiography predicts the likelihood of recovery of function and beneficial reverse remodeling with revascularization, beta blockade, and cardiac resynchronization therapy. Exercise stress testing should ideally be used because dobutamine reduces preload, afterload, and, hence, MR and is, therefore, not useful for assessing the dynamic component of MR.

When present, secondary ischemic MR may exhibit a broad range of severities and conveys a dismal prognosis,[19] doubling the risk of death following myocardial infarction.[18] The increased mortality risk relates not only to the presence of MR but also, more importantly, to the severity of the MR.[20,21] Several methods can be used to determine the severity of secondary MR. Semi-quantitative approaches, such as color flow mapping of the regurgitant jet, vena contracta width, and both the Doppler and the PISA methods, can provide some objective measure of the severity of the secondary MR; but the most robust measurement is the EROA. In the setting of ischemic heart disease, an EROA of 20 mm^2 or more is considered severe and associated with excess mortality.[22] The evaluation of functional ischemic MR only under resting conditions might underestimate the full impact of the lesion and its clinical effects. Indeed, secondary MR is a dynamic lesion (see **Fig. 1**) and its severity may vary over time.[23,24] The second major role of stress echocardiography in secondary ischemic MR is to examine possible dynamic changes in MR severity and in hemodynamics. In this context, dobutamine stress echocardiography is not suitable to assess the dynamic component of MR. Indeed, the direct effect of dobutamine on loading conditions is a major confounding variable because it leads almost systematically to a decrease in mitral regurgitant orifice size. Instead, exercise Doppler echocardiography has recently emerged as a well-suited method to quantitate the dynamic component of secondary ischemic MR. There is a good correlation between EROA measured during exercise by the PISA method and that obtained by the quantitative Doppler volumetric method.[24]

Dynamic Secondary MR: Determinants and Mechanisms

The exercise-induced change in secondary MR severity (**Fig. 3**) is likely determined by the complex interaction between mitral valve leaflets, mitral annulus dimension, LA compliance and pressure, LV systolic dimension, function, pressure, and chronotropy and the exercise-induced changes in these parameters.[23,25] The strongest correlation is observed with changes in the mitral valve configuration. The increase in EROA during exercise results from bulging in the systolic tenting area (the area enclosed between the mitral leaflets and the annulus plane), an increase in coaptation distance (apical displacement of the coaptation leaflet tips), and a systolic expansion of the mitral annulus. Importantly, such changes occur without detectable ischemia during exercise echocardiography and are independent of exercise-induced changes in hemodynamic parameters (arterial

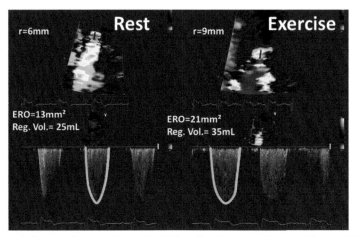

Fig. 3. Exercise-induced changes in secondary MR. ERO, effective regurgitant orifice; r, PISA radius; Reg Vol, regurgitant volume.

pressure, heart rate). Changes in regional loading conditions and a more spherical LV shape during exercise also contribute to changes in the mitral valve configuration. Dynamic secondary MR also occurs in the context of LV dyssynchrony.[26] The decrease in EROA during exercise is mainly observed in patients with inferior myocardial infarction who have non transmural necrosis and contractile reserve in the basal LV segments. Such a reduction in EROA is possibly related to the reduction of the tethering forces and can be interpreted in light of an experiment model of reverse remodeling induced by repositioning the papillary muscles.

In Which Patients Should Exercise Stress Echocardiography be Performed?

Exercise echocardiography can unmask hemodynamically significant MR in patients with LV systolic dysfunction and only mild to moderate secondary MR at rest, hence, identifying patients at higher risk for heart failure and death (see **Table 1**). Exercise Doppler echocardiography can provide useful information in the following patients with secondary MR: (1) those with exertional dyspnea out of proportion to the severity of resting LV dysfunction or MR, (2) those in whom acute pulmonary edema occurs without an obvious contributing factor, (3) those with moderate MR before surgical revascularization, (4) those in whom individual risk stratification is requested, and (5) those who have had a mitral valve surgery but with persistent postoperative pulmonary hypertension.

IMPACT OF DYNAMIC SECONDARY MR ON EXERCISE TOLERANCE

Exertional dyspnea is a cardinal symptom in patients with ischemic LV dysfunction[27] and can occur out of proportion to the degree of LV dysfunction, the degree of secondary MR at rest, or transient diastolic dysfunction. In such a situation, exercise-induced increases in secondary ischemic MR severity might limit the stroke volume adaptation during exercise and contribute in part to the limitation of exercise capacity.[28] Secondary MR can be the additional factor that, together with LV systolic dysfunction, results in impaired exercise tolerance. Backward flow from the LV to the left atrium during systole limits stroke volume, resulting in reduced cardiac output and impaired exercise tolerance. If sufficient contractile reserve is maintained, cardiac output may be increased during exercise and the severity of MR does not increase and may even diminish. With severe LV dysfunction, the increase in contractility during stress is limited, and any increase in afterload

results in a marked decrease in cardiac output and more severe MR. Even mild to moderate MR at rest may become a significant factor that limits stroke volume during stress and leads to the impairment of exercise tolerance. Hence, the severity of MR assessed by Doppler echocardiography at rest is unrelated to exercise MR severity. Indeed, most patients exhibit small increases in the amount of MR, whereas others have either a large increase or a significant decrease in the effective regurgitant orifice (EROA).

Clinical and Prognostic Impacts of Dynamic Secondary MR

Intermittent increases in secondary MR severity during daily life activities could also raise left atrial and pulmonary vascular pressures acutely, generating pulmonary congestion and contributing to worsening dyspnea or flash pulmonary edema.[27] The relationship between dynamic secondary MR and these clinical spectrums has been confirmed recently. Exercise-induced changes in regurgitant volume and in SPAP are larger in patients who stop their exercise because of dyspnea as compared with those who stop for fatigue.[29] The magnitude of increase in regurgitant volume is also greater in patients hospitalized for pulmonary edema in the context of chronic systolic LV dysfunction.[27] Dynamic changes in secondary MR provide additional prognostic information over resting evaluation and unmask patients at high risk for a poor outcome.[12,13] A large exercise-induced increase in secondary MR and an increase in ERO of 13 mm^2 or more (see **Table 1**) are associated with increased mortality, morbidity, and hospital admissions for worsening heart failure and major cardiac events.[13] Many patients with dynamic secondary MR die of refractory heart failure. Repetitive transient increases in MR may accentuate the chronic volume overload induced by secondary MR and contribute to progressive LV dilation and dysfunction, leading to end-stage heart failure. Dynamic secondary MR is also a determinant of rapid QRS widening and may subsequently lead to permanent electromechanical dyssynchrony, which further deteriorates the LV systolic function.

MS

Rheumatic fever is the main cause of MS worldwide, even in industrialized countries. The second most frequent cause of MS in developed countries is degenerative MS or calcific MS. Other causes are rare and include congenital anomalies (parachute valve, cor triatriatum), infiltrative diseases, inflammatory diseases (erythematous lupus or rheumatoid arthritis), carcinoid disease, or tumors (myxoma).

The primary hemodynamic consequence of MS is the obstruction of the LV inflow caused by the restricted mitral valve opening, which is caused by an abnormal mitral valve and/or subvalvular apparatus. When the mitral valve area (MVA) starts to decrease (<2.5 cm^2), the transvalvular pressure gradient increases, leading to LA pressure overload. Left atrium (LA) compliance acts as a compensatory mechanism helping to limit the pressure overload to LA chamber. However, with time, LA dilates and compliance is no longer sufficient to compensate allowing pressure to be passively transmitted to the pulmonary veins. Long-standing pulmonary venous hypertension can, in turn, cause changes in the pulmonary arterioles, including intimal hyperplasia and medial hypertrophy leading to PHT, RV dysfunction, and congestive heart failure.

The ESC's current guidelines[1] recommend surgery for all patients with significant MS (MVA <1.5 cm^2) and symptoms. Symptomatic patients with mild MS (mean transmitral pressure gradient <5 mm Hg, valve area >1.5 cm^2) should be followed up on an annual basis but do not require further evaluation from the initial workup. All other categories of patients with MS could benefit from stress echocardiography. When MS is significant (valve area <1.5 cm^2), a hemodynamic stress test should be performed, especially in sedentary patients. This test could also be helpful in patients with apparently mild MS but who describe limiting symptoms, such as dyspnea. The assessment of exercise tolerance is of high clinical interest for the management of these patients. The data regarding the use of stress testing in mitral stenosis are rather limited.

Stress-Induced Changes in Transmitral Mean Pressure Gradient

Because the exercise stress test is more physiologic, it should be preferably recommended. Nonetheless, dobutamine stress testing may also be performed[30,31] and seems to provide similar hemodynamic results (ie, changes in transmitral mean pressure gradient, MVA, and SPAP) and impact on the occurrence of dyspnea during stress. In a study including 53 patients with various degrees of MS (ranging from 2.6 cm^2–0.7 cm^2), Reis and colleagues[14] have demonstrated that dobutamine stress echocardiography may be performed safely, without major complications. The normal dose dobutamine infusion protocol test was applied to all patients starting at 10 μg/kg/min for 5 minutes and then increasing by 10 μg/kg/min every 3 minutes, to a maximum of 40 μg/kg/min.

For a given diastolic mitral flow, patients (n = 29) with cardiovascular events during the follow-up (including hospitalization, acute pulmonary edema, or supraventricular arrhythmias) had significantly higher transmitral mean pressure gradient at peak dose dobutamine infusion and a steeper increase than patients without an event. They also found that a peak dobutamine transmitral mean pressure gradient more than 18 mm Hg was significantly and independently associated with reduced event-free survival.

In 1991, Leavitt and colleagues[32] reported exercise stress echocardiography feasibility in patients with MS. In this study, all patients with MS exhibited an exercise-induced increase in transmitral mean pressure gradient, even in the presence of a concomitant increase in MVA. Furthermore, a paralleled marked increase in SPAP accompanied these exercise hemodynamic changes. For a given mitral antegrade flow, the presence of a marked increase in the mean pressure gradient during exercise despite a concomitant increase in MVA, leading to a marked increase in SPAP, underlines the important role of LA compliance (**Fig. 4**). Noninvasively, only the net atrioventricular compliance (Cn) can be measured. The impact of Cn on exercise mitral hemodynamic changes was emphasized in the elegant study of Schwammenthal and colleagues[33] whereby patients with low Cn represented an important clinical entity, with symptoms corresponding to severe increases in SPAP during stress echocardiography. The close relationship between Cn and SPAP was also confirmed at rest.[34]

Stress-Induced Changes in SPAP

According to the American College of Cardiology/American Heart Association's guidelines,[35] intervention is recommended in asymptomatic patients with an SPAP of more than 60 mm Hg (ie, PHT) at peak exercise. However, the additional value of peak hemodynamic parameters over exercise-induced symptoms for decision making remains controversial, and limited data are available on the pattern of progression of hemodynamic variables at each level of effort and its potential additional value in tolerance evaluation. Furthermore, the clinical interpretation of the development of exercise PHT should be performed cautiously. Indeed, according to exercise load and time, some patients may reach the threshold of PHT, whereas their functional capacity and pulmonary function are not impaired. Furthermore, there is a lack of studies assessing pulmonary compliance and vascular resistance, which play an important role in the development of PHT, during exercise.

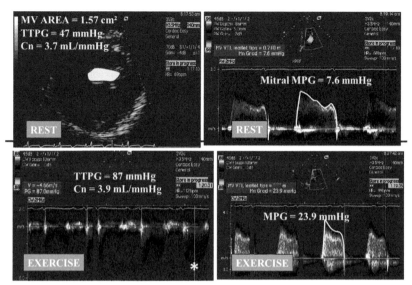

Fig. 4. Exercise-induced changes in transmitral mean pressure gradient (MPG) in asymptomatic patient with moderate resting MS. The significant increase in MPG without parallel improvement in net atrioventricular compliance (Cn) leads to marked increase in transtricuspid pressure gradient (TTPG). The *asterisk* indicates peak tricuspid regurgitation velocity. MV, mitral valve.

It was recently emphasized that the serial measurement of SPAP at each step of exercise (ie, evaluation of the patterns of increase in SPAP) may overcome this issue and seems to provide more useful information than the simple measurement of peak exercise SPAP.[36,37] Recent studies report that during exercise, SPAP generally increases by 2 main patterns: (1) takeoff pattern and (2) *plateau* pattern.[36] The takeoff pattern displays a progressive and slow increase in SPAP during exercise, with a steeper increase in the final stage, which mimics normal subjects, indicating good prognosis. The *plateau* pattern represents an early steep increase with no or a mild further increase in SPAP, which is typically associated with more severely compromised exercise PHT and frequently seen in patients with resting PHT, and correlates with reduced survival.[37]

In asymptomatic patients with MS, the study from Brochet and colleagues[15] provides interesting new insights regarding the exercise-induced changes in SPAP. In their study, they investigated 48 asymptomatic patients with at least moderate MS who performed exercise echocardiography. During exercise, 22 (46%) patients developed dyspnea. No difference was noted in both resting and exercise mitral valve hemodynamics between these patients and those without exercise dyspnea. Surprisingly, the 2 groups of patients had similar exercise SPAP (69 ± 10 vs 68 ± 11 mm Hg, $P = .58$) and no statistically different frequency of exercise-induced PHT (83% vs 73%, $P = .26$). Nevertheless, the kinetics of exercise-induced changes in SPAP were significantly different between patients who developed exercise dyspnea and those who did not. Indeed, patients with dyspnea exhibited an early steep and marked relative increase in SPAP. An early (ie, 60 W) exercise-induced increase in SPAP of 90% or more was associated with more than a 2-fold increase in the risk to develop dyspnea during exercise or to require mitral valve intervention during the follow-up. To summarize, these data suggest that early hemodynamic changes during exercise and not only peak exercise values have an important adjunct value to the assessment of exercise tolerance.

Management of Patients with MS

The assessment of mitral valve morphology is key in the management of patients with MS. In the presence of suitable mitral valve morphology for percutaneous balloon valvotomy, patients who deny symptoms but have an objective significant limitation of exercise tolerance may be considered for percutaneous valvotomy. This procedure can also be proposed in patients with a valve area of 1.5 cm^2 or more who, during exercise, exhibit a transmitral mean gradient of more than 15 mm Hg, pulmonary artery wedge pressure of 25 mm Hg or more, or pulmonary artery systolic pressure of more than 60 mm Hg.[35] **Table 1** summarizes cut-off values for different criteria obtained during dobutamine stress echocardiography or exercise stress echocardiography. In the presence of such criteria, close follow-up and reference to a dedicated heart valve clinic[38] should be recommended.

SUMMARY

Exercise stress echocardiography has utility in the evaluation of patients with both primary and secondary MR, whereas dobutamine stress echocardiography should only be used in limited cases, notably in patients in whom exercise is not possible. Worsening of MR severity, a marked increase in pulmonary arterial pressure, limited contractile reserve, impaired exercise capacity, together with the occurrence of symptoms during exercise echocardiography provide diagnostic and prognostic information that can contribute toward the identification of a subset of patients at higher risk who may benefit from mitral valve surgery (see **Table 1**). Despite limited data in this population, exercise or dobutamine stress echocardiography may also have clinical utility in patients with MS, specifically in the absence of symptoms or in patients with equivocal symptoms. Clinicians should, therefore, not hesitate to refer patients for a complete evaluation, especially when surgery is contemplated. The stress echocardiography examination is a cost-effective, safe, and widely available test that does not expose patients to radiation. Hence, exercise echocardiography, currently only a recommended diagnostic modality in patients with mitral valve disease, may become an integral, standard tool in the evaluation of patients with mitral heart valve disease.

REFERENCES

1. Vahanian A, Alfieri O, Andreotti F, et al. Guidelines on the management of valvular heart disease (version 2012): the Joint Task Force on the Management of Valvular Heart Disease of the European Society of Cardiology (ESC) and the European Association for Cardio-Thoracic Surgery (EACTS). Eur Heart J 2012;33:2451–96.
2. Pierard LA, Lancellotti P. Stress testing in valve disease. Heart 2007;93:766–72.
3. Gibbons RJ, Balady GJ, Beasley JW, et al. ACC/AHA guidelines for exercise testing. A report of the American College of Cardiology/American Heart Association Task Force on practice guidelines (Committee on Exercise Testing). J Am Coll Cardiol 1997;30:260–311.
4. Lee R, Haluska B, Leung DY, et al. Functional and prognostic implications of left ventricular contractile reserve in patients with asymptomatic severe mitral regurgitation. Heart 2005;91:1407–12.
5. Leung DY, Griffin BP, Stewart WJ, et al. Left ventricular function after valve repair for chronic mitral regurgitation: predictive value of preoperative assessment of contractile reserve by exercise echocardiography. J Am Coll Cardiol 1996;28:1198–205.
6. Lancellotti P, Cosyns B, Zacharakis D, et al. Importance of left ventricular longitudinal function and functional reserve in patients with degenerative mitral regurgitation: assessment by two dimensional speckle tracking. J Am Soc Echocardiogr 2008;21:1331–6.
7. Magne J, O'Connor K, Mahjoub H, et al. Evaluation and impact on outcome of left ventricular contractile reserve in asymptomatic degenerative mitral regurgitation. Eur Heart J 2011;32(Suppl):170.
8. Stoddard MF, Prince CR, Dillon S, et al. Exercise-induced mitral regurgitation is a predictor of morbid events in subjects with mitral valve prolapse. J Am Coll Cardiol 1995;25:693–9.
9. Messika-Zeitoun D, Johnson BD, Nkomo V, et al. Cardiopulmonary exercise testing determination of functional capacity in mitral regurgitation: physiologic and outcome implications. J Am Coll Cardiol 2006;47:2521–7.
10. Magne J, Lancellotti P, Pierard LA. Exercise-induced changes in degenerative mitral regurgitation. J Am Coll Cardiol 2010;56:300–9.
11. Magne J, Lancellotti P, Pierard LA. Exercise pulmonary hypertension in asymptomatic degenerative mitral regurgitation. Circulation 2010;122:33–41.
12. Lancellotti P, Troisfontaines P, Toussaint AC, et al. Prognostic importance of exercise-induced changes in mitral regurgitation in patients with chronic ischemic left ventricular dysfunction. Circulation 2003;108:1713–7.
13. Lancellotti P, Gerard PL, Pierard LA. Long-term outcome of patients with heart failure and dynamic functional mitral regurgitation. Eur Heart J 2005;26:1528–32.
14. Reis G, Motta MS, Barbosa MM, et al. Dobutamine stress echocardiography for noninvasive assessment and risk stratification of patients with rheumatic mitral stenosis. J Am Coll Cardiol 2004;43:393–401.
15. Brochet E, Detaint D, Fondard O, et al. Early hemodynamic changes versus peak values: what is more useful to predict occurrence of dyspnea during stress echocardiography in patients with asymptomatic mitral stenosis? J Am Soc Echocardiogr 2011;24:392–8.
16. Kusunose K, Popovic ZB, Motoki H, et al. Prognostic significance of exercise induced right ventricular dysfunction in asymptomatic degenerative mitral regurgitation. Circ Cardiovasc Imaging 2013;6(2):167–76.
17. Magne J, Mahjoub H, Pibarot P, et al. Prognostic importance of exercise brain natriuretic peptide in asymptomatic degenerative mitral regurgitation. Eur J Heart Fail 2012;14:1293–302.

18. Magne J, Senechal M, Dumesnil JG, et al. Ischemic mitral regurgitation: a complex multifaceted disease. Cardiology 2009;112:244–59.

19. Lamas G, Mitchell G, Flaker G, et al. Clinical significance of mitral regurgitation after acute myocardial infarction. Circulation 1997;96:827–33.

20. Grigioni F, Enriquez-Sarano M, Zehr KJ, et al. Ischemic mitral regurgitation. Long-term outcome and prognostic implications with quantitative Doppler assessment. Circulation 2001;103:1759–64.

21. Grigioni F, Detaint D, Avierinos JF, et al. Contribution of ischemic mitral regurgitation to congestive heart failure after myocardial infarction. J Am Coll Cardiol 2005;45:260–7.

22. Lancellotti P, Moura L, Pierard LA, et al. European Association of Echocardiography recommendations for the assessment of valvular regurgitation. Part 2: mitral and tricuspid regurgitation (native valve disease). Eur J Echocardiogr 2010;11:307–32.

23. Lancellotti P, Lebrun F, Pierard LA. Determinants of exercise-induced changes in mitral regurgitation in patients with coronary artery disease and left ventricular dysfunction. J Am Coll Cardiol 2003;42:1921–8.

24. Lebrun F, Lancellotti P, Pierard LA. Quantitation of functional mitral regurgitation during bicycle exercise in patients with heart failure. J Am Coll Cardiol 2001;38:1685–92.

25. Giga V, Ostojic M, Vujisic-Tesic B, et al. Exercise-induced changes in mitral regurgitation in patients with prior myocardial infarction and left ventricular dysfunction: relation to mitral deformation and left ventricular function and shape. Eur Heart J 2005; 26:1860–5.

26. Lancellotti P, Melon P, Sakalihasan N, et al. Effect of cardiac resynchronization therapy on functional mitral regurgitation in heart failure. Am J Cardiol 2004;94:1462–5.

27. Pierard LA, Lancellotti P. The role of ischemic mitral regurgitation in the pathogenesis of acute pulmonary edema. N Engl J Med 2004;351:1627–34.

28. Szymanski C, Levine RA, Tribouilloy C, et al. Impact of mitral regurgitation on exercise capacity and clinical outcomes in patients with ischemic left ventricular dysfunction. Am J Cardiol 2011;108:1714–20.

29. Tumminello G, Lancellotti P, Lempereur M, et al. Determinants of pulmonary artery hypertension at rest and during exercise in patients with heart failure. Eur Heart J 2007;28:569–74.

30. Cheitlin MD. Stress echocardiography in mitral stenosis: when is it useful? J Am Coll Cardiol 2004;43: 402–4.

31. Hecker SL, Zabalgoitia M, Ashline P, et al. Comparison of exercise and dobutamine stress echocardiography in assessing mitral stenosis. Am J Cardiol 1997;80:1374–7.

32. Leavitt JI, Coats MH, Falk RH. Effects of exercise on transmitral gradient and pulmonary artery pressure in patients with mitral stenosis or a prosthetic mitral valve: a Doppler echocardiographic study. J Am Coll Cardiol 1991;17:1520–6.

33. Schwammenthal E, Vered Z, Agranat O, et al. Impact of atrioventricular compliance on pulmonary artery pressure in mitral stenosis: an exercise echocardiographic study. Circulation 2000;102:2378–84.

34. Li M, Déry JP, Dumesnil JG, et al. Usefulness of measuring net atrioventricular compliance by Doppler echocardiography in patients with mitral stenosis. Am J Cardiol 2005;96:432–5.

35. Bonow RO, Carabello BA, Kanu C, et al. ACC/AHA 2006 guidelines for the management of patients with valvular heart disease: a report of the American College of Cardiology/American Heart Association Task Force on Practice Guidelines (writing committee to revise the 1998 guidelines for the management of patients with valvular heart disease): developed in collaboration with the Society of Cardiovascular Anesthesiologists: endorsed by the Society for Cardiovascular Angiography and Interventions and the Society of Thoracic Surgeons. Circulation 2006;114: e84–231.

36. Tolle JJ, Waxman AB, Van Horn TL, et al. Exercise-induced pulmonary arterial hypertension. Circulation 2008;118:2183–9.

37. Lewis GD, Murphy RM, Shah RV, et al. Pulmonary vascular response patterns during exercise in left ventricular systolic dysfunction predict exercise capacity and outcomes. Circ Heart Fail 2011;4:276–85.

38. Lancellotti P, Rosenhek R, Pibarot P, et al. ESC Working Group on Valvular Heart Disease position paper–heart valve clinics: organization, structure, and experiences. Eur Heart J 2013. [Epub ahead of print].

Index

Note: Page numbers of article titles are in **boldface** type.

A

Acute rheumatic fever (ARF)
   clinical manifestations of, 179
Anatomic regurgitant orifice area
   in MR evaluation
      in mitral valve disease, 211
ARF. See Acute rheumatic fever (ARF)

B

Balloon valvotomy
   three-dimensional echocardiography in
      preoperative mitral valve evaluation for, 275
Barlow's disease, 203–204
   causes of, 203–204
   fibroelastic deficiency vs., 203–204
Bioprosthetic heart valves
   assessment of
      echocardiography in, 290–291

C

Cardiomyopathy
   hypertrophic, 159
Chordae tendineae
   anatomy of, 155
Color flow area
   in MR grading, 170
Continuous-wave (CW) Doppler profile
   in MR grading, 171
CW Doppler profile. See Continuous-wave (CW)
   Doppler profile

D

Doppler evaluation
   in mitral stenosis assessment, 180–184
      mitral valve area, 181–184
      pulmonary artery pressure estimation, 180–181
      transmitral pressure gradient, 180
   in prosthetic heart valve assessment, 294–295
Doppler integrated approach
   in MR grading, 174

E

Echocardiography. See also specific types, e.g.,
   Stress echocardiography
   of calcific mitral stenosis, 196–198
   exercise

in MR assessment and severity in myxomatous
      disease, 223
   in mitral stenosis assessment, **179–191**. See also
      Mitral stenosis, echocardiographic
      assessment of
   during mitral valve percutaneous interventions,
      237–270. See also specific interventions, e.g.,
      Percutaneous mitral balloon valvuloplasty
      (PMBV)
      complications of, 256–264
         PVLs, 256–264
      introduction, 237
      MitraClip system, 243–256
      PMBV, 237–243
   in MR assessment, **165–168**
   in myxomatous disease management, **217–229**.
      See also Myxomatous disease, management of
   in prosthetic mitral valve assessment, **287–309**.
      See also Prosthetic mitral valves,
      echocardiographic assessment of
   three-dimensional
      in MR grading, 172–174
Endocarditis
   prosthetic mitral valve–related
      echocardiographic assessment of, 301–305
Exercise echocardiography
   in MR assessment and severity in myxomatous
      disease, 223

F

Fibroelastic deficiency
   Barlow's disease vs., 203–204
Functional/ischemic mitral regurgitation (MR), 159

G

Gorlin hydraulic orifice equation, 170
Group A streptococcal infections
   RHD and, 179

H

HCM. See Hypertrophic cardiomyopathy (HCM)
Hypertrophic cardiomyopathy (HCM), 159

I

Ischemic mitral regurgitation (MR), **231–236**
   acute and chronic

Cardiol Clin 31 (2013) 323–326
http://dx.doi.org/10.1016/S0733-8651(13)00026-X
0733-8651/13/$ – see front matter © 2013 Elsevier Inc. All rights reserved.

cardiology.theclinics.com

Moving?

Make sure your subscription moves with you!

To notify us of your new address, find your **Clinics Account Number** (located on your mailing label above your name), and contact customer service at:

Email: journalscustomerservice-usa@elsevier.com

800-654-2452 (subscribers in the U.S. & Canada)
314-447-8871 (subscribers outside of the U.S. & Canada)

Fax number: 314-447-8029

Elsevier Health Sciences Division
Subscription Customer Service
3251 Riverport Lane
Maryland Heights, MO 63043

*To ensure uninterrupted delivery of your subscription, please notify us at least 4 weeks in advance of move.

Printed and bound by CPI Group (UK) Ltd, Croydon, CR0 4YY

03/10/2024

01040347-0014